Cholera Control in 2021: Bioecology, Immunology, Current and Future Vaccines and Treatment Options

Cholera Control in 2021: Bioecology, Immunology, Current and Future Vaccines and Treatment Options

Editor

David Nalin

MDPI • Basel • Beijing • Wuhan • Barcelona • Belgrade • Manchester • Tokyo • Cluj • Tianjin

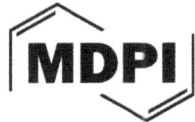

Editor
David Nalin
Center for Immunology and
Microbial Diseases, Albany
Medical College
USA

Editorial Office
MDPI
St. Alban-Anlage 66
4052 Basel, Switzerland

This is a reprint of articles from the Special Issue published online in the open access journal *Tropical Medicine and Infectious Disease* (ISSN 2414-6366) (available at: https://www.mdpi.com/journal/tropicalmed/special_issues/cholera_tropicalmed).

For citation purposes, cite each article independently as indicated on the article page online and as indicated below:

LastName, A.A.; LastName, B.B.; LastName, C.C. Article Title. *Journal Name* **Year**, *Volume Number*, Page Range.

ISBN 978-3-0365-4239-3 (Hbk)
ISBN 978-3-0365-4240-9 (PDF)

Cover image courtesy of David Nalin

© 2022 by the authors. Articles in this book are Open Access and distributed under the Creative Commons Attribution (CC BY) license, which allows users to download, copy and build upon published articles, as long as the author and publisher are properly credited, which ensures maximum dissemination and a wider impact of our publications.

The book as a whole is distributed by MDPI under the terms and conditions of the Creative Commons license CC BY-NC-ND.

Contents

About the Editor vii

Preface to "Cholera Control in 2021: Bioecology, Immunology, Current and Future Vaccines and Treatment Options" ix

Moiz Usmani, Kyle D. Brumfield, Yusuf Jamal, Anwar Huq, Rita R. Colwell and Antarpreet Jutla
A Review of the Environmental Trigger and Transmission Components for Prediction of Cholera
Reprinted from: *Trop. Med. Infect. Dis.* **2021**, 6, 147, doi:10.3390/tropicalmed6030147 1

Amanda K. Debes, Allison M. Shaffer, Thaddee Ndikumana, Iteka Liesse, Eric Ribaira, Clement Djumo, Mohammad Ali and David A. Sack
Cholera Hot-Spots and Contextual Factors in Burundi, Planning for Elimination
Reprinted from: *Trop. Med. Infect. Dis.* **2021**, 6, 76, doi:10.3390/tropicalmed6020076 15

Thomas J. Bollyky
Oral Rehydration Salts, Cholera, and the Unfinished Urban Health Agenda
Reprinted from: *Trop. Med. Infect. Dis.* **2022**, 7, 67, doi:10.3390/tropicalmed7050067 27

Jan Holmgren
An Update on Cholera Immunity and Current and Future Cholera Vaccines
Reprinted from: *Trop. Med. Infect. Dis.* **2021**, 6, 64, doi:10.3390/tropicalmed6020064 33

Jacqueline Deen and John D. Clemens
Licensed and Recommended Inactivated Oral Cholera Vaccines: From Development to Innovative Deployment
Reprinted from: *Trop. Med. Infect. Dis.* **2021**, 6, 32, doi:10.3390/tropicalmed6010032 53

Edward T. Ryan, Daniel T. Leung, Owen Jensen, Ana A. Weil, Taufiqur Rahman Bhuiyan, Ashraful Islam Khan, Fahima Chowdhury, Regina C. LaRocque, Jason B. Harris, Stephen B. Calderwood, Firdausi Qadri and Richelle C. Charles
Systemic, Mucosal, and Memory Immune Responses following Cholera
Reprinted from: *Trop. Med. Infect. Dis.* **2021**, 6, 192, doi:10.3390/tropicalmed6040192 65

David R. Nalin
The History of Intravenous and Oral Rehydration and Maintenance Therapy of Cholera and Non-Cholera Dehydrating Diarrheas: A Deconstruction of Translational Medicine: From Bench to Bedside?
Reprinted from: *Trop. Med. Infect. Dis.* **2022**, 7, 50, doi:10.3390/tropicalmed7030050 77

Richard A. Cash
Using Oral Rehydration Therapy (ORT) in the Community
Reprinted from: *Trop. Med. Infect. Dis.* **2021**, 6, 92, doi:10.3390/tropicalmed6020092 105

David Nalin
Issues and Controversies in the Evolution of Oral Rehydration Therapy (ORT)
Reprinted from: *Trop. Med. Infect. Dis.* **2021**, 6, 34, doi:10.3390/tropicalmed6010034 111

David Nalin
Correction: Nalin, D. Issues and Controversies in the Evolution of Oral Rehydration Therapy (ORT). *Trop. Med. Infect. Dis.* 2021, 6, 34
Reprinted from: *Trop. Med. Infect. Dis.* **2022**, 7, 103, doi:10.3390/tropicalmed7060103 127

Farzana Afroze, Steven Bloom, Paul Bech, Tahmeed Ahmed, Shafiqul Alam Sarker, John D. Clemens, Farhana Islam and David Nalin
Cholera and Pancreatic Cholera: Is VIP the Common Pathophysiologic Factor?
Reprinted from: *Trop. Med. Infect. Dis.* **2020**, 5, 111, doi:10.3390/tropicalmed5030111 . . . . **129**

David Nalin
Eliminating Cholera Incidence and Mortality: Unfulfilled Tasks
Reprinted from: *Trop. Med. Infect. Dis.* **2022**, 7, 69, doi:10.3390/tropicalmed7050069 . . . . **141**

About the Editor

David R. Nalin

David R Nalin, MD, Dr.Sci.HC, Professor Emeritus, Center for Immunology and Microbial Diseases, Albany Medical College, Albany NY. After internship and medical residency (Montefiore, NYC) and senior residency (Harvard Service, BCH), Dr. Nalin attained the rank of Senior Surgeon In the U.S. Public Health Service, serving in Dhaka, Bangladesh (then E. Pakistan) as Research Associate, Office of International Research, NIH, and later Assistant Professor, medicine and pathobiology at Johns Hopkins Center for Medical Research and Associate Professor of medicine, international medicine and epidemiology and Director, U. Md. Pakistan Medical Research Center, Lahore. He is currently Professor Emeritus, Center for Immunology and Microbial Diseases, AMC.

Dr. Nalin led the team that first demonstrated that oral glucose-electrolyte solutions(ORS) reduced maintenance intravenous fluid needs by 80% in severe cholera, and published numerous studies demonstrating ORS effectiveness for most acute life-threatening watery diarrhoeal diseases for both rehydration and maintenance therapy. The BMJ estimated that by 1999 ORS saved over 70,000,000 lives.

As Director, Clinical Research, Vaccines and Infectious Diseases and Director, Vaccine Scientific Affairs at Merck (1983–2002) he designed and monitored studies of imipenem-cilastatin, norfloxacin and ivermectin, M-M-R® II, hepatitis A and HPV vaccines.

He has published over 100 peer-reviewed articles, over 200 letters, reviews, book chapters, and abstracts and holds three patents for new vaccination methods. His awards include the Pollin Prize for Pediatric Research and the Prince Mahidol Award 2006, recognizing his development of ORS; the AMC Humanitarian award (2010), the Friends of Liberation War Award Bangladesh (2013) and the Dr. Sci. H.C. degree from the University of Vermont (2017).

Preface to "Cholera Control in 2021: Bioecology, Immunology, Current and Future Vaccines and Treatment Options"

In 2017, the Global Task Force on Cholera Control launched an initiative to reduce cholera deaths by 90% in at least 20 countries by 2030 [1]. This Special Issue focuses on the search for strategies to control cholera and non-cholera dehydrating diarrheas, including vaccinology and therapeutics, and provides the opportunity to release these ten original papers in book form as an overview of the current control options for cholera and related diseases. The papers include 7 original reports, 2 reviews and 1 perspective article.

Moiz Usmani and colleagues[1] discuss climate variables' influence on epidemics and the role of trigger and transmission components in relation to pathogens' environmental distribution. The extra-human bioecologic cycle of V. cholerae (and related organisms) shifts the focus from eradication, which is not possible, to control. Instead, effective control is likely to require improved environmental risk modeling and the identification of trigger components and their role in transmission and transition from endemic to epidemic form.

In this context, the study of Amanda Debes and colleagues on cholera "hot-spots" and contextual factors in Burundi [2] can provide a useful approach to the improved control developing from oral vaccination and comprehensive community-based WASH and treatment modules to eliminate ongoing high case-fatality rates in affected African Nations.

Thomas Bollyky [3] discusses the challenges posed by shifting demographics and urbanization regarding the impact of planning and control programs on both vaccine-based and treatment-based components. Effective control measures will require careful attention to gaps in the urban health agenda.

Jan Holmgren [4] discusses the expanded research on cholera immunity leading to oral cholera vaccines (OCV), which have improved prospects for a reduction in clinical disease burden and deaths, as well as cross-protection against severe ETEC disease in both endemic and epidemic situations. Although contaminated water (imbibed or contaminating food) is key to cholera transmission, a surprising added benefit of OCV, noted in several trials in endemic areas, is the protection of unvaccinated family or community members when vaccine coverage exceeds 50%.

Novel deployment strategies for inactivated oral cholera vaccines are discussed by Jacqueline Dean and John Clemens [5] in a review of follow-up data from single-dose, targeted deployment ring vaccination trials and other new delivery strategies, as well as indirect effects such as herd immunity.

The limitations of current vaccines require solutions based on continued research on human local and humoral responses to *V. cholera* antigens. The provision of adequately protective vaccines for immune-naïve individuals (young children and natives of non-endemic regions) remains a future goal. Achieving long-term protection with (preferably) single-dose vaccines and the role of memory immune responses and questions regarding correlates of protection are discussed in detail in the article by Edward Ryan and co-workers [6].

Focusing on the treatment arm of control measures, the history of progress (and regress) in transitional medicine regarding intravenous and oral therapy for cholera and related diseases is comprehensively reviewed in the article by David Nalin [7] on the "Bench to Bedside" vs. "Bedside to Bench" perspectives.

The essentials when delivering oral rehydration therapy (ORT) at the community level are reviewed by Richard Cash [8] based on his experience in the programs conducted by BRAC in Bangladesh villages.

Current controversies in ORT are discussed in David Nalin's review [9] of ongoing modifications to oral solution composition in relation to electrolyte balance, efficacy during rehydration and maintenance phases, and potential safety issues, with a special focus on safety concerns and the differences between cholera and non-cholera dehydrating diarrheas.

Farzana Afroze and co-workers [10] report on the confirmation of a role for Vasoactive Intestinal Polypeptide (VIP) in human cholera pathogenesis, potentially pointing the way to new therapies aiming to quickly stop cholera diarrhea.

References

1. Usmani, M.; Brumfield, K.D.; Jamal, Y.; Huq, A.; Colwell, R.R.; Jutla, A. A Review of the Environmental Trigger and Transmission Components for Prediction of Cholera. *Trop. Med. Infect. Dis.* **2021**, *6*, 147. https://doi.org/10.3390/tropicalmed6030147.
2. Debes, A.K.; Shaffer, A.M.; Ndikumana, T.; Liesse, I.; Ribaira, E.; Djumo, C.; Ali, M.; Sack, D.A. Cholera Hot-Spots and Contextual Factors in Burundi, Planning for Elimination. *Trop. Med. Infect. Dis.* **2021**, *6*, 76. https://doi.org/10.3390/tropicalmed6020076.
3. Bollyky, T.J. Oral Rehydration Salts, Cholera, and the Unfinished Urban Health Agenda. *Trop. Med. Infect. Dis.* **2022**, *7*, 67. https://doi.org/10.3390/tropicalmed7050067.
4. Holmgren, J. An Update on Cholera Immunity and Current and Future Cholera Vaccines. *Trop. Med. Infect. Dis.* **2021**, *6*, 64. https://doi.org/10.3390/tropicalmed6020064.
5. Deen, J.; Clemens, J.D. Licensed and Recommended Inactivated Oral Cholera Vaccines: From Development to Innovative Deployment. *Trop. Med. Infect. Dis.* **2021**, *6*, 32. https://doi.org/10.3390/tropicalmed6010032.
6. Ryan, E.T.; Leung, D.T.; Jensen, O.; Weil, A.A.; Bhuiyan, T.R.; Khan, A.I.; Chowdhury, F.; LaRocque, R.C.; Harris, J.B.; Calderwood, S.B.; Qadri, F.; Charles, R.C. Systemic, Mucosal, and Memory Immune Responses following Cholera. *Trop. Med. Infect. Dis.* **2021**, *6*, 192. https://doi.org/10.3390/tropicalmed6040192.
7. Nalin, D.R. The History of Intravenous and Oral Rehydration and Maintenance Therapy of Cholera and Non-Cholera Dehydrating Diarrheas: A Deconstruction of Translational Medicine: From Bench to Bedside? *Trop. Med. Infect. Dis.* **2022**, *7*, 50. https://doi.org/10.3390/tropicalmed7030050.
8. Ryan, E.T.; Leung, D.T.; Jensen, O.; Weil, A.A.; Bhuiyan, T.R.; Khan, A.I.; Chowdhury, F.; LaRocque, R.C.; Harris, J.B.; Calderwood, S.B.; Qadri, F.; Charles, R.C. Systemic, Mucosal, and Memory Immune Responses following Cholera. *Trop. Med. Infect. Dis.* **2021**, *6*, 192. https://doi.org/10.3390/tropicalmed6040192.
9. Nalin, D. Issues and Controversies in the Evolution of Oral Rehydration Therapy (ORT). *Trop. Med. Infect. Dis.* **2021**, *6*, 34. https://doi.org/10.3390/tropicalmed6010034.
10. Afroze, F.; Bloom, S.; Bech, P.; Ahmed, T.; Sarker, S.A.; Clemens, J.D.; Islam, F.; Nalin, D. Cholera and Pancreatic Cholera: Is VIP the Common Pathophysiologic Factor? *Trop. Med. Infect. Dis.* **2020**, *5*, 111. https://doi.org/10.3390/tropicalmed5030111

David Nalin
Editor

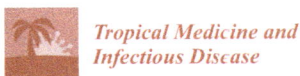

Review

A Review of the Environmental Trigger and Transmission Components for Prediction of Cholera

Moiz Usmani [1], Kyle D. Brumfield [2,3], Yusuf Jamal [1], Anwar Huq [2], Rita R. Colwell [2,3,*] and Antarpreet Jutla [1]

- [1] Geohealth and Hydrology Laboratory, Department of Environmental Engineering Sciences, University of Florida, Gainesville, FL 32603, USA; moiz.usmani@ufl.edu (M.U.); yjamal@ufl.edu (Y.J.); antar.jutla@essie.ufl.edu (A.J.)
- [2] Maryland Pathogen Research Institute, University of Maryland, College Park, MD 20742, USA; kbrum@umd.edu (K.D.B.); huq@umd.edu (A.H.)
- [3] University of Maryland Institute for Advanced Computer Studies, University of Maryland, College Park, MD 20742, USA
- * Correspondence: rcolwell@umd.edu

Abstract: Climate variables influence the occurrence, growth, and distribution of *Vibrio cholerae* in the aquatic environment. Together with socio-economic factors, these variables affect the incidence and intensity of cholera outbreaks. The current pandemic of cholera began in the 1960s, and millions of cholera cases are reported each year globally. Hence, cholera remains a significant health challenge, notably where human vulnerability intersects with changes in hydrological and environmental processes. Cholera outbreaks may be epidemic or endemic, the mode of which is governed by trigger and transmission components that control the outbreak and spread of the disease, respectively. Traditional cholera risk assessment models, namely compartmental susceptible-exposed-infected-recovered (SEIR) type models, have been used to determine the predictive spread of cholera through the fecal–oral route in human populations. However, these models often fail to capture modes of infection via indirect routes, such as pathogen movement in the environment and heterogeneities relevant to disease transmission. Conversely, other models that rely solely on variability of selected environmental factors (i.e., examine only triggers) have accomplished real-time outbreak prediction but fail to capture the transmission of cholera within impacted populations. Since the mode of cholera outbreaks can transition from epidemic to endemic, a comprehensive transmission model is needed to achieve timely and reliable prediction with respect to quantitative environmental risk. Here, we discuss progression of the trigger module associated with both epidemic and endemic cholera, in the context of the autochthonous aquatic nature of the causative agent of cholera, *V. cholerae*, as well as disease prediction.

Keywords: environmental parameters; cholera; *Vibrio cholerae*; trigger; transmission; prediction

Citation: Usmani, M.; Brumfield, K.D.; Jamal, Y.; Huq, A.; Colwell, R.R.; Jutla, A. A Review of the Environmental Trigger and Transmission Components for Prediction of Cholera. *TMID* 2021, 6, 147. https://doi.org/10.3390/tropicalmed6030147

Academic Editor: David Nalin

Received: 14 June 2021
Accepted: 31 July 2021
Published: 5 August 2021

Publisher's Note: MDPI stays neutral with regard to jurisdictional claims in published maps and institutional affiliations.

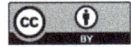

Copyright: © 2021 by the authors. Licensee MDPI, Basel, Switzerland. This article is an open access article distributed under the terms and conditions of the Creative Commons Attribution (CC BY) license (https://creativecommons.org/licenses/by/4.0/).

1. Introduction

Cholera is transmitted primarily by ingestion of contaminated water containing the bacterium *Vibrio cholerae* and has plagued the world for centuries. The ongoing cholera pandemic, the seventh, which started in the 1960s, continues to claim millions of victims every year and is considered the world's longest-running pandemic [1–3]. This acute diarrheal disease remains one of the most significant public health burdens in many regions globally, notably in Latin America, sub-Saharan Africa, and Southern Asia [4,5], where an estimated one million cases are reported every year [6]. The World Health Organization estimates that up to four million reported cholera cases occur across the world annually [4]. However, the actual number of cholera cases is likely much higher as many cases go unreported, especially in developing countries

In recent years, cholera outbreaks have originated primarily in coastal areas [7,8]. The disease is prevalent in parts of the world where human vulnerability (i.e., lack of access to clean water and appropriate sanitation) intersects with changes in hydrological and environmental processes, which provide conditions favorable for the occurrence and growth of *V. cholerae* in the aquatic environment. Furthermore, massive cholera outbreaks are often associated with natural and anthropogenic disasters. A recent example is one of the largest cholera outbreaks in 2016 during the months following Hurricane Matthew [9], which lashed rains over the southwestern coast of Haiti. Damage to water, sanitation, and hygiene (WASH) infrastructure coupled with elevated air temperatures and above-average rainfall promoted exposure of the population to contaminated water. An outbreak of cholera was reported subsequently.

Throughout history, during periods of active conflict and raging wars, infectious diseases have claimed more lives than actual war-induced injuries [10]. Since March 2015, Yemen, a coastal Middle Eastern country, has experienced surges of violent civil unrest. In October 2016, Yemen reported the first of a series of sporadic cholera outbreaks. After the initial reports, the number of cases declined briefly for a few months until the WASH infrastructure failed, resulting in a severe spike in the number of reported cholera cases. The resurgence of the disease and continued environmental exposure of the population proved disastrous to public health. By the end of 2017, Yemen was experiencing the largest cholera outbreak in recorded history [11], which ultimately accounted for an estimated 80% of the globally reported cholera cases that had been recorded since 2015 [12]. While natural disasters can be catalytic for cholera, the Yemen cholera outbreak demonstrates the enormous potential for an anthropogenic catastrophe to affect public health similarly and perhaps even more devastatingly.

Cholera occurs predominantly in two forms: epidemic, characterized either by the sporadic or rampant occurrence of cases in an outbreak; and endemic, defined as cases occurring annually at a continuous level, often with distinct seasonal peaks in the number of cases. Data from epidemiological surveillance suggest that the Yemen cholera outbreak began in the epidemic mode [13]. The dominant hypothesis for epidemic cholera is related to conditions when the air temperature is suddenly anomalously high and excess rainfall occurs with insufficient and/or damaged WASH infrastructure in the region. Human populations will then be at higher risk of exposure to cholera bacteria, hence the disease [14,15]. Per contra, endemic cholera has been shown to occur in a region where *V. cholerae* is constant, even at low abundance, and circulating in the aquatic environment (e.g., rivers, estuaries, and coastal aquatic ecosystems providing conditions favorable for the bacterium). Often, environmental factors influencing endemic cholera will result in cyclical or seasonal recurrence of the disease [16,17]. A sustained epidemic mode of cholera can evolve to become endemic in regions, with the potential for enhanced and continued exposure to, and transmission of, *V. cholerae* [18]. From our previous research [2,19–23], it is understood that *V. cholerae* ecology must be viewed in the context of its natural aquatic environment and a changing climate driving cholera as a potential re-emerging infectious disease.

The dominant forms of cholera (epidemic and endemic) are guided by two components that are key to a disease outbreak, namely trigger and transmission. The trigger module (TM) comprises those mechanisms that support the growth, multiplication, persistence, and distribution of *V. cholerae* in the environment. That is, when TM indicates conditions are favorable for the high abundance of the bacterium and is coincident with insufficient WASH infrastructure, there will be increased interaction between *V. cholerae* and the human population. Following a prevailing TM, the transmission component (TrM) comprises pathways by which an outbreak of cholera will occur and engages complex interactions between humans and contaminated water. The foundational theory of TrM is that humans can accelerate the spread of cholera via intestinal colonization and shedding of cholera bacteria into the environment, thereby contaminating drinking water systems [18]. Given favorable environmental conditions, the bacterium multiplies and can infect a population through the fecal–environmental–oral transmission route. Here, we discuss progression of the TM underlying epidemic cholera, and the TrM associated with both epidemic and endemic cholera, in the context of *V. cholerae* as a bacterium autochthonous to the aquatic habitat and prediction of cholera in the human population.

2. *Vibrio cholerae* and Its Natural Habitat

Vibrio cholerae, the causative agent of the acute diarrheal disease cholera, is a Gram-negative bacterium native to the aquatic environment. Historically, detection of *V. cholerae* was achieved by determining its presence clinically during cholera outbreaks [24]. However, before the advent of epifluorescent microscopy [25,26] and molecular markers [27–31], detection of the presence of *V. cholerae* in the environment was accomplished by employing culture-based techniques [32]. Such investigations significantly underestimated *V. cholerae* populations in the environment, namely because the bacterium can enter a viable but non-culturable (VBNC) state [33]. In the environment and between outbreaks, when environmental conditions are unfavorable for growth and reproduction, the VBNC state allows the bacterium to become metabolically dormant [34,35]. When environmental conditions again become favorable, VBNC cells regain cultivability, having retained virulence potential [36,37]. Furthermore, *V. cholerae* attaches to zooplankton by switching from motile to biofilm lifestyles, which enhances long-term survivability of the bacterium in the environment [38]. Zooplankton, namely copepods, feed on components of the phytoplankton population. Hence, an association between the occurrence of copepods and phytoplankton blooms has been observed [19]. In nutrient-rich water, the increase in the phytoplankton population followed by a zooplankton bloom results in an abundance of *V. cholerae* in coastal waters [16,22]. Because a single copepod can carry up to 10^4 *V. cholerae* cells [19,39], ingestion of untreated drinking water containing a small number of copepods can increase the risk of infection significantly [40–42]. Thus, copepods are a major host and vector of disease. *V. cholerae* has also been observed at high densities attached to abiotic substrates, such as sediment, and associated with various aquatic organisms (e.g., crustaceans, arthropods, fishes, waterfowl, and aquatic plants) [20]. Conversely, in the environment, *V. cholerae*, in association with phages and protozoa, can form antagonistic relationships that reduce microbial populations and shape evolution [20,43].

V. cholerae shares many genotypic and phenotypic characteristics with other bacterial taxa, namely Enterobacteriaceae, and toxigenic strains of *V. cholerae* have acquired the ability to produce cholera toxin, a primary virulence factor, via horizontal gene transfer mediated by a lysogenic bacteriophage [44]. The presence and broad distribution of its virulence genes in the environment have been well documented, and such genes that play a role in the pathogenicity of *V. cholerae* for humans may, at the same time, have environmental relevance (e.g., allowing for metabolic processes, establishing symbiosis, and/or modulating predator/prey relationships in the natural aquatic environment) [45–47]. In the environment, novel phylogenetic lineages of *V. cholerae* have emerged, carrying mutations potentially involved in adapting to aquatic ecosystems [48–50]. Environmental factors, such as the presence of chitin and/or nutrient limitation, can influence horizontal gene transfer [51]. Because many environmental *V. cholerae* isolates have been shown to encode various virulence factors [52] and genetic mutations, some of which have the potential to alter virulence factor production [53], horizontally acquire additional pathogenicity genes [54,55], and even undergo serogroup conversion [55], it is important to determine the total number of *V. cholerae* present in given samples.

Changes in the aquatic environment can have an impact on the intensity of a cholera outbreak [2,23,56–58], and seasonal outbreaks occur annually in regions where the disease is endemic [16,17,59–61]. During outbreaks, the reported number of cholera cases generally peaks during warmer months of the year, notably in Latin America and Africa, but bi-modal peaks are typical in the Bengal Delta region, related to the hydroclimatic influence on the environment in which the bacterium occurs [62]. In Northern Europe and the Atlantic coast of the United States, heatwaves and warming sea temperatures (up to ~1.5 °C over the past half-century) have been associated with long-term increases in abundance of certain pathogenic *Vibrio* spp., namely *V. cholerae*, *V. parahaemolyticus*, and *V. vulnificus* [21]. While it is worth noting that other *Vibrio* spp., such as *Vibrio splendidus*, express virulence factors at low temperatures [63], observed increases in *Vibrio* spp. abundance in Northern Europe and the US were associated with an unprecedented occurrence of environmentally acquired *Vibrio* infections in the human population [21]. Moreover, a changing climate, namely increased sea temperature, could lead to prolonged seasonal abundance of *V. cholerae*, with profound public health implications [64].

Since *V. cholerae* is autochthonous to the aquatic environment, playing an essential role in nutrient cycling [65,66], cholera cannot be eradicated. Therefore, the ecology of *V. cholerae* must be understood in terms of those environmental parameters that drive cholera, especially as a re-emerging infectious disease and in constructing risk prediction models. Furthermore, early warning systems will be needed to safeguard public health in geographical regions vulnerable to natural disasters such as hurricanes and earthquakes or active conflict, namely social strife or civil war, with resultant damage to safe water and sanitation infrastructure.

3. Trigger and Transmission Components for Prediction of Cholera

Traditionally, the spread of cholera has been associated with human activity, notably travel [24] and not hydroclimatic processes. Hydroclimatic processes control the distribution, growth, and incidence of *V. cholerae* in aquatic ecosystems [2] and contribute to genetic diversity and epidemic potential [48]. Therefore, the spread of cholera is a complex function of global travel coupled with climatic processes and the subsequent potential exposure of populations to new spatial and temporal disease outbreaks. Thus, epidemiological research can improve public health interventions aimed at controlling cholera by employing environmental predictive modeling. In 1996, Colwell [2] reported that environmental variables were linked to cholera epidemics and could be evaluated using remote sensing and utilized to develop predictive cholera models. Subsequently, several investigators have confirmed the association of *V. cholerae* with environmental parameters, including sea surface temperature [67–69], sea surface height [67–69], chlorophyll [23,68,70], precipitation [14,71,72], water storage [73], and salinity [74,75], and suggested their use in cholera risk prediction. Accordingly, a mechanistic understanding of environmental factors in the trigger and transmission of cholera has been developed [9,15,76]. While both TM and TrM are important in understanding the global persistence of cholera, high mortality rates observed in epidemic regions (>3%) compared to the endemic areas (<1%) [15] have caused intervention efforts to focus essentially on the TM of predictive cholera modeling systems.

In 2013, Jutla et al. [15] proposed the hypothesis for an epidemic cholera trigger risk prediction system whereby anomalously high (defined as more than one standard positive deviation above the long-term average (>30 years)) temperatures followed by anomalously high precipitation, over a period of four weeks, in a region of damaged or compromised WASH infrastructure, facilitated interaction between contaminated water and the human population and comprised an environment favorable for triggering an epidemic cholera outbreak. With this hypothesis, if one or more of the respective conditions are not satisfied, the region has a lower risk of experiencing an outbreak. Initial support of this hypothesis was obtained from analysis of an earthquake that struck Nepal in 2015 [76], and the hypothesis was validated spatially and temporally for several geographic regions, including South Sudan, Cameroon, Zimbabwe, Haiti, Mozambique, Rwanda, Central African Republic, Nepal, and Bangladesh [9,14,15,70,76] Subsequently, the hypothesis was extended to predict the impact of a disaster (natural or anthropogenic) in triggering a cholera outbreak [9,76]. Results showed that natural and anthropogenic disasters that damaged WASH facilities in a region were generally accompanied by high precipitation, collectively making the environment strongly favorable for the growth of *V. cholerae* and increasing human interaction with contaminated water sources. Thus, policy makers and health professionals are now able to use predictive environmental TMs as a tool to prevent, control, and eliminate cholera. It is worth noting, however, that once an outbreak occurs, the TM should be employed in conjunction with TrM to fully capture the progression of cholera in a given region. The transmission component is more broadly useful compared to the TM since TrM largely relates to the mechanism governing the disease dynamics in a human population and is often employed for forecasting the spread of cholera and public health decision-making [77,78]. Many modeling efforts have been made to reduce the disparity between the actual number of cases in a region and the number predicted by the model (i.e., the forecasted number of cases) [72,79,80]. The compartmental model is the most common type of TrM, mainly because it is simple and easy to use [81]. Compartmental models generally divide a given population into three compartments: Susceptible (S), Exposed (E), Infected (I), and Recovered (R) The four compartments collectively comprise the basic SEIR transmission model [18], a frequently used approach in the epidemiological research domain. Typically, disease dynamics are captured by the rates at which individuals of a population transition between each state (i.e., S, E, I, and R). In Figure 1, we extend the presentation of a basic SIR model to S-E-I-R, accounting for the pathway between the susceptible and exposed populations that have the potential to become infected.

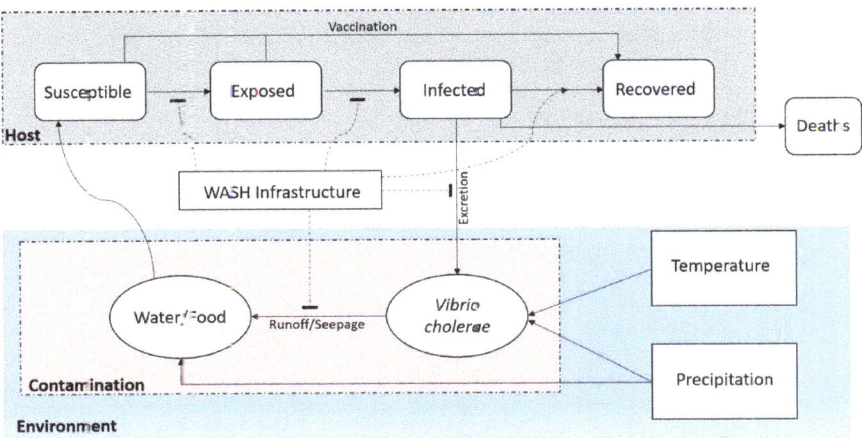

Figure 1. Fundamental cholera susceptible-exposed-infected-recovered (SEIR) transmission model. Susceptible (S) individuals of a population who have been exposed to *Vibrio cholerae* have the potential to acquire the disease from infected (I) individuals. At that point, they also have the potential to become infected (i.e., enter the infectious state), until eventual recovery from the disease (R) or death. Grey shading depicts the SEIR model, which also highlights the potential use of vaccines in curtailing the disease. Water, sanitation, and hygiene (WASH) infrastructure is a critical factor influencing cholera transmission at every stage of the model, from infected to susceptible individuals. Blue represents environmental factors, namely temperature and precipitation, that promote the growth and distribution of *Vibrio cholerae*, the causative agent of cholera, in aquatic reservoirs. Pink shows the potential transmission route from the environment to humans via contaminated food or water containing the *V. cholerae*. Arrow: positive effect; block: negative effect.

The fundamental theory of the SEIR model is presented as the simultaneous presence of four entities (i.e., S, E, I, and R) required for a cholera outbreak. That is, there must be a sufficient quantity of *V. cholerae* circulating within a population, including a large enough number of susceptible individuals. If any of the four entities is missing, the number of cases in an outbreak is reduced, thereby preventing a sporadic outbreak from becoming epidemic in scale. With respect to the dynamics of cholera, there are cyclic interactions between the human population and the pathogen. The robustness of an SEIR-based TrM relies heavily on the extent to which the module is capable of capturing the interactions. Accordingly, a number of studies have employed various mathematical and biological concepts to modify the basic SEIR model in order to incorporate complex interactions associated with modeling cholera outbreaks [82–85]. Table 1 summarizes a few key studies utilizing the SEIR model in cholera outbreaks.

More sophisticated SEIR modeling concepts have been proposed with varying constraints of population structure [86], socio-economic factors [86,87], and other critical factors relevant to the transmission dynamics of cholera. Primarily, mathematical sophistication introduced into a SEIR model aims to address the environmental, biological, and behavioral stochasticity inherent in the mechanism of cholera transmission [56]

However, in some cases, rigorous mathematical complexity may impart problems in evaluating the success of intervention strategies and in assessing the effectiveness of behavioral changes in the human population [80]. In contrast, assumptions made to reduce complexity bring major drawbacks also introduce uncertainty, with respect to overall predictive power. Infection with *V. cholerae* O1, the primary pandemic serogroup, results in protective immunity (i.e., vibriocidal antibodies) that decrease the risk of future infection [88]. Modeling cholera vaccines usually require an assumption that vaccinated individuals share the same protective rate as those naturally infected, and therefore the vaccinated susceptible individuals are treated as 'resistant' [89]. Age has been shown to be important, as children under the age of 5 and the elderly have the highest disease burden of cholera [90,91], but models typically assume that the population age is constant. Attempts to integrate human behavior into the SEIR model typically include the assumption that humans will behave rationally in response to the disease [83]. In practice, this assumption requires the susceptible population to be adequately informed regarding the severity of the cholera outbreak, take necessary measures to reduce contact with contaminated water/food, such as boiling or filtering water, cleaning food preparation areas, and cooking food (especially seafood) properly, and exercise appropriate sanitation practices, including the appropriate disposal of excreta. The assumption of rationality is associated with SEIR models, but it is challenging to quantify the inherent characteristics of human behavior to achieve a realistic representation of the human component in the model. While this assumption eases the model sophistication, it fails to capture the heterogeneities of cholera transmission, increasing the difference between reality and model prediction [80]. Moreover, elucidation of the human factor in cholera modeling is aggravated by the assumption that the mixing of susceptible and infectious individuals will be homogeneous. However, in reality, it has been observed that individuals move within a strong influence of socio-economic factors [92–94]. Hence, various methods have been used to avoid the problematic assumption of homogenous mixing, which includes dividing the susceptible population into low- and high-risk groups or into various categories, based on age, neighborhood, and behavioral risk [86,95]. In addition to these factors, education is considered to be the most cost-effective intervention strategy to prevent the transmission of cholera within at-risk populations [96].

While these methods help to improve the prediction of cholera transmission within well-mixed populations, they fail to capture cholera modes of infection via indirect routes, such as pathogen movement via the environment, or heterogeneities relevant to disease transmission. Interaction between environment and humans is of paramount importance for predictive modeling of cholera [87]. Traditional SEIR models are less successful in dealing with indirect modes of cholera transmission, most likely explaining why they are successful in predicting highly infectious human pathogen spread via direct human-to-human contact (e.g., for viruses causing influenza and coronavirus disease 2019, COVID-19) compared to cholera, where indirect transmission plays a more important role [80]. The importance of indirect transmission routes has encouraged the incorporation of water quality models, seasonality, and climate-driven concepts into SEIR models [58,97–100]. Seasonality is more often analyzed in regions prone to flooding after heavy precipitation, such as Bangladesh [57] and Yemen [101], where monsoons promote a bimodal peak of reported cholera cases [13,17]. The integration of environmental variables into SEIR models will therefore be expected to yield better performance. Given the complex nature of *V. cholerae* in the aquatic environment, an individual environmental variable is insufficient to capture the indirect mode of cholera transmission. That is, to understand the complete dynamics of a cholera outbreak, predictive models need to capture both the direct, namely pathogen movement via humans, and indirect transmission routes. In contrast to SEIR models, models relying solely on the variability of environmental factors have shown remarkable success in real-time cholera prediction [102], suggesting that indirect transmission routes also must be monitored. Furthermore, sensitivity analysis has shown parameter uncertainty in SEIR models, implying small uncertainties in the model parameters (e.g., infection rate) may result in large variations in overall performance [80,103]. Due to parameter uncertainties with respect to cholera and an inability to incorporate indirect transmission routes, SEIR models have been less successful in modeling cholera than other infectious diseases.

Table 1. Cholera prediction using variants of susceptible-infectious-recovered models.

Author(s)	Study Descriptions/Methodology	Important Findings and Outcomes
Codeço 2001 [18]	Proposed mathematical model to explain the dynamics of epidemic and endemic cholera. This study is one of the first applications of the SIR model for cholera transmission.	• Cholera epidemiology depends on social and environmental factors. • Complex interaction between host and pathogen is difficult to model.
Wang et al., 2015 [83]	Separated ordinary differential equation (ODE) and reaction-convection-diffusion partial differential equation (PDE) models to examine the homogeneous and heterogeneous environments associated with cholera transmission.	• Basic reproduction number (R_0) remains a sharp threshold for disease dynamics even when human behavior is considered. • Proposed mathematical justification of several consequences associated with human behavior.
Meszaros et al., 2020 [84]	Proposed a mathematical model for cholera incorporating transmission within and between households.	• Vaccine interventions appeared more effective than water treatment or antibiotic administration to control household cholera.
Abrams et al., 2013 [85]	Developed three cholera surveillance models to forecast the expected number of cases in Haiti during the 2010–2011 cholera epidemic.	• Models increased in complexity as more information became available: first projection estimated 105,000 cholera cases the first year; subsequent projections using different methods estimated up to 652,000 cases. • Timely and realistic projections are crucial in areas with limited resources: real-time projections allowed public health officials to plan and implement response measures better.
Torres et al., 2018 [82]	Proposed and analyzed a SITRV (susceptible-infectious-treated-recovered-vaccinated) type model for cholera.	• The SITRV type model fits well for the cholera outbreak in Yemen April 2017–2018. • The model provides important conclusions concerning vaccination campaigns during a cholera outbreak.
Che et al., 2020 [86]	Used a "fitted" demographic equation (i.e., disease-free equation) to capture total population and a fitted low-high risk structured cholera differential equation model to study reported cholera cases in Cameroon 1987–2004.	• Dual strategies of either vaccination and treatment or vaccination and improved sanitation or combined strategy of vaccination, treatment, and improved sanitation reduce the basic reproductive number of cholera cases. • Rates of scaled contact and the vaccination of susceptible populations are important parameters for cholera prediction.

Table 1. *Cont.*

Author(s)	Study Descriptions/Methodology	Important Findings and Outcomes
Dangbé et al., 2018 [87]	Proposed a model considering climatic factors and human behavior on the spread of cholera	• The transmission and spread of cholera can be affected by climatic factors, the proportion of malnourished individuals, and the number of individuals practicing proper hygiene. • Disease-free equilibrium stability depends on the basic reproduction number (R_0).
Baracchini et al., 2017 [56]	Proposed a stochastic, rainfall–temperature driven model to examine the seasonality of cholera in Bangladesh.	• Rainfall buffers disease transmission in wet regions while enhancing cholera resurgence in dry regions. • Local variation of temperature and rainfall can be used to explain seasonal patterns.
Koepke et al., 2016 [97]	Proposed a predictive 'susceptible-infected-recovered-susceptible' (SIRS) type model in the form of continuous-time hidden Markov states to estimate the contribution of water depth and water temperature on the spread of cholera.	• Hidden states can be used to predict an increase in infected individuals weeks before the observed number of cholera cases increases, thereby providing early notification of the epidemic. • Added support to the hypothesis that environmental forces influence the trigger of a cholera outbreak.
Perez-Saez et al., 2017 [58]	Proposed a probabilistic spatial model to investigate the role human mobility plays in cholera transmission.	• With respect to cholera risk, highly populated urban centers are more sensitive to El Niño/Southern Oscillation than rural periphery. • Cholera risk is largely transmitted from a climate-sensitive core to the periphery. • Included human mobility as a model parameter to improve outbreak prediction performance.

4. Discussion

Climate variability has had a dramatic impact on marine animal and plant communities, as well as marine prokaryotes, all of which play fundamental roles in maintaining life on Earth. Over the past half-century, changes in precipitation and temperature [104] have promoted the emergence and re-emergence of infectious diseases globally [105]. The Fourth Assessment Report of the Intergovernmental Panel on Climate Change (IPCC) suggested that the world will experience enhanced climate variability, including long-term increases in precipitation, temperature, and the number of extreme events, including droughts, floods, hurricanes, and tornadoes [106]. The complex interactions between and among various environmental conditions influence the ecological niche of disease agents. For example, a number of studies have documented a pattern of poleward spreading of *V. cholerae*, demonstrating geographic expansion [21,107–109]. Historically, only *V. cholerae* serogroup O1 was associated with pandemic cholera. However, non-O1 *V. cholerae* are causative agents of sporadic, yet significant, infections ranging in severity from mild to life-threatening. It has recently been reported that *V. cholerae* non-O1 infections are on the rise and represent one of the most striking examples of emerging human diseases linked to climate change [109].

On both local and global scales, climate variability has the potential to significantly affect the emergence, distribution, and prevalence of infectious disease agents and thereby impose a significant burden on public health [110]. One such observation was the massive cholera outbreak in Haiti during the months following Hurricane Matthew [9]. More recently, a cholera outbreak occurred in Yemen following civil unrest in 2016. Cholera appears to be transitioning towards endemicity in that country. In both Haiti and Yemen, cholera occurred during anomalously high temperatures and precipitation, lending support to the trigger hypothesis. Despite the advances made to date, an effective cholera predictive modeling system capable of effectively capturing the transmission of disease through compartmental models has yet to be developed. The transition of cholera from epidemic to endemic in Haiti and Yemen underscores the urgent need for environmental quantitative risk models. On a global scale, it will be necessary for future models to incorporate comparative data baselines with real-time data to improve model output and prediction.

Since it is now well established that *V. cholerae* is ubiquitous in the aquatic environment and plays a critical role in nutrient cycling and in environmental homeostasis, cholera cannot be eradicated, but it can be successfully controlled. Predictive models for cholera risk assessment will be critical in the future to safeguard public health. There is much greater interest in predictive modeling, and the transmission components of such models are receiving greater attention. However, emphasis on trigger components is needed to improve our understanding of the dynamics and progression of cholera. Trigger components have been described that improve quantitative risk modeling as well as disease intervention measures. Yet, most studies of cholera transmission are mechanistic and employ compartmental models, namely the susceptible-exposed-infectious-recovered model. The limitation of mechanistically driven compartmental models is their inability to quantify the uncertainty associated with the spread of cholera. The evolution of the quantitative risk modeling associated with the trigger module is highly promising, but greater success is expected with improved transmission modeling for quantitative risk prediction. With new information from satellite remote sensing, a comprehensive transmission component for the reliable and timely prediction of cholera will surely be available in the near future.

Author Contributions: Conceptualization: M.U., K.D.B., Y.J., A.J., A.H. and R.R.C.; Methodology: M.U., K.D.B. and Y.J.; Software: M.U., K.D.B. and Y.J.; Validation: M.U., K.D.B. and Y.J.; Formal Analysis: M.U., K.D.B. and Y.J.; Investigation: M.U., K.D.B. and Y.J.; Resources: A.J., A.H. and R.R.C.; Data Curation: M.U., K.D.B. and Y.J.; Writing—Original Draft Preparation: M.U., K.D.B. and Y.J.; Writing—Review and Editing: M.U., K.D.B., Y.J., A.J., A.H. and R.R.C.; Visualization: M.U., K.D.B. and Y.J.; Supervision: A.J., A.H. and R.R.C.; Project Administration: M.U., K.D.B., Y.J., A.J., A.H. and R.R.C.; Funding Acquisition: A.J., A.H. and R.R.C. All authors have read and agreed to the published version of the manuscript.

Funding: This research was funded by the National Institute of Environmental Health Sciences, National Institutes of Health (NIH) under award number R01ES030317A and the National Science Foundation (NSF) under award number OCE1839171 to Anwar Huq and Rita Colwell (University of Maryland, College Park, MD) with Antarpreet Jutla (University of Florida, Gainesville, FL). Further support was supplied by NSF under award number CCF1918749 to Rita Colwell. Colwell and Jutla gratefully acknowledge support from NASA award 80NSSC20K0814.

Conflicts of Interest: The sponsors had no role in the design, execution, interpretation, or writing of the study.

References

1. Oprea, M.; Njamkepo, E.; Cristea, D.; Zhukova, A.; Clark, C.G.; Kravetz, A.N.; Monakhova, E.; Ciontea, A.S.; Cojocaru, R.; Rauzier, J.; et al. The seventh pandemic of cholera in Europe revisited by microbial genomics. *Nat. Commun.* **2020**, *11*, 5347. [CrossRef] [PubMed]
2. Colwell, R.R. Global Climate and Infectious Disease: The Cholera Paradigm. *Science* **1996**, *274*, 2025–2031. [CrossRef]
3. Cholera. Available online: https://www.who.int/news-room/fact-sheets/detail/cholera (accessed on 29 June 2021).
4. Ali, M.; Nelson, A.R.; Lopez, A.L.; Sack, D.A. Updated global burden of cholera in endemic countries. *PLoS Negl. Trop. Dis.* **2015**, *9*, e0003832. [CrossRef] [PubMed]
5. Jutla, A.S.; Akanda, A.S.; Islam, S. Tracking Cholera in Coastal Regions using Satellite Observations. *J. Am. Water Resour. Assoc.* **2010**, *46*, 651–662. [CrossRef]
6. WHO; UNICEF. *Progress on Sanitation and Drinking Water: 2010 Update*; WHO: Geneva, Switzerland; UNICEF: New York, NY, USA, 2010. Available online: https://www.who.int/water_sanitation_he (accessed on 5 June 2021).
7. Griffith, D.C.; Kelly-Hope, L.A.; Miller, M.A. Review of reported cholera outbreaks worldwide, 1995–2005. *Am. J. Trop. Med. Hyg.* **2006**, *75*, 973–977. [CrossRef] [PubMed]
8. Huq, A.; Colwell, R. Vibrios in the marine and estuarine environment: Tracking *Vibrio cholerae*. *Ecosyst. Health* **1996**, *2*, 198–214.

9. Khan, R.; Anwar, R.; Akanda, S.; McDonald, M.D.; Huq, A.; Jutla, A.; Colwell, R. Assessment of Risk of Cholera in Haiti following Hurricane Matthew. *Am. J. Trop. Med. Hyg.* **2017**, *97*, 896–903. [CrossRef] [PubMed]
10. Connolly, M.A.; Heymann, D.L. Deadly comrades: War and infectious diseases. *Lancet* **2002**, *360*, s23–s24. [CrossRef]
11. Federspiel, F.; Ali, M. The cholera outbreak in Yemen: Lessons learned and way forward. *BMC Public Health* **2018**, *18*, 1338. [CrossRef]
12. Republic, S.A. WHO Alliance for the Global Elimination of Trachoma by 2020: Progress report on elimination of trachoma, 2014–2016. *Relev. Epidemiol. Hebd.* **2017**, *92*, 359–368.
13. Camacho, A.; Bouhenia, M.; Alyusfi, R.; Alkohlani, A.; Naji, M.A.M.; de Radiguès, X.; Abubakar, A.M.; Almoalmi, A.; Seguin, C.; Sagrado, M.J.; et al. Cholera epidemic in Yemen, 2016–2018: An analysis of surveillance data. *Lancet. Glob. Health* **2018**, *6*, e680–e690. [CrossRef]
14. Jutla, A.; Aldaach, H.; Billian, H.; Akanda, A.; Huq, A.; Colwell, R. Satellite Based Assessment of Hydroclimatic Conditions Related to Cholera in Zimbabwe. *PLoS ONE* **2015**, *10*, e0137828. [CrossRef]
15. Jutla, A.; Whitcombe, E.; Hasan, N.; Haley, B.; Akanda, A.; Huq, A.; Alam, M.; Sack, R.B.; Colwell, R. Environmental factors influencing epidemic cholera. *Am. J. Trop. Med. Hyg.* **2013**, *89*, 597–607. [CrossRef] [PubMed]
16. Alam, M.; Hasan, N.A.; Sadique, A.; Bhuiyan, N.A.; Ahmed, K.U.; Nusrin, S.; Nair, G.B.; Siddique, A.K.; Sack, R.B.; Sack, D.A.; et al. Seasonal cholera caused by *Vibrio cholerae* serogroups O1 and O139 in the coastal aquatic environment of Bangladesh. *Appl. Environ. Microbiol.* **2006**, *72*, 4096–4104. [CrossRef] [PubMed]
17. Alam, M.; Islam, A.; Bhuiyan, N.A.; Rahim, N.; Hossain, A.; Khan, G.Y.; Ahmed, D.; Watanabe, H.; Izumiya, H.; Faruque, A.S.G.; et al. Clonal transmission, dual peak, and off-season cholera in Bangladesh. *Infect. Ecol. Epidemiol.* **2011**, *1*. [CrossRef]
18. Codeço, C.T. Endemic and epidemic dynamics of cholera: The role of the aquatic reservoir. *BMC Infect. Dis.* **2001**, *1*, 1. [CrossRef] [PubMed]
19. Huq, A.; Small, E.B.; West, P.A.; Huq, M.I.; Rahman, R.; Colwell, R.R. Ecological relationships between *Vibrio cholerae* and planktonic crustacean copepods. *Appl. Environ. Microbiol.* **1983**, *45*, 275–283. [CrossRef]
20. Almagro-Moreno, S.; Taylor, R.K. Cholera: Environmental Reservoirs and Impact on Disease Transmission. *Microbiol. Spectr.* **2013**, *1*. [CrossRef]
21. Vezzulli, L.; Grande, C.; Reid, P.C.; Hélaouët, P.; Edwards, M.; Höfle, M.G.; Brettar, I.; Colwell, R.R.; Pruzzo, C. Climate influence on *Vibrio* and associated human diseases during the past half-century in the coastal North Atlantic. *Proc. Natl. Acad. Sci. USA* **2016**, *113*, E5062–E5071. [CrossRef]
22. Vezzulli, L.; Pezzati, E.; Brettar, I.; Höfle, M.; Pruzzo, C. Effects of Global Warming on *Vibrio* Ecology. *Microbiol. Spectr.* **2015**, *3*. [CrossRef]
23. Constantin de Magny, G.; Murtugudde, R.; Sapiano, M.R.P.; Nizam, A.; Brown, C.W.; Busalacchi, A.J.; Yunus, M.; Nair, G.B.; Gil, A.I.; Lanata, C.F.; et al. Environmental signatures associated with cholera epidemics. *Proc. Natl. Acad. Sci. USA* **2008**, *105*, 17676–17681. [CrossRef] [PubMed]
24. Pollitzer, R. Cholera studies. 1. History of the disease. *Bull. World Health Organ.* **1954**, *10*, 421–461. [PubMed]
25. Hasan, J.A.; Bernstein, D.; Huq, A.; Loomis, L.; Tamplin, M.L.; Colwell, R.R. Cholera DFA: An improved direct fluorescent monoclonal antibody staining kit for rapid detection and enumeration of *Vibrio cholerae* O1. *FEMS Microbiol. Lett.* **1994**, *120*, 143–148. [CrossRef] [PubMed]
26. Lowenhaupt, E.; Huq, A.; Colwell, R.R.; Adingra, A.; Epstein, P.R. Rapid detection of *Vibrio cholerae* O1 in west Africa. *Lancet* **1998**, *351*, 34. [CrossRef]
27. Fykse, E.M.; Skogan, G.; Davies, W.; Olsen, J.S.; Blatny, J.M. Detection of *Vibrio cholerae* by real-time nucleic acid sequence-based amplification. *Appl. Environ. Microbiol.* **2007**, *73*, 1457–1466. [CrossRef]
28. Nandi, B.; Nandy, R.K.; Mukhopadhyay, S.; Nair, G.B.; Shimada, T.; Ghose, A.C. Rapid method for species-specific identification of *Vibrio cholerae* using primers targeted to the gene of outer membrane protein OmpW. *J. Clin. Microbiol.* **2000**, *38*, 4145–4151. [CrossRef]
29. Bauer, A.; Rørvik, L.M. A novel multiplex PCR for the identification of *Vibrio vulnificus*, *Vibrio cholerae* and *Vibrio vulnificus*. *Lett. Appl. Microbiol.* **2007**, *45*, 371–375. [CrossRef]
30. Hoshino, K.; Yamasaki, S.; Mukhopadhyay, A.K.; Chakraborty, S.; Basu, A.; Bhattacharya, S.K.; Nair, G.B.; Shimada, T.; Takeda, Y. Development and evaluation of a multiplex PCR assay for rapid detection of toxigenic *Vibrio cholerae* O1 and O139. *FEMS Immunol. Med. Microbiol.* **1998**, *20*, 201–207. [CrossRef] [PubMed]
31. Brumfield, K.D.; Carignan, B.M.; Ray, J.N.; Jumpre, P.E.; Son, M.S. Laboratory Techniques Used to Maintain and Differentiate Biotypes of *Vibrio cholerae* Clinical and Environmental Isolates. *J. Vis. Exp.* **2017**. [CrossRef]
32. Thompson, F.L.; Swings, J. Taxonomy of the Vibrios. In *The Biology of Vibrios*; ASM Press: Washington, DC, USA, 2014; pp. 27–43.
33. Colwell, R.R.; Grimes, D.J. *Nonculturable Microorganisms in the Environment*; Springer: Boston, MA, USA, 2000; ISBN 978-1-4757-0273-6. [CrossRef]
34. Oliver, J.D. Recent findings on the viable but nonculturable state in pathogenic bacteria. *FEMS Microbiol. Rev.* **2010**, *34*, 415–425. [CrossRef]
35. Colwell, R.R. Viable but nonculturable bacteria: A survival strategy. *J. Infect. Chemother.* **2000**, *6*, 121–125. [CrossRef]
36. Colwell, R.R.; Brayton, P.; Herrington, D.; Tall, B.; Huq, A.; Levine, M.M. Viable but non-culturable *Vibrio cholerae* O1 revert to a cultivable state in the human intestine. *World J. Microbiol. Biotechnol.* **1996**, *12*, 28–31. [CrossRef]

37. Senoh, M.; Ghosh-Banerjee, J.; Ramamurthy, T.; Colwell, R.R.; Miyoshi, S.-I.; Nair, G.B.; Takeda, Y. Conversion of viable but nonculturable enteric bacteria to culturable by co-culture with eukaryotic cells. *Microbiol. Immunol.* **2012**, *56*, 342–345. [CrossRef]
38. Alam, M.; Sultana, M.; Nair, G.B.; Siddique, A.K.; Hasan, N.A.; Sack, R.B.; Sack, D.A.; Ahmed, K.U.; Sadique, A.; Watanabe, H.; et al. Viable but nonculturable *Vibrio cholerae* O1 in biofilms in the aquatic environment and their role in cholera transmission. *Proc. Natl. Acad. Sci. USA* **2007**, *104*, 17801–17806. [CrossRef] [PubMed]
39. Colwell, R.R.; Spira, W.M. *Cholera*; Barua, D., Greenough, W.B., Eds.; Springer: Boston, MA, USA, 1992; ISBN 973-1-4757-9690-2. [CrossRef]
40. Huq, A.; Xu, B.; Chowdhury, M.A.; Islam, M.S.; Montilla, R.; Colwell, R.R. A simple filtration method to remove plankton-associated *Vibrio cholerae* in raw water supplies in developing countries. *Appl. Environ. Microbiol.* **1996**, *62*, 2508–2512. [CrossRef] [PubMed]
41. Colwell, R.R.; Huq, A.; Islam, M.S.; Aziz, K.M.A.; Yunus, M.; Khan, N.H.; Mahmud, A.; Sack, R.B.; Nair, G.B.; Chakraborty, J.; et al. Reduction of cholera in Bangladeshi villages by simple filtration. *Proc. Natl. Acad. Sci. USA* **2003**, *100*, 1051–1055. [CrossRef]
42. Cash, R.A.; Music, S.I.; Libonati, J.P.; Snyder, M.J.; Wenzel, R.P.; Hornick, R.B. Response of Man to Infection with *Vibrio cholerae*. I. Clinical, Serologic, and Bacteriologic Responses to a Known Inoculum. *J. Infect. Dis.* **1974**, *129*, 45–52. [CrossRef]
43. Silva-Valenzuela, C.A.; Camilli, A. Niche adaptation limits bacteriophage predation of *Vibrio cholerae* in a nutrient-poor aquatic environment. *Proc. Natl. Acad. Sci. USA* **2019**, *116*, 1627–1632. [CrossRef] [PubMed]
44. Faruque, S.M.; Mekalanos, J.J. Phage-bacterial interactions in the evolution of toxigenic *Vibrio cholerae*. *Virulence* **2012**, *3*, 556–565. [CrossRef] [PubMed]
45. Vezzulli, L.; Guzmán, C.A.; Colwell, R.R.; Pruzzo, C. Dual role colonization factors connecting *Vibrio cholerae*'s lifestyles in human and aquatic environments open new perspectives for combating infectious diseases. *Curr. Opin. Biotechnol.* **2008**, *19*, 254–259. [CrossRef] [PubMed]
46. McFall-Ngai, M. Divining the Essence of Symbiosis: Insights from the Squid-*Vibrio* Model. *PLoS Biol.* **2014**, *12*, e1001783. [CrossRef]
47. Martínez, J.L. Bacterial pathogens: From natural ecosystems to human hosts. *Environ. Microbiol.* **2013**, *15*, 325–333. [CrossRef]
48. Mavian, C.; Paisie, T.K.; Alam, M.T.; Browne, C.; de Rochars, V.M.B.; Nembrini, S.; Cash, M.N.; Nelson, E.J.; Azarian, T.; Ali, A.; et al. Toxigenic *Vibrio cholerae* evolution and establishment of reservoirs in aquatic ecosystems. *Proc. Natl. Acad. Sci. USA* **2020**, *117*, 7897–7904. [CrossRef]
49. Hasan, N.A.; Choi, S.Y.; Eppinger, M.; Clark, P.W.; Chen, A.; Alam, M.; Haley, B.J.; Taviani, E.; Hine, E.; Su, Q., et al. Genomic diversity of 2010 Haitian cholera outbreak strains. *Proc. Natl. Acad. Sci. USA* **2012**, *109*, E2010–E2017. [CrossRef] [PubMed]
50. Conner, J.G.; Teschler, J.K.; Jones, C.J.; Yildiz, F.H. Staying Alive: *Vibrio cholerae*'s Cycle of Environmental Survival, Transmission, and Dissemination. *Microbiol. Spectr.* **2016**, *4*. [CrossRef]
51. Meibom, K.L.; Blokesch, M.; Dolganov, N.A.; Wu, C.-Y.; Schoolnik, G.K. Chitin induces natural competence in *Vibrio cholerae*. *Science* **2005**, *310*, 1824–1827. [CrossRef] [PubMed]
52. Ceccarelli, D.; Chen, A.; Hasan, N.A.; Rashed, S.M.; Huq, A.; Colwell, R.R. Non-O1/non-O139 *Vibrio cholerae* carrying multiple virulence factors and *V. cholerae* O1 in the Chesapeake Bay, Maryland. *Appl. Environ. Microbiol.* **2015**, *81*, 1909–1918. [CrossRef] [PubMed]
53. Carignan, B.M.; Brumfield, K.D.; Son, M.S. Single Nucleotide Polymorphisms in Regulator-Encoding Genes Have an Additive Effect on Virulence Gene Expression in a *Vibrio cholerae* Clinical Isolate. *Msphere* **2016**, *1*, e00253-16. [CrossRef]
54. Blokesch, M.; Schoolnik, G.K. Serogroup Conversion of *Vibrio cholerae* in Aquatic Reservoirs. *PLoS Pathog.* **2007**, *3*, e81. [CrossRef] [PubMed]
55. Colwell, R.R.; Huq, A.; Chowdhury, M.A.; Brayton, P.R.; Xu, B. Serogroup conversion of *Vibrio cholerae*. *Can. J. Microbiol.* **1995**, *41*, 946–950. [CrossRef] [PubMed]
56. Baracchini, T.; King, A.A.; Bouma, M.J.; Rodó, X.; Bertuzzo, E.; Pascual, M. Seasonality in cholera dynamics: A rainfall-driven model explains the wide range of patterns in endemic areas. *Adv. Water Resour.* **2017**, *108*, 357–366. [CrossRef]
57. Martinez, P.P.; Reiner, R.C.; Cash, B.A.; Rodó, X.; Shahjahan Mondal, M.; Roy, M.; Yunus, M.; Faruque, A.S.G.; Huq, S.; King, A.A.; et al. Cholera forecast for Dhaka, Bangladesh, with the 2015–2016 El Niño: Lessons learned. *PLoS ONE* **2017**, *12*, e0172355. [CrossRef] [PubMed]
58. Perez-Saez, J.; King, A.A.; Rinaldo, A.; Yunus, M.; Faruque, A.S.G.; Pascual, M. Climate-driven endemic cholera is modulated by human mobility in a megacity. *Adv. Water Resour.* **2017**, *108*, 367–376. [CrossRef]
59. Deen, J.; Mengel, M.A.; Clemens, J.D. Epidemiology of cholera. *Vaccine* **2020**, *38* (Suppl. 1), A31–A40. [CrossRef]
60. Glass, R.I.; Becker, S.; Huq, M.I.; Stoll, B.J.; Khan, M.U.; Merson, M.H.; Lee, J.V.; Black, R.E. Endemic cholera in rural Bangladesh, 1966–1980. *Am. J. Epidemiol.* **1982**, *116*, 959–970. [CrossRef]
61. Shears, P. Recent developments in cholera. *Curr. Opin. Infect. Dis.* **2001**, *14*, 553–558. [CrossRef] [PubMed]
62. Akanda, A.S.; Jutla, A.S.; Islam, S. Dual peak cholera transmission in Bengal Delta: A hydroclimatological explanation. *Geophys. Res. Lett.* **2009**, *36*, L19401. [CrossRef]
63. Lattos, A.; Bitchava, K.; Giantsis, I.A.; Theodorou, J.A.; Batargias, C.; Michaelidis, B. The implication of *Vibrio* bacteria in the winter mortalities of the critically endangered pinna nobilis. *Microorganisms* **2021**, *9*, 922. [CrossRef] [PubMed]
64. Baker-Austin, C.; Stockley, L.; Rangdale, R.; Martinez-Urtaza, J. Environmental occurrence and clinical impact of *Vibrio vulnificus* and *Vibrio vulnificus*: A European perspective. *Environ. Microbiol. Rep.* **2010**, *2*, 7–18. [CrossRef]

65. Ceccarelli, D.; Colwell, R.R. *Vibrio* ecology, pathogenesis, and evolution. *Front. Microbiol.* **2014**, *5*. [CrossRef]
66. Thompson, J.R.; Polz, M.F. Dynamics of *Vibrio* Populations and Their Role in Environmental Nutrient Cycling. In *The Biology of Vibrios*; ASM Press: Washington, DC, USA, 2014; pp. 190–203. [CrossRef]
67. Lobitz, B.; Beck, L.; Huq, A.; Wood, B.; Fuchs, G.; Faruque, A.S.G.; Colwell, R. Climate and infectious disease: Use of remote sensing for detection of *Vibrio cholerae* by indirect measurement. *Proc. Natl. Acad. Sci. USA* **2000**, *97*, 1438–1443. [CrossRef]
68. Emch, M.; Feldacker, C.; Yunus, M.; Streatfield, P.K.; DinhThiem, V.; Canh, D.G.; Ali, M. Local environmental predictors of cholera in Bangladesh and Vietnam. *Am. J. Trop. Med. Hyg.* **2008**, *78*, 823–832. [CrossRef] [PubMed]
69. Xu, M.; Cao, C.X.; Wang, D.C.; Kan, B.; Xu, Y.F.; Ni, X.L.; Zhu, Z.C. Environmental factor analysis of cholera in China using remote sensing and geographical information systems. *Epidemiol. Infect.* **2016**, *144*, 940–951. [CrossRef]
70. Jutla, A.S.; Akanda, A.S.; Islam, S. A framework for predicting endemic cholera using satellite derived environmental determinants. *Environ. Model. Softw.* **2013**, *47*, 148–158. [CrossRef]
71. Kirpich, A.; Weppelmann, T.A.; Yang, Y.; Ali, A.; Morris, J.G.; Longini, I.M. Cholera Transmission in Ouest Department of Haiti: Dynamic Modeling and the Future of the Epidemic. *PLoS Negl. Trop. Dis.* **2015**, *9*, e0004153. [CrossRef] [PubMed]
72. Eisenberg, M.C.; Kujbida, G.; Tuite, A.R.; Fisman, D.N.; Tien, J.H. Examining rainfall and cholera dynamics in Haiti using statistical and dynamic modeling approaches. *Epidemics* **2013**, *5*, 197–207. [CrossRef]
73. Jutla, A.; Akanda, A.; Unnikrishnan, A.; Huq, A.; Colwell, R. Predictive Time Series Analysis Linking Bengal Cholera with Terrestrial Water Storage Measured from Gravity Recovery and Climate Experiment Sensors. *Am. J. Trop. Med. Hyg.* **2015**, *93*, 1179–1186. [CrossRef] [PubMed]
74. Huq, A.; West, P.A.; Small, E.B.; Huq, M.I.; Colwell, R.R. Influence of water temperature, salinity, and pH on survival and growth of toxigenic *Vibrio cholerae* serovar 01 associated with live copepods in laboratory microcosms. *Appl. Environ. Microbiol.* **1984**, *48*, 420–424. [CrossRef]
75. Singleton, F.L.; Attwell, R.; Jangi, S.; Colwell, R.R. Effects of temperature and salinity on *Vibrio cholerae* growth. *Appl. Environ. Microbiol.* **1982**, *44*, 1047–1058. [CrossRef] [PubMed]
76. Khan, R.; Nguyen, T.H.; Shisler, J.; Lin, L.-S.; Jutla, A.; Colwell, R.R. Evaluation of Risk of Cholera after a Natural Disaster: Lessons Learned from the 2015 Nepal Earthquake. *J. Water Resour. Plan. Manag.* **2018**, *144*, 04018044. [CrossRef]
77. Heesterbeek, H.; Anderson, R.M.; Andreasen, V.; Bansal, S.; De Angelis, D.; Dye, C.; Eames, K.T.D.; Edmunds, W.J.; Frost, S.D.W.; Funk, S.; et al. Modeling infectious disease dynamics in the complex landscape of global health. *Science* **2015**, *347*, aaa4339. [CrossRef] [PubMed]
78. Chowell, G.; Sattenspiel, L.; Bansal, S.; Viboud, C. Mathematical models to characterize early epidemic growth: A review. *Phys. Life Rev.* **2016**, *18*, 66–97. [CrossRef]
79. Andrews, J.R.; Basu, S. Transmission dynamics and control of cholera in Haiti: An epidemic model. *Lancet* **2011**, *377*, 1248–1255. [CrossRef]
80. Grad, Y.H.; Miller, J.C.; Lipsitch, M. Cholera modeling: Challenges to quantitative analysis and predicting the impact of interventions. *Epidemiology* **2012**, *23*, 523–530. [CrossRef] [PubMed]
81. Brauer, F. *Compartmental Models in Epidemiology BT—Mathematical Epidemiology*; Brauer, F., van den Driessche, P., Wu, J., Eds.; Springer: Berlin/Heidelberg, Germany, 2008; pp. 19–79, ISBN 978-3-540-78911-6. [CrossRef]
82. Lemos-Paião, A.P.; Silva, C.J.; Torres, D.F.M. A cholera mathematical model with vaccination and the biggest outbreak of world's history. *AIMS Math.* **2019**, *3*, 448–463. [CrossRef]
83. Wang, X.; Gao, D.; Wang, J. Influence of human behavior on cholera dynamics. *Math. Biosci.* **2015**, *267*, 41–52. [CrossRef] [PubMed]
84. Meszaros, V.A.; Miller-Dickson, M.D.; Baffour-Awuah, F.; Almagro-Moreno, S.; Ogbunugafor, C.B. Direct transmission via households informs models of disease and intervention dynamics in cholera. *PLoS ONE* **2020**, *15*, e0229837. [CrossRef]
85. Abrams, J.Y.; Copeland, J.R.; Tauxe, R.V.; Date, K.A.; Belay, E.D.; Mody, R.K.; Mintz, E.D. Real-time modelling used for outbreak management during a cholera epidemic, Haiti, 2010–2011. *Epidemiol. Infect.* **2013**, *141*, 1276–1285. [CrossRef]
86. Che, E.N.; Kang, Y.; Yakubu, A.-A. Risk structured model of cholera infections in Cameroon. *Math. Biosci.* **2020**, *320*, 108303. [CrossRef] [PubMed]
87. Dangbé, E.; Irépran, D.; Perasso, A.; Békollé, D. Mathematical modelling and numerical simulations of the influence of hygiene and seasons on the spread of cholera. *Math. Biosci.* **2018**, *296*, 60–70. [CrossRef]
88. Glass, R.I.; Svennerholm, A.M.; Khan, M.R.; Huda, S.; Imdadul Huq, M.; Holmgren, J. Seroepidemiological studies of El tor cholera in bangladesh: Association of serum antibody levels with protection. *J. Infect. Dis.* **1985**, *151*, 236–242. [CrossRef] [PubMed]
89. Chao, D.L.; Longini, I.M.; Morris, J.G. Modeling Cholera Outbreaks. In *Cholera Outbreaks*; Nair, G.B., Takeda, Y., Eds.; Springer: Berlin/Heidelberg, Germany, 2014; pp. 195–209. ISBN 978-3-642-55404-9. [CrossRef]
90. Ritter, A.S.; Chowdhury, F.; Franke, M.F.; Becker, R.L.; Bhuiyan, T.R.; Khan, A.I.; Saha, N.C.; Ryan, E.T.; Calderwood, S.B.; LaRocque, R.C.; et al. Vibriocidal titer and protection from cholera in children. *Open Forum Infect. Dis.* **2019**, *6*. [CrossRef]
91. Faruque, A.S.G.; Malek, M.A.; Khan, A.I.; Huq, S.; Salam, M.A.; Sack, D.A. Diarrhoea in elderly people: Aetiology, and clinical characteristics. *Scand. J. Infect. Dis.* **2004**, *36*, 204–208. [CrossRef] [PubMed]
92. Cassiers, T.; Kesteloot, C. Socio-spatial Inequalities and Social Cohesion in European Cities. *Urban. Stud.* **2012**, *49*, 1909–1924. [CrossRef]

93. Najib, K. Socio-spatial inequalities and dynamics of rich and poor enclaves in three French cities: A policy of social mixing under test. *Popul. Space Place* **2020**, *26*. [CrossRef]
94. Gerometta, J.; Haussermann, H.; Longo, G. Social Innovation and Civil Society in Urban Governance: Strategies for an Inclusive City. *Urban. Stud.* **2005**, *42*, 2007–2021. [CrossRef]
95. Al-Arydah, M.; Mwasa, A.; Tchuenche, J.M.; Smith, R.J. Modeling cholera disease with education and chlorination. *J. Biol. Syst.* **2013**, *21*, 1340007. [CrossRef]
96. Einarsdóttir, J.; Passa, A.; Gunnlaugsson, G. Health education and cholera in rural Guinea-Bissau. *Int. J. Infect. Dis.* **2001**, *5*, 133–138. [CrossRef]
97. Koepke, A.A.; Longini, I.M., Jr.; Halloran, M.E.; Wakefield, J.; Minin, V.N. Predictive modeling of cholera outbreaks in Bangladesh. *Ann. Appl. Stat.* **2016**, *10*. [CrossRef] [PubMed]
98. Kulinkina, A.V.; Mohan, V.R.; Francis, M.R.; Kattula, D.; Sarkar, R.; Plummer, J.D.; Ward, H.; Kang, G.; Balraj, V.; Naumova, E.N. Seasonality of water quality and diarrheal disease counts in urban and rural settings in south India. *Sci. Rep.* **2016**, *6*, 20521. [CrossRef]
99. Altizer, S.; Dobson, A.; Hosseini, P.; Hudson, P.; Pascual, M.; Rohani, P. Seasonality and the dynamics of infectious diseases. *Ecol. Lett.* **2006**, *9*, 467–484. [CrossRef]
100. Ruiz-Moreno, D.; Pascual, M.; Bouma, M.; Dobson, A.; Cash, B. Cholera Seasonality in Madras (1901–1940): Dual Role for Rainfall in Endemic and Epidemic Regions. *Ecohealth* **2007**, *4*, 52–62. [CrossRef]
101. Nishiura, H.; Tsuzuki, S.; Yuan, B.; Yamaguchi, T.; Asai, Y. Transmission dynamics of cholera in Yemen, 2017: A real time forecasting. *Theor. Biol. Med. Model.* **2017**, *14*, 14. [CrossRef] [PubMed]
102. Predicting Cholera Risk in Yemen. Available online: https://earthobservatory.nasa.gov/images/147101/predicting-cholera-risk-in-yemen (accessed on 5 June 2021).
103. van den Driessche, P. Reproduction numbers of infectious disease models. *Infect. Dis. Model.* **2017**, *2*, 288–303. [CrossRef] [PubMed]
104. Aguilar, E.; Peterson, T.C.; Obando, P.R.; Frutos, R.; Retana, J.A.; Solera, M.; Soley, J.; García, I.G.; Araujo, R.M. Santos, A.R.; et al. Changes in precipitation and temperature extremes in Central America and northern South America, 1961–2003. *J. Geophys. Res. Atmos.* **2005**, *110*, 1–15. [CrossRef]
105. El-Sayed, A.; Kamel, M. Climatic changes and their role in emergence and re-emergence of diseases. *Environ. Sci. Pollut. Res.* **2020**, *27*, 22336–22352. [CrossRef]
106. AR4 Climate Change 2007: The Physical Science Basis—IPCC. Available online: https://www.ipcc.ch/report/ar4/wg1/ (accessed on 29 June 2021).
107. Baker-Austin, C.; Trinanes, J.; Gonzalez-Escalona, N.; Martinez-Urtaza, J. Non-Cholera Vibrios: The Microbial Barometer of Climate Change. *Trends Microbiol.* **2017**, *25*, 76–84. [CrossRef]
108. Baker-Austin, C.; Trinanes, J.A.; Taylor, N.G.H.; Hartnell, R.; Siitonen, A.; Martinez-Urtaza, J. Emerging Vibrio risk at high latitudes in response to ocean warming. *Nat. Clim. Chang.* **2013**, *3*, 73–77. [CrossRef]
109. Vezzulli, L.; Baker-Austin, C.; Kirschner, A.; Pruzzo, C.; Martinez-Urtaza, J. Global emergence of environmental non-O1/O139 *Vibrio cholerae* infections linked with climate change: A neglected research field? *Environ. Microbiol.* **2020**, *22*, 4342–4355. [CrossRef]
110. Anderson, P.K.; Cunningham, A.A.; Patel, N.G.; Morales, F.J.; Epstein, P.R.; Daszak, P. Emerging infectious diseases of plants: Pathogen pollution, climate change and agrotechnology drivers. *Trends Ecol. Evol.* **2004**, *19*, 535–544. [CrossRef]

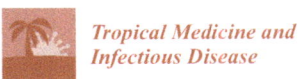

Article

Cholera Hot-Spots and Contextual Factors in Burundi, Planning for Elimination

Amanda K. Debes [1,*], Allison M. Shaffer [1], Thaddee Ndikumana [2], Iteka Liesse [2], Eric Ribaira [3], Clement Djumo [3], Mohammad Ali [1] and David A. Sack [1]

1. Department of International Health, Johns Hopkins School of Public Health, Baltimore, MD 21205, USA; Allisonshaffer94@gmail.com (A.M.S.); moali.jhsph@gmail.com (M.A.); dsack1@jhu.edu (D.A.S.)
2. Ministry of Public Health, Rue Pierre Ngendandumwe, Bujumbura B.P. 1650, Burundi; ndikumanathaddee@gmail.com (T.N.); iteka.liesse5@gmail.com (I.L.)
3. UNICEF Burundi Country Office, Bujumbura B.P. 1650, Burundi; eribaira@unicef.org (E.R.); cdjumo@unicef.org (C.D.)
* Correspondence: adebes1@jhu.edu

Abstract: The Republic of Burundi first reported cholera cases in 1978 and outbreaks have been occurring nearly every year since then. From 2008–2020, 6949 cases and 43 deaths were officially reported. To evaluate Burundi's potential to eliminate cholera, we identified hotspots using cholera incidence and disease persistence as suggested by the Global Task Force for Cholera Control. The mean annual incidence for each district that reported cholera ranged from 0.29 to 563.14 cases per 100,000 population per year from 2014–2020. Ten of 12 Health Districts which recorded cholera cases reported a mean annual incidence ≥5 per 100,000 for this time period. Cholera cases occur during the second half of the year in the areas near Lake Tanganyika and along the Ruzizi River, with the highest risk district being Bujumbura Centre. Additional research is needed to understand the role of Lake Tanganyika; risks associated with fishing; migration patterns; and other factors that may explain cholera's seasonality. Due to the consistent epidemiological pattern and the relatively small area affected by cholera, control and elimination are feasible with an integrated program of campaigns using oral cholera vaccine over the short term and community-based interventions including WASH activities for sustained control.

Keywords: cholera; diarrhea; Burundi; hot spot; oral cholera vaccine

1. Introduction

1.1. Background Information Regarding Burundi

The Republic of Burundi is a landlocked country in the Great Lakes region of Africa which has outbreaks of cholera regularly every year. It lies between Rwanda to the north, Tanzania to the south and east, the Democratic Republic of the Congo (DRC) to the northwest, and Lake Tanganyika to the southwest. The Ruzizi River (also spelled Rusizi River), which flows into Lake Tanganyika from Lake Kivu, serves as the border between the DRC and Burundi. The capital of the country, Bujumbura, is located near the northern part of Lake Tanganyika. The total land area is 27,830 sq km, and the country is divided into 18 provinces which are further divided into 47 districts and 119 communes. The smallest subdivision is the colline, of which there are 2638.

Some of the factors in Burundi that relate to cholera patterns include seasonality, population density, insufficient water-sanitation infrastructure, considerable internal and external migration, poverty, and the relationship of people to Lake Tanganyika.

Burundi has two rainy seasons, a major one from February to May and a lesser one between September and November. The dry seasons are from June to August and December to January. Minimum monthly temperatures appear to be constant throughout the year, but higher maximal temperatures occur from July to October [1].

While the country is geographically small, it is among the top five most densely populated countries in Africa with 463 inhabitants per square kilometers [2]. It has a high fertility rate (about 5.4 children per woman), an infant mortality ratio estimated to be 42 per 1000 live births and a maternal mortality ratio estimated to be 548 per 100,000 live births [2]. Over 90% are employed in agriculture and about 85% of the people are rural subsistence farmers [1], and 65% of the population are living in poverty, or less than USD 1.90 per day per person [3,4].

Indicators of water and sanitation for Burundi demonstrate the need for major improvements. According to the Joint Monitoring Project of the WHO and UNICEF [5], 20% of the population use unimproved or surface water for drinking, and another 20% use water sources that are too far away from their homes. Less than half of the population (46%) has access to basic sanitation, and 40% use unimproved latrines. Handwashing with soap appears to be practiced regularly by only 6% of the population. Thus, many households still rely on unsafe sources for drinking water and lack basic sanitation and hygiene facilities. This is especially true for the lowest quintile and for the rural populations, where the percentages are more worrisome.

Burundi has a long history of both natural disasters and civil conflict, both of which have contributed to its high degree of migration. Within Burundi, people are often displaced because of natural disasters such as landslides, flooding and high winds [6]. When persons are displaced, they are less likely to have access to basic water and hygiene infrastructure. According to a report by the International Organization of Migration (IOM)(7), 90% of 15,000 Internally Displaced People (IDPs) in one area (Bubanza and Kirundo) did not have access to a latrine [7]. Nationally, approximately 42% of collines report that IDP households do not have access to latrines. Further, handwashing systems with soap are not present in 81% of collines, and concerns about the drinking water were reported in 37% of collines. When natural disasters destroy infrastructure such as water sources, roads, etc., people who are not displaced are still affected by the natural disasters and are also at higher risk for cholera. Many displaced persons settle in the provinces along Lake Tanganyika and the Ruzizi River, which our analysis identifies as cholera hotspots.

Migration to and from neighboring countries arise due to violent conflicts, but sometimes are related to the search for employment. As of 31 January 2021, 306,000 people have fled Burundi (almost 3% of the population), with over half of the refugees traveling to Tanzania (148,000) and many others traveling to Rwanda (62,000), the DRC (47,000), and Uganda (50,000) [8]. Since 2017, 125,063 individuals have been repatriated to Burundi as of 31 January 2021, with nearly all of those individuals returning from Tanzania. Returning migrants often have difficulty reintegrating because of the population density, lack of employment and loss of land that they formerly owned. The UNHCR does support their right to return if the decision to return is voluntary, but its stated policy is to not actively promote returning.

Lake Tanganyika plays a critical role in the life and economy of Burundi. The lake is an extremely large, deep, freshwater lake with an alkaline pH (pH 8.5–9); the surface temperature ranges between 25 and 28 °C [9,10] without major differences in characteristics in the water's physical or chemical properties during the seasons. There have been few publications describing epidemic cholera in Burundi; however, in the late 1990s, *V. cholerae* was isolated from the water of Lake Tanganyika and cholera cases were associated with exposure to or drinking lake water in case control studies [11].

1.2. Study Background Information

In East and Central Africa, Burundi is one of the countries where cholera is endemic. Burundi first reported cholera cases to the World Health Organization (WHO) in 1978 and cases have been reported in Burundi every year, except during 1986–1989 [12]. Compared to neighboring countries such as the DRC or Tanzania with much larger populations, Burundi reports fewer annual numbers of cholera cases and deaths; still, these outbreaks have a major impact on the country. The reported cases are typically concentrated along

Lake Tanganyika, near the border with the DRC. The provinces with cholera cases, unofficially called the "cholera belt", are usually along the "plain d'Imbo", which includes the northeast bordering the DRC (Cibitoke, Bubanza) and the provinces along Lake Tanganyika (Rumonge, Makamba, and Bujumbura Mairie/Rural). Interestingly, this pattern has persisted for several decades [11]. In addition to the outbreaks within Burundi, in 2015 a large cholera outbreak occurred in a Burundian refugee settlement in Kigoma, Tanzania, with over 3000 cases and 30 deaths. It is not clear if the refugees from Burundi introduced cholera into the camps or were susceptible because of the conditions in the camps [13].

Cholera cases that were reported to the World Health Organization (WHO) from 2008 through 2018 are shown in Table 1. It should be noted that many countries, especially in Asia, known to have large number of cholera cases do not report or severely under-report cases to the WHO.

Table 1. Number of cholera cases reported to the World Health Organization annually between 2008 and 2018. The totals for the "World" include all cases reported to WHO.

	2008	2009	2010	2011	2012	2013	2014	2015	2016	2017	2018
Burundi	234	355	333	1072	214	1557	582	442	434	300	92
Tanzania	2911	7700	4469	942	286	270	0	11,563	11,360	4895	4777
Uganda	3726	1095	2341	0	6326	748	309	1461	516	292	4440
DRC	30,150	22,899	18,384	21,700	33,661	26,944	22,203	19,182	28,093	56,190	30,768
Rwanda	23	0	0	0	9	0	0	0	355	0	0
All Africa	179,323	217,333	115,106	188,678	117,570	0	105,287	71,176	71,058	179,385	120,652
World	190,130	221,226	317,106	589,854	245,393	129,064	190,549	172,454	132,121	1,227,391	499,447

Cases of cholera, both suspected and confirmed, are recorded using Burundi's Integrated Disease Surveillance and Response (IDSR) system [14]. According to the Burundian National Cholera Plan, a "suspected" case, outside of an outbreak, is a patient with acute watery diarrhea, five years or older with severe dehydration, or one who dies from the diarrhea. If a cholera outbreak is ongoing, a suspected cholera patient is one aged five years or older with acute watery diarrhea. During an outbreak, this definition includes diarrhea patients two years or older. A case is "confirmed" when a microbiological culture from the fecal specimen of a suspected case is positive for *Vibrio cholerae* O1 or O139 (Serotype O139 has never been isolated in Burundi). Generally, the National Reference Laboratory in Bujumbura is the laboratory that confirms the case. One case of suspected cholera signifies the alert threshold, while a case must be confirmed before declaring an outbreak, signifying the "action threshold." The first ten suspected cases are to be cultured, but after one or more are culture-confirmed, it is not necessary to confirm each case.

This epidemiological analysis is intended to provide an overview of the burden of cholera. A principal objective of this analysis was to identify cholera hotspots in Burundi since these are the areas where interventions should focus. A secondary objective was the identification of other factors that may assist in informing intervention and cholera control decisions. Per the GTFCC guidance on developing a national cholera control plan, countries should conduct a situational analysis to include an assessment of the country's cholera epidemiological situation. This includes the review of historical cholera burden data to identify cholera hotspots and to review contextual factors of hotspots, including population mobility, vulnerability, weather patterns, access to WaSH, among potential other contextual factors [15]. Burundi last updated their National Cholera Control Plan (NCP) in 2012; thus, this analysis may provide information relevant to the National Plan.

2. Materials and Methods

2.1. Cholera Case Data

Weekly reported suspected cholera case data from Burundi for the years 2014–2020 were obtained from the IDSR surveillance system conducted by the Ministry of Public Health of Burundi (MOPH). Cholera cases are reported at the Health District level. Burundi is divided into 47 Health Districts, and each Health District consists of 2–4 communes. The names of these Health Districts were matched with the names in the reference mapping file. The duration of each outbreak was calculated by comparing the start and end week of reported cases in each Health District. Outbreaks that might have continued across Health District borders were considered as two separate outbreaks.

2.2. Population Data

The population data were obtained at the commune level from the most recent census, in 2008. Although the population has increased since then, we assumed this growth was occurring at a similar rate in the different commune [16]. The Health District populations were calculated by adding together the populations of the communes in the Health District.

2.3. Geographic Information Systems (GIS) Data

The Health District boundary map of Burundi was obtained from the United Nations Office for the coordination of Human Affairs. The maps were projected in WGS84 UTM coordinates system Zone 37S (http://geokov.com/education/utm.aspx, accessed on 16 February 2021). Data for cholera hotspots were analyzed using the second administrative boundary level as the geographic unit of analysis.

2.4. Identification of Hotspots

Hotspots are defined by the GTFCC as a geographically limited area where environmental, cultural and/or socioeconomic conditions facilitate the transmission of the disease in that cholera persists or reappears regularly [15]. We then applied the GTFCC definition which utilizes mean annual incidence and persistence to differentiate low, medium and high-risk districts to identify priority areas/hotspots [17].

This analysis used the method for hotspot analysis recommended by the Global Task Force on Cholera Control (GTFCC), which is based on the mean annual incidence of cholera cases and the persistence of the disease [18]. Ideally, this analysis is based on a minimum of five years of weekly or monthly district or administrative level-2 data. As data for more than seven years were available for this analysis, we conducted the analysis to determine if the hotspots are consistent over time, depicting the hotspots for the first 5-year period and compared to the latter 5-year period. Districts were excluded from the analysis if they reported a very low mean annual incidence (less than 5 cases per 100,000 population per year) since these very low rates likely represented falsely reported cases or, if they represented true cases, the low rates suggest the absence of onward transmission.

2.5. Definitions in Data Management

The end of a discrete outbreak is defined, per the GTFCC, as the point when two weeks have passed with no further suspected cases [18]. Persistence is measured by the proportion (or percentage) of weeks with cholera being reported in the district. Annual incidence is determined by the total number of cases reported per year divided by the population, the sum of which is multiplied by 100,000 persons. The mean annual incidence is subsequently determined as the average of the time period considered for the analysis (in this case, 5 years). This calculation is further defined in the GTFCC tool [17].

Ethical Considerations: As this study only uses secondary, aggregated, de-identified data, the Ministry of Public Health of Burundi determined that ethical approval was unnecessary. Additionally, the IRB at the Johns Hopkins Bloomberg School of Public Health Institutional Review Board determined that this activity was exempt.

3. Results

3.1. Weekly Number of Cases

Cholera cases were reported every year between 2008 and 2020. Over this 13-year span, 6949 cases and 43 deaths were reported. A more detailed analysis was conducted for two five-year periods for which we had data at district level to facilitate the use of the GTFCC tool. The 7 years of total data were divided into two 5-year periods of analysis, overlapping in years 2016–2018, but facilitating the assessment of whether the hotspots were consistent over time. From 2014 to 2018, 575, 423, 434, 344, and 92 cases were reported for these years, respectively, for a total of 1868 cases and 14 deaths. The second analysis was from 2016–2020, during which 1195 cases and 3 deaths, and 139 cases and 1 death, were reported in 2019 and 2020, respectively. These cases were reported from 12 Health Districts, all on the western side of the country near Lake Tanganyika, or along the Ruzizi River near the border with the DRC.

Cases occurred during discrete outbreaks within individual districts experiencing from one to eleven such outbreaks during the 7 years (median of 4.5 outbreaks). The outbreaks lasted from 1 to 24 weeks, with most lasting fewer than 3 weeks. The distribution of the number of outbreaks per district is shown in Figure 1.

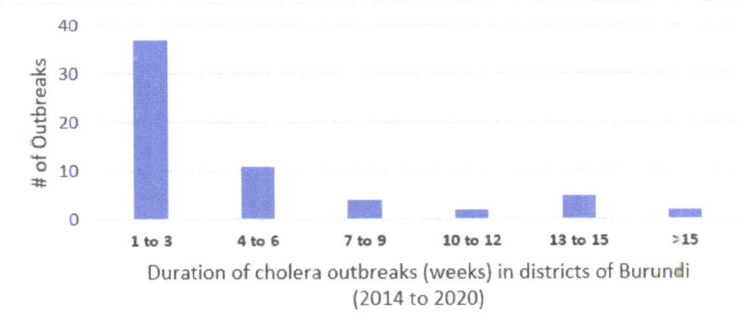

Figure 1. Duration of cholera outbreaks (weeks) in districts of Burundi (2014–2020).

The weekly number of cases during the surveillance period showed a seasonal pattern, with most cases occurring during the second half of the year (Figure 2). The pattern in 2018 was unusual in that the outbreak started very late in the year, during the last week of 2018, and this outbreak continued into 2019. This was followed by a more typical wave starting in June 2019. Outbreaks tended to start at the end of the dry season but continued into the rainy season.

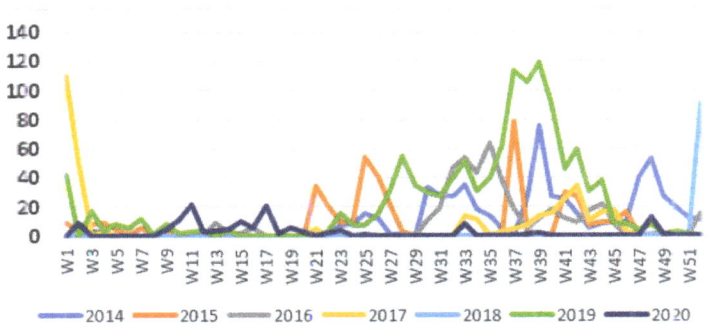

Figure 2. Weekly cases of cholera, 2014–2020.

3.2. Hotspot Classification–Mean Annual Incidence and Persistence

Cholera occurred annually in Burundi during the timeframe of this analysis (Figure 3). The mean annual incidence for each district that reported cholera ranged from 0.29 to 563.14 cases per 100,000 population per year.

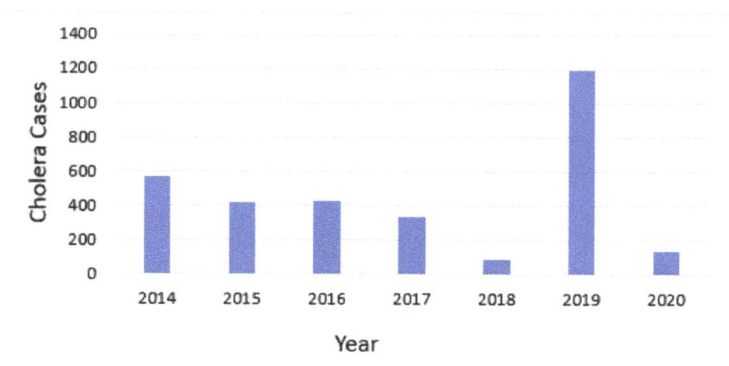

Figure 3. Annual number of cholera cases.

Of 12 Health Districts that reported cholera, ten reported a mean annual incidence ≥5 per 100,000 during the time period of 2014–2020. The cutoff values for determining the magnitude of the cholera risk include applying the median annual incidence (23/100,000) and the median proportion (percentage) of weeks with cholera, defined as persistence (8%), among the nine districts included in the analysis for 2014–2018. For the time period of 2016–2020, the median annual incidence was 13/100,000 and persistence was 5% among the nine districts included in the analysis for this time period. The districts reporting cholera were subsequently grouped into high, medium, and lower risk among the identified hotspots according to the criteria in Table 2.

Table 2. Thresholds of mean annual incidence and stability of cases applied per hotspot type.

Type of Hotspots	Mean Annual Incidence Per 100,000 Population (70th percentile value)		Proportion of Weeks with Cholera Reported (60th Percentile Value)	
	2014–2018	2016–2020	2014–2018	2016–2020
High	>23	>13	>8%	>5%
Medium	>23	>13	≤8%	≤5%
Medium	≤23	≤13	>8%	>5%
Lower	≤23	≤13	≤8%	≤5%

When applying the combination of the two cutoffs in Table 2 for the 2014–2018 time period, there were four high-risk districts, one medium-risk district and four low-risk districts. Applying the same cutoffs to the most recent time period of 2016–2020, three health districts were considered as high risk, three were considered medium risk and three were low risk. When applying the cut-offs, other districts in the country were below the threshold for the analysis. The populations of these districts according to the 2008 census are shown in Table 3, and the hotspot districts for the 2014–2018 and 2016–2020 time periods are mapped and shown graphically in Figure 4.

Table 3. Health Districts categorized by the type of hotspots, based on thresholds of the mean annual incidence and persistence of cholera, defined as the proportion of total weeks during two overlapping time periods.

Type of Hotspot	District	2014–2018		2016–2020		Population (Refers to Groups 2016–2020)
		Mean Annual Incidence/100,000	Proportion of Weeks with Cholera Reported (%)	Mean Annual Incidence/100,000	Proportion of Weeks with Cholera Reported (%)	
High	Bujumbura centre	57.37	16.92	142.12	21.92	123,415
	Cibitoke	50.89	14.23	42.20	16.15	229,867
	Kabezi	37.05	10.38	31.22	6.54	171,665
	Total high					524,947
Medium	Mpanda	15.57	8.08	8.02	5.38	172,138
	Bujumbura nord *	-	-	12.70	3.92	248,915
	Rumonge Φ	29.55	10	18.85	4.62	203,744
	Total Medium					624,797
Lower	Bubanza	6.1	3.1	5.55	1.92	165,885
	Bujumbura sud	5.3	4.2	5.93	4.23	124,836
	Nyanza-Lac Ψ	5.77	4.51	4.51	2.31	203,811
	Mabayi δ	6.2	0.4	-	-	230568
	Total Lower					494,532
Total Hotspots						1,644,276

* Did not appear in earlier analysis but was medium in later analysis. Φ High in earlier analysis, medium in later analysis. Ψ Medium in earlier, low in later analysis. δ Low in earlier analysis, did not appear in later analysis.

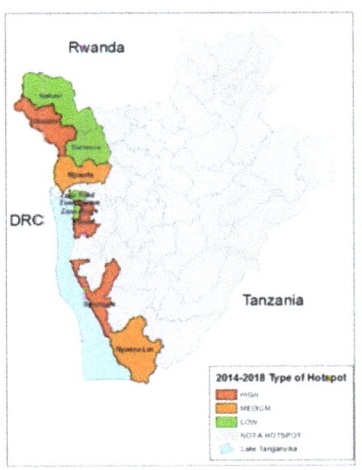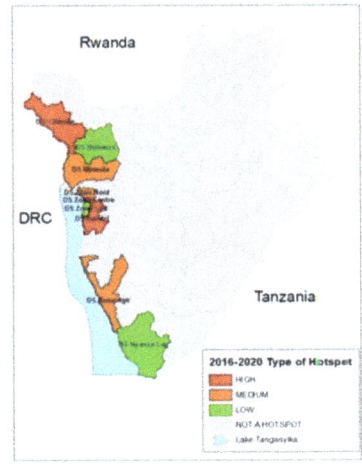

Figure 4. 2014–2018 Hotspot classification map as compared to 2016–2020 Hotspot classification map.

4. Discussion

4.1. Hotspots and Contextual Factor Findings

This analysis demonstrates that cholera occurred every year in Burundi from 2014 through 2020 and the hotspot pattern proved to be consistent during the period 2014 to 2020. Although there was some variability between the districts in their rank order, the same areas along Lake Tanganyika and along the Ruzizi River, bordering the DRC, were the districts which reported cholera. Other parts of Burundi away from the Lake or the River rarely reported cholera. The designation of high, medium and lower risk hotspots are designations suggested by the GTFCC, and national policy makers will use this information, along with other factors, as they develop plans for cholera control.

Since cholera was first reported in Burundi in 1978, it has remained consistent with very few exceptions. The regular pattern of yearly outbreaks is highlighted further by the striking seasonal pattern in which cholera outbreaks start in the second half of the calendar year and by the consistent locations where the outbreaks occur. The outbreaks occur along the edge of Lake Tanganyika or north of the Lake along the Ruzizi River, which forms the border with the DRC.

During these outbreaks, several hundred cases are reported. These numbers are smaller than the numbers of cases in neighboring countries with much larger populations, such as the DRC or Tanzania, but they do constitute a great threat to the people of Burundi. Cholera outbreaks require many resources and require the need for very rapid and vigorous response limited health workers to avoid cholera deaths.

The two time periods of hotspot analysis identified three of the same Health Districts with consistent high priority risk, with a fourth identified in the 2014–2018 time period which remained medium risk in the most recent time period. Both analyses identified additional Health Districts with heightened risk but at a somewhat lower level. The identification of these districts and the predictable nature of the time and place of the outbreaks provide valuable information with which to focus prevention efforts. Such preventive efforts should, of course, include improving water and sanitation infrastructure. For the short term, campaigns to provide oral cholera vaccine to the people living in the highest risk health districts might quickly eliminate these seasonal outbreaks. As the cholera pattern is so consistent, the effectiveness of the OCV campaigns could quickly be evaluated. Being a relatively small country, this would require vaccinating about 1.6 million people living in the districts at risk, or if one were to be more selective, 728,000 living in the highest risk districts identified in either time period. While the maps identify the districts at highest risk, additional local knowledge should be added to provide a more comprehensive understanding of the actual areas at risk. For example, if cases from Bujumbura Centre are actually from the urban area, specific evaluations may be needed to address municipal water and sanitation needs and also consider the specific neighborhoods from which cases arise.

4.2. Planning for Elimination

Vaccination campaigns in Burundi would be logistically feasible because the high-risk districts are geographically close to the capital, Bujumbura, where the vaccine could be stored and teams mobilized. The national laboratory is also located in Bujumbura, which simplifies the confirmation of cases following the vaccine campaign; this is important to document the vaccine's effectiveness.

With financial support from GAVI (Geneva, Switzerland), OCV campaigns have been carried out in several African countries including Malawi [19–21], Uganda [22,23], Zambia [24] and South Sudan [25], among others. African countries that have used the largest number of doses include the DRC, Nigeria, Zambia, South Sudan, and Malawi, but 16 African countries have now used OCV [26].

OCV is recommended as a two-dose vaccine with an interval of about 2 to 4 weeks between vaccine rounds. Campaigns using a two-week immunization strategy are possible in Burundi; however, cholera's unique epidemiology in Burundi suggests consideration of other vaccination strategies. Specifically, the first round should be given prior to the expected cholera season (e.g., the month of May). The second round could be given two weeks later, but another option is to wait until the following May to give the second round. The consideration of a delayed second round relates to the protection provided by a single dose [27,28] and the potential that two rounds of vaccine over two years may extend protection because the campaign provided during the second round will immunize additional people who have moved into the area in the intervening year, thus increasing vaccine coverage over a longer period.

In addition to using OCV to prevent cholera, enhanced surveillance would improve the understanding of cholera's epidemiology in Burundi and would be needed to monitor and evaluate the effectiveness of interventions such as vaccine campaigns and WASH improvements. Rapid diagnostic tests (RDTs) are now available that allow the detection of a case within 15 min. If these were made available in the health facilities in the hotspot districts, outbreaks could be detected rapidly, and samples could be sent to the National Laboratory to declare the outbreak even more quickly. The RDTs can then be used to monitor the course of the outbreak while determining the proportion of cases which are true cases and determine when the outbreak is over. Isolates that are detected at the National Lab should be saved so that molecular testing can confirm their relation to isolates from neighboring countries, especially the DRC and Tanzania.

Reasons for the consistent cholera season in Burundi were not identified. The association of the hotspots being adjacent to Lake Tanganyika and to the border with the DRC suggests the infection may be transmitted from the DRC where cholera is known to be endemic [29]. During the years 2014–2018, over 150,000 cases were reported to the WHO from the DRC, and most of these cases occurred in Eastern DRC. Molecular studies of the strains in the DRC and Burundi would need to be conducted to validate this assumption. Transmission pattern studies and hotspot analyses have been completed in the neighboring country of Uganda [22,30]. Cross-border spread was demonstrated in a study comparing the borders of neighboring countries of Uganda–DRC as well as Malawi–Mozambique, describing how to work to control this risk area [31]. The identification of cholera hotspots near the African Great Lakes is similar to findings from previous studies in the DRC, Uganda, and Malawi [8,21–23].

Some suggest that a high-risk group are the fishermen who often travel back and forth across the lake. Certainly, fishing villages have been identified as having a higher cholera risk in Uganda [32] and Malawi [33]. The chemistry of lake water is favorable to the maintenance of *V. cholerae*, having an alkaline pH, and *V. cholerae* has been recovered from lake water in the past during an outbreak. If so, it is possible that the domestic use of lake water may be a vehicle of transmission, but this does not explain cholera's seasonality in Burundi.

The strong seasonality suggests that climate changes may also be related to the timing of outbreaks. During most years, the outbreaks start during the hotter drier months, but then accelerate during the rainy season. It may be that certain climate factors help to initiate an outbreak, but then the rainy season leads to more environmental contamination leading to increased transmission. In endemic areas of Bangladesh and West Bengal, cholera rates have a strong seasonality [34].

Safe water and improved sanitation will be critical for cholera control, and certainly the national indicators for water and sanitation demonstrate the need for much improvement. We did not, however, identify specific WASH indicators that would explain the higher risk observed in the hotspot districts. Nevertheless, if RDT and OCV are used in these districts, increased emphasis for improving safe water and sanitation should focus on these districts. The lack of correlation between WASH indicators and cholera risk suggests that data on these risk factors need to be collected from specific subgroups who have had cholera rather than a representative sample of households in the district, most of whom have not had cholera.

4.3. Limitations

This analysis had certain limitations. Since this analysis assumes that each district is distinct, the spread of outbreaks between Health Districts is not easily shown and likely under-estimates the true duration of the outbreaks. In fact, many outbreaks did occur simultaneously in different districts and their duration would have extended if the spread between districts was considered. Secondly, only some of the cases were confirmed; however, this method of confirming initial cases and then counting clinically determined cases is consistent with WHO recommendations. Thirdly, we did not have migration histories of the cases to understand where the infection may have been acquired, nor was DNA from Burundian strains available to determine their relation to strains from the DRC or Tanzania. Fourthly, the analysis of hotspots would have benefited if precise GIS points of the actual cases were available. This would have been especially helpful to differentiate urban and rural cases. Fifthly, declaring an outbreak depends on sending samples to the lab in Bujumbura to confirm *V. cholerae*. If rapid tests were used in the field, these might detect outbreaks more quickly. Finally, we used population data from the 2008 census, and we assumed that the increase in numbers would be similar in the different Health Areas. Plans for interventions will need to use updated population numbers when determining the requirements for vaccines and for WASH interventions in these Health Districts.

5. Conclusions

Several factors suggest that cholera could be quickly eliminated as a public health problem in Burundi using an integrated program with OCV for the short term and WASH interventions for the longer term. (1) The country and specifically the hotspot districts are of sufficient size to vaccinate in an organized campaign; (2) the hotspot districts demonstrate consistent cholera persistence over an extended time period; and (3) they are geographically close to the capital of Bujumbura, simplifying logistical requirements for OCV campaigns and follow-up evaluations.

The GTFCC has set a goal of eliminating cholera from at least 20 countries by 2030, and Burundi should be included on this list. Due to the consistency of cholera patterns, Burundi is unique in that the impact of such an integrated intervention will be apparent very quickly. This epidemiological analysis of Burundi includes the assessment of hotspots and an overview of contextual/risk factors, based on the data available, which may be used in concert with the GTFCC's framework to update Burundi's national cholera control plan and plan for elimination [31].

Author Contributions: Con-ceptualization, A.K.D., A.M.S., E.R., C.D., and D.A.S.; methodology, A.K.D., A.M.S., M.A., and D.A.S.; validation, A.K.D., E.R., and D.A.S.; formal analysis, A.K.D., M.A., and D.A.S.; investigation, A.K.D., A.M.S., E.R., C.D., and D.A.S.; resources, A.K.D., A.M.S., T.N., I.L., E.R., C.D., and D.A.S.; data curation, A.K.D., T.N., I.L., E.R., C.D., M.A. and D.A.S.; writing—original draft preparation, A.K.D. and D.A.S.; writing—review and editing, A.K.D., A.M.S., T.N., I.L., E.R., C.D., M.A., and D.A.S.; visualization, A.K.D., E.R., C.D. and D.A.S.; supervision, A.K.D., T.N., I.L., E.R., and D.A.S.; project administration, A.K.D. and E.R.; funding acquisition, A.K.D. All authors have read and agreed to the published version of the manuscript.

Funding: This work was supported in part, by a grant from UNICEF AN# 43264783, by the Bill & Melinda Gates Foundation [OPP1148763] and a grant from the National institute of Allergy and Infectious Disease [NIAID] (5R01AI123422).

Institutional Review Board Statement: Ethical review and approval were waived for this study as it was deemed to not qualify as human subjects research as defined by the DHHS regulations 45 CFR 46.102 and does not require IRB oversight (JHSPH IRB #00009628, 31 May 2019).

Data Availability Statement: The data presented in this study are available on request from the corresponding author. The data are not publicly available but have been submitted to the GTFCC cholera data collection.

Conflicts of Interest: The authors declare no conflict of interest.

References

1. Information WWC. Average Monthly Snow And Rainfall In Bujumbura In Millimeter 2019. Available online: https://weather-and-climate.com/average-monthly-precipitation-Rainfall,Bujumbura,Burundi (accessed on 18 March 2021).
2. United_Nations_Statistics_Division. UN Data. A World of Informations. 2021. Available online: http://data.un.org/default.aspx (accessed on 1 March 2021).
3. World_Food_Program. Where We Work/Burundi Italy: World Food Program. 2020. Available online: https://www.wfp.org/countries/burundi (accessed on 2 March 2021).

4. Joint_Monitoring_Project_(JMP). WHO/UNICEF. 2021. Available online: https://washdata.org/data/household#!/ (accessed on 16 February 2021).
5. UNICEF. UNICEF Burundi Humanitarian Situation Report No. 4 - Reporting Period: 1 January to 31 December 2020 New York: UNICEF. 2021. Available online: https://reliefweb.int/report/burundi/unicef-burundi-humanitarian-situation-report-no-4-reporting-period-01-january-31-0 (accessed on 6 February 2021).
6. International_Organization_for_Migration. OM Burundi Emergency Tracking Overview—Natural Disasters: October 2018–June 2019. International Organization for Migration. 2019. Available online: https://reliefweb.int/report/burundi/iom-burundi-emergency-tracking-overview-natural-disasters-october-2018-june-2019 (accessed on 12 June 2019).
7. UNHCR. Burundi Situation 2021. Available online: https://data2.unhcr.org/en/situations/burundi (accessed on 16 February 2021).
8. De Wever, A.; Muylaert, K.; Van der Gucht, K.; Pirlot, S.; Cocquyt, C.; Descy, J.P. Bacterial community composition in Lake Tanganyika: Vertical and horizontal heterogeneity. *Appl. Environ. Microbiol.* **2005**, *71*, 5029–5037. [CrossRef] [PubMed]
9. Nkoko, D.B.; Giraudoux, P.; Plisnier, P.D.; Tinda, A.M.; Piarroux, M.; Sudre, B. Dynamics of cholera outbreaks in Great Lakes region of Africa, 1978–2008. *Emerg. Infect. Dis.* **2011**, *17*, 2026–2034. [CrossRef] [PubMed]
10. Birmingham, M.; Lee, L.; Ndayimirije, N.; Nkurikiye, S.; Hersh, B.S.; Wells, J.G.; Deming, M.S. Epidemic cholera in Burundi: Patterns of transmission in the Great Rift Valley Lake region. *Lancet* **1997**, *349*, 981–985. [CrossRef]
11. World_Health_Organization. Global Health Observatory, Number of Reported Cholera Cases Geneva: WHO. 2016. Available online: https://www.who.int/gho/epidemic_diseases/cholera/cases/en/ (accessed on 16 February 2021).
12. MSF. Cholera Outbreak among Burundian Refugees 2015. Available online: https://www.msf.org/tanzania-cholera-outbreak-among-burundian-refugees (accessed on 8 September 2019).
13. AFRO. Status of the Implementation of the IDSR Second Edition in 2010 in the WHO African Region: AFRO. 2016. Available online: https://www.afro.who.int (accessed on 16 September 2019).
14. OCHA. Burundi–Subnational Population Statistics New York. 2018. Available online: http://ghdx.healthdata.org/organizations/central-bureau-census-burundi (accessed on 16 February 2021).
15. Global Task Force on Cholera Control G. *Framework for the Development and Monitoring of a Multisectoral National Cholera Plan*; WHO: Geneva, Switzerland, 2019.
16. Humanitarian_Data_Exchange. Burundi–Health District Boundaries (2017) OCHA. 2017. Available online: https://data.humdata.org/dataset/burundi-health-district-boundaries-2017 (accessed on 16 February 2021).
17. GTFCC. Guidance and tool for countries to identify priority areas for intervention Geneva: GTFCC. Available online: https://www.gtfcc.org/resources/guidance-and-tool-for-countries-to-identify-priority-areas-for-intervention/ (accessed on 16 February 2021).
18. Global Task Force on Cholera Control. *Interim Guidance Document on Cholera Surveillance*; WHO: Geneva, Switzerland, 2017.
19. M'Bangombe, M.; Pezzoli, L.; Reeder, B.; Kabuluzi, S.; Msyamboza, K.; Masuku, H.; Ngwira, B.; Cavailler, P.; Grandesso, F.; Palomares, A.; et al. Oral cholera vaccine in cholera prevention and control, Malawi. *Bull. World Health Organ* **2018**, *96*, 428–435. [CrossRef] [PubMed]
20. Grandesso, F.; Kasambara, W.; Page, A.-L.; Debes, A.K.; M'Bang'Ombe, M.; Palomares, A.; Lechevalier, P.; Pezzoli, L.; Alley, I.; Salumu, L.; et al. Effectiveness of oral cholera vaccine in preventing cholera among fishermen in Lake Chilwa, Malawi: A case-control study. *Vaccine* **2019**, *37*, 3668–3676. [CrossRef] [PubMed]
21. Sauvageot, D.; Saussier, C.; Gobeze, A.; Chipeta, S.; Mhango, I.; Kawalazira, G.; Mengel, M.A.; Legros, D.; Cavailler, P.; M'Bang'Ombe, M. Oral cholera vaccine coverage in hard-to-reach fishermen communities after two mass Campaigns, Malawi, 2016. *Vaccine* **2017**, *35*, 5194–5200. [CrossRef] [PubMed]
22. Bwire, G.; Ali, M.; Sack, D.A.; Nakinsige, A.; Naigaga, M.; Debes, A.K.; Ngwa, M.C.; Brooks, W.A.; Orach, C.G. Identifying cholera "hotspots" in Uganda: An analysis of cholera surveillance data from 2011 to 2016. *PLoS Negl. Trop. Dis.* **2017**, *11*, e0006118. [CrossRef] [PubMed]
23. Bwire, G. Lessons and challenges of implementing an integrated oral cholera vaccine and WaSH response to a cholera epidemic in Hoima district, Uganda. *BMJ Open* **2019**. under review.
24. Ferreras, E.; Matapo, B.; Chizema-Kawesha, E.; Chewe, O.; Mzyece, H.; Blake, A.; Moonde, L.; Zulu, G.; Poncin, M.; Sinyange, N.; et al. Delayed second dose of oral cholera vaccine administered before high-risk period for cholera transmission: Cholera control strategy in Lusaka, 2016. *PLoS ONE* **2019**, *14*, e0219040. [CrossRef] [PubMed]
25. Iyer, A.S.; Bouhenia, M.; Rumunu, J.; Abubakar, A.; Gruninger, R.J.; Pita, J.; Lino, R.L.; Deng, L.L.; Wamala, J.F.; Ryan, E.T.; et al. Immune Responses to an Oral Cholera Vaccine in Internally Displaced Persons in South Sudan. *Sci. Rep* **2016**, *6*, 35742. [CrossRef] [PubMed]
26. Bouhenia, M. Overview of the CCV Campaigns in 2020. In Proceedings of the 7th Meeting of the GTFCC Working Group on Oral Cholera, Virtual Event, 19 November–10 December 2020.
27. Azman, A.S.; Luquero, F.J.; Ciglenecki, I.; Grais, R.F.; Sack, D.A.; Lessler, J. Correction: The Impact of a One-Dose versus Two-Dose Oral Cholera Vaccine Regimen in Outbreak Settings: A Modeling Study. *PLoS Med.* **2015**, *12*, e1001867. [CrossRef] [PubMed]
28. Qadri, F.; Ali, M.; Lynch, J.; Chowdhury, F.; Khan, A.I.; Wierzba, T.F.; Excler, J.-L.; Saha, A.; Islam, T.; Begum, Y.; et al. Efficacy of a single-dose regimen of inactivated whole-cell oral cholera vaccine: Results from 2 years of follow-up of a randomised trial. *Lancet Infect. Dis.* **2018**, *18*, 666–674. [CrossRef]

29. Ingelbeen, B.; Hendrickx, D.; Miwanda, B.; Van Der Sande, M.A.; Mossoko, M.; Vochten, H.; Riems, B.; Nyakio, J.-P.; Vanlerberghe, V.; Lunguya, O.; et al. Recurrent Cholera Outbreaks, Democratic Republic of the Congo, 2008–2017. *Emerg. Infect. Dis.* **2019**, *25*, 856–864. [CrossRef] [PubMed]
30. Bwire, G.; Sack, D.A.; Almeida, M.; Li, S.; Voeglein, J.B.; Debes, A.K.; Kagirita, A.; Buyinza, A.W.; Orach, C.G.; Stine, O.C. Molecular characterization of Vibrio cholerae responsible for cholera epidemics in Uganda by PCR, MLVA and WGS. *PLoS Negl. Trop. Dis.* **2018**, *12*, e0006492. [CrossRef] [PubMed]
31. Bwire, G.; Mwesawina, M.; Baluku, Y.; Kanyanda, S.S.E.; Orach, C.G. Cross-Border Cholera Outbreaks in Sub-Saharan Africa, the Mystery behind the Silent Illness: What Needs to Be Done? *PLoS ONE* **2016**, *11*, e0156674. [CrossRef] [PubMed]
32. Bwire, G.; Munier, A.; Ouedraogo, I.; Heyerdahl, L.; Komakech, H.; Kagirita, A.; Wood, R.; Mhlanga, R.; Njanpop-Lafourcade, B.; Malimbo, M.; et al. Epidemiology of cholera outbreaks and socio-economic characteristics of the communities in the fishing villages of Uganda: 2011–2015. *PLoS Negl. Trop. Dis.* **2017**, *11*, e0005407. [CrossRef] [PubMed]
33. Khonje, A.; Metcalf, C.A.; Diggle, E.; Mlozowa, D.; Jere, C.; Akesson, A.; Corbet, T.; Chimanga, Z. Cholera outbreak in districts around Lake Chilwa, Malawi: Lessons learned. *Malawi Med. J.* **2012**, *24*, 29–33. [PubMed]
34. Sack, R.B.; Siddique, A.K.; Longini, I.M., Jr.; Nizam, A.; Yunus, M.; Islam, M.S. A 4-year study of the epidemiology of Vibrio cholerae in four rural areas of Bangladesh. *J. Infect. Dis.* **2003**, *187*, 96–101. [CrossRef] [PubMed]

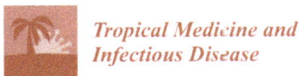

Tropical Medicine and Infectious Disease

Perspective

Oral Rehydration Salts, Cholera, and the Unfinished Urban Health Agenda

Thomas J. Bollyky

Council on Foreign Relations, Washington, DC 20006, USA; tbollyky@cfr.org

Abstract: Cholera has played an outsized role in the history of how cities have transformed from the victims of disease into great disease conquerors. Yet the current burden of cholera and diarrheal diseases in the fast-urbanizing areas of low-income nations shows the many ways in which the urban health agenda remains unfinished and must continue to evolve.

Keywords: cholera; urban health; oral rehydration

Citation: Bollyky, T.J. Oral Rehydration Salts, Cholera, and the Unfinished Urban Health Agenda. *TMID* 2022, 7, 67. https://doi.org/10.3390/tropicalmed7050067

Academic Editor: David Nalin

Received: 14 March 2022
Accepted: 27 April 2022
Published: 29 April 2022

Publisher's Note: MDPI stays neutral with regard to jurisdictional claims in published maps and institutional affiliations.

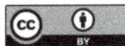

Copyright: © 2022 by the author. Licensee MDPI, Basel, Switzerland. This article is an open access article distributed under the terms and conditions of the Creative Commons Attribution (CC BY) license (https://creativecommons.org/licenses/by/4.0/).

Cholera has played an outstanding role in the history of how cities, to quote the great urbanist Jane Jacobs, stopped being "helpless and devastated victims of disease," and "became great disease conquerors". Yet, the current burden of cholera and diarrheal diseases in the fast-urbanizing areas of low-income nations shows the many ways in which the urban health agenda remains unfinished and must continue to evolve.

A Simple Solution

Cholera and other diarrheal diseases have long been terrible killers of children in poor countries. During the 1970s, World Health Organization (WHO) officials estimated that there were about 500 million cases of diarrhea in children under the age of five each year, resulting in at least five million deaths annually [1].

In 1968, two young researchers, Richard Cash and David Nalin, were working on cholera treatments at the Pakistan Cholera Research Lab in Dhaka, Bangladesh [2]. There, Nalin and Cash successfully tested an oral solution of glucose and salt with 29 patients, building upon earlier scientific findings that sugar helps the gut to absorb new fluid. They would later conduct further tests to show that the same is true for children [3]. A few years later, an Indian physician named Dilip Mahalanabis demonstrated, in a West Bengal refugee camp, that oral rehydration was effective in responding to a cholera outbreak even outside a hospital or clinical setting, preventing the need for intravenous liquids in emergency relief circumstances [3–5].

Those results set in motion the development of an oral rehydration solution, which now costs a few cents per packet. This therapy may be administered at home, without the help of a nurse or physician, and has replaced the indiscriminate and unnecessary administration of antibiotics to treat diarrhea. Starting in 1979, employees at the Bangladesh Rural Advancement Committee (BRAC), a nongovernmental organization, went door-to-door in rural Bangladesh and taught 12 million mothers how to make and use the life-saving salt solution [6]. This effort took ten years and, in more recent years, the BRAC has extended the program to other poor nations [7]. WHO, UNICEF, and the U.S. Centers for Disease Control and Prevention have included oral rehydration solution in their protocols as an essential medicine to treat diarrhea [5].

As a result of these collective efforts, oral rehydration solution has saved the lives of an estimated 50 million people worldwide, the vast majority of them children in poor nations [8]. The treatment has helped reduce annual diarrheal deaths from five million to an estimated 500,000 in 2017, despite a significant percentage increase in the world's population. Much of this decline is attributable to decades-old interventions, such as oral rehydration solution, the promotion of exclusive breastfeeding, and the more recent recommendation to use zinc for diarrhea treatment. A new oral cholera vaccine, which requires clean water and two doses given two weeks apart, has helped reduce massive outbreaks in Somalia and Yemen and the high burden of disease in the Democratic Republic of Congo (DRC) and South Sudan. In 2018, Bangladesh and India reported not a single death from the disease [9].

More than 50 years after its development, oral rehydration solution (ORS) is recognized as an important treatment for other forms of dehydration as well, including dehydration-induced kidney injury and Ebola virus disease. Much more remains to be done, however. The global adoption of ORS slowed after 1995, and more than half of the world's children in low- and middle-income countries still do not receive cost-effective and easy-to-administer treatment [10,11]. Still, it is hard to disagree with the prestigious British medical journal *Lancet*, which in 1978, called oral rehydration treatment "potentially the most important medical advance of the twentieth century" [12].

The oral rehydration solution first pioneered by Nalin and Cash and distributed by Bangladesh's innovative nongovernmental organizations has not only prevented millions of unnecessary deaths, but they—along with antibiotics and childhood vaccines—have also been one of a handful of cheap, lifesaving interventions that have enabled cities in developing countries to grow beyond the limits of their poverty and infrastructure [13]. This progress has occurred despite many poor countries being unable to make the same heavy investment in clean water and sanitation that accompanied earlier urbanization in wealthier nations. In doing so, these humble salts have contributed to the rise of a new phenomenon in human history: large, low-income country cities.

Large Cities Were Once a Rich Country Phenomenon

For most of human history, the only large cities were either wealthy industrial centers, such as Liverpool or London, or the capitals of empires, such as Rome, which could draw enough migrants from the countryside to compensate for the loss of city dwellers due to the unrelenting assault of viruses, bacteria, and parasites that accompanied crowds of people. Great epidemics like the Plague of Athens are famous for ravaging the urban centers of antiquity, but it was the everyday killers—tuberculosis, dysentery, and other intestinal and diarrheal diseases—that kept large cities deadly for millennia. As recently as 1800, only 3 percent of humanity lived in cities.

Scientific advancements, such as germ theory, and industrial and consumer demands for clean water and fire protection, all contributed to the public health revolution that followed [14,15], but it was the repeated pandemics of cholera in the 19th century that demonstrated that selective sanitation only for the wealthy was insufficient to prevent the heavy toll of water-borne disease [16]. The first municipal and national boards of health in Britain and the United States were established after repeated outbreaks of cholera [17–19]. Access to municipal waterworks increased exponentially, from low levels to widespread coverage over a few decades [20]. The percentage of urban American households supplied with filtered water grew from 0.3 percent in 1880 to 93 percent in 1940 [21]. In 1857, no U.S. city had a sanitary sewer system; by 1900, 80 percent of U.S. city residents were served by one [22]. Life expectancy at birth for males in New York City rose from 29 years in 1880 to 45 years in 1910 [23]. Improved access to filtered and chlorinated water alone accounted for nearly half of the decline in mortality in U.S. cities between 1900 and 1936 [24]. Similar advances were seen elsewhere in the cities of Europe and other industrializing nations [25,26].

As the relentless toll of everyday plagues and parasites lessened, more big cities emerged, but only in wealthy, industrialized nations. When the United Kingdom became one-third urbanized in 1861, the average income of its citizens was around USD 5000 (measured in 2005 dollars) [27]. The United States became a majority urban country in 1920 with a per capita income, in contemporary terms, of about USD 7500 [28].

It was not until 1960 that growth in cities started to shift to poorer nations. No low-income country with a per capita income below USD 1250 (measured again in 2005 dollars) was more than one-third urbanized in 1960; six nations with per capita incomes between

USD 1500 and USD 2500 reached that threshold, almost all in Latin America [27]. Over time, the level of the wealth of nations urbanizing progressively declined, and urban population growth shifted to South Asia and sub-Saharan Africa [29]. In some cases, this urbanization has occurred ahead of the industrialization that prompted migration to cities in wealthier nations [30]. With the decline in endemic infectious diseases and child mortality, the natural growth rate has contributed a larger share to the overall increase in urbanization in low- and middle-income nations [31]. The population of city dwellers globally is projected to grow by 2.5 billion by 2050, with nearly 90 percent in lower-income nations in Africa and Asia.

The Global Geography of Cities and the Unfinished Urban Health Agenda

Urbanization in lower-income nations could offer billions of people better access to jobs and healthcare services and a gateway to the world economy. No country has ever become wealthy without urbanizing first. To reap those benefits, those nations will have to confront the looming health and environmental challenges of urban life [32].

Population growth is outpacing city infrastructure and the expansion of public services in the fastest-urbanizing nations, especially in sub-Saharan Africa. The availability of piped water in cities in the region fell by 10 percent between 1990 and 2015, and only four out of ten new city residents had access to improved sanitation, as defined by the World Health Organization [33]. The construction of adequate housing and paved roads is likewise not keeping up with urbanization in many poor cities in the region. Nigeria, the most populous nation in sub-Saharan Africa, is projected to have a shortfall of 20 million urban housing units by 2030 [34].

The results of urban population growth outpacing city infrastructure are slums, informal settlements where 880 million people live worldwide [35]. Poor, crowded cities with limited health systems have also been the ideal incubators for outbreaks of emerging infections, like the Ebola epidemics in West Africa in 2014 and the Democratic Republic of Congo in 2018. Both SARS-CoV-1 and SARS-CoV-2 might have originated from uncontrolled urban wet markets. Modern cities are often larger and denser than Athens and the other urban centers of antiquity; outbreaks that occur in today's cities can spread internationally faster and with greater ease via global trade and air travel. Higher levels of air pollution are also a threat, responsible for killing an estimated 6.1 million people prematurely in 2016 [36].

The slums in lower-income nations today are considerably healthier than slums in the 19th century cities of the United States and Europe, where between 200 and 300 out of every 1000 children under the age of five died. There is limited health data on modern slums, however, and much progress is reported in averages that may mask disparities. There is some indication that the health benefits of urban life may not be equally distributed among the poor residents of cities like Cairo, Dhaka, or Nairobi [37,38].

A recent study found that cities offer greater access to piped water and sanitation, but that reported rates of diarrhea increase with greater urban density in lower-income nations [30]. Municipal water systems in dense urban areas are older, poorly maintained, and suffer from low or intermittent water pressure, which reduces the effectiveness of chlorination [39,40]. Many cities in low-income countries supply water on a rotating basis for a limited number of hours at a time [41]. Moreover, urban water systems are only effective in fighting water-borne disease when paired with street cleaning and well-functioning sewer systems, which many lower-income country cities still lack [42,43]. Waste treatment plants are rare in Africa and Asia, and treat only 15 percent of municipal wastewater in Latin America [44]. Deaths from cholera and other diarrheal illnesses in lower-income countries are generally decreasing much faster than the incidence of these diseases, suggesting that treatment is playing a large role than effective prevention [45]. Other rising health concerns also increase with urban density in lower-income nations, such as obesity, high blood pressure, and diabetes [30].

It may be time to think about the urban health agenda more as being more about economic geography than cityscapes per se [46]. This insight rings true to the lived experience of this COVID-19 pandemic. The most devastated areas in wealthy and poor nations alike have often been those with crowded living conditions, poor and socially marginalized residents, workplaces with few provisions for worker safety, and inadequate access to public services such as effective sanitation and safe water [47]. This is a particular concern in the fast-urbanizing regions where ORS is lowest in central sub-Saharan Africa, parts of western and eastern sub-Saharan Africa, the Middle East, and South America [5].

Societal and medical responses to cholera have helped shaped the history of cities, but it is cities that will define the future burden of cholera, diarrheal disease, and global health more broadly.

Funding: This research was funded by Bloomberg Philanthropies.

Institutional Review Board Statement: Not applicable.

Informed Consent Statement: Not applicable.

Data Availability Statement: Not applicable.

Conflicts of Interest: The author declares no conflict of interest.

References

1. Control of Diarrhoeal Diseases: WHO's Programme Takes Shape. *WHO Chron.* **1978**, *32*, 369–372.
2. Woodward, B. *Scientists Greater than Einstein*; Quill Driver Books: Fresno, CA, USA, 2009; p. 113.
3. Ruxin, J.N. Magic Bullet: The History of Oral Rehydration Therapy. *Med. Hist.* **1994**, *38*, 363–397. [CrossRef] [PubMed]
4. Gawande, A. Slow Ideas. The New Yorker. Available online: http://www.newyorker.com/magazine/2013/07/29/slow-ideas (accessed on 11 March 2022).
5. Wiens, K.E.; Lindstedt, P.A.; Blacker, B.F.; Johnson, K.B.; Baumann, M.M.; Schaeferr, L.E.; Abbastabar, H., Sr.; Abd-Allah, F.; Abdelalim, A.; Abdollahpour, I.; et al. Mapping Geographical Inequalities in Oral Rehydration Therapy Coverage in Low-Income and Middle-Income Countries, 2000–2017. *Lancet Glob. Health* **2020**, *8*, e1038–e1060. [CrossRef]
6. Koehlmoos, T.; Islam, Z.; Anwar, S.; Hossain, S.; Gazi, R.; Streatfield, P.K.; Bhuiya, A. Health Transcends Poverty: The Bangladesh Experience. In *'Good Health at Low Cost' 25 Years on: What Makes a Successful Health System*; Balabanova, D., McKee, M., Mills, A., Eds.; The London School of Hygiene and Tropical Medicine: London, UK, 2011.
7. Yee, A. The Power, and Process, of a Simple Solution. *The New York Times*. Available online: https://opinionator.blogs.nytimes.com/2014/08/14/the-power-and-process-of-a-simple-solution/ (accessed on 11 March 2022).
8. Fontaine, O.; Garner, P.; Bhan, M.K. Oral Rehydration Therapy: The Simple Solution for Saving Lives. *BMJ* **2007**, *334*, s14. [CrossRef] [PubMed]
9. World Health Organization. *Wkly. Epidemiol. Rec.* **2019**, *94*, 561–580.
10. UNICEF. Diarrhoea Remains a Leading Killer of Young Children, Despite the Availability of a Simple Treatment Solution. Available online: https://data.unicef.org/topic/child-health/diarrhoeal-disease/# (accessed on 7 December 2017).
11. Khan, A.M.; Wright, J.E.; Bhutta, Z.A. A Half Century of Oral Rehydration Therapy in Childhood Gastroenteritis: Toward Increasing Uptake and Improving Coverage. *Dig. Dis. Sci.* **2020**, *65*, 355–360. [CrossRef]
12. Water with Sugar and Salt. *Lancet* **1978**, *312*, 300–301. [CrossRef]
13. Leon, D.A. Cities, Urbanization and Health. *Int. J. Epidemiol.* **2008**, *37*, 4–8. [CrossRef]
14. Brown, J.C. Coping with Crisis? The Diffusion of Waterworks in Late Nineteenth-Century German Towns. *J. Econ. Hist.* **1988**, *48*, 307–318. [CrossRef]
15. Hamlin, C. Cholera Forcing: The Myth of the Good Epidemic and the Coming of Good Water. *Am. J. Public Health* **2009**, *99*, 1946–1954. [CrossRef]
16. Szereter, S. *Health and Wealth: Studies in History and Policy*; University of Rochester: Rochester, NY, USA, 2007; p. 119.
17. Porter, D. *Health, Civilization, and the State: A History of Public Health from Ancient to Modern Times*; Routledge Books: New York, NY, USA, 1999; p. 153.
18. Duffy, J. *The Sanitarians: A History of American Public Health*; University of Illinois Press: Champaign, IL, USA, 1992; p. 53.
19. Jackson, L. *Dirty Old London: The Victorian Fight Against Filth*; Yale University Press: New Haven, CT, USA, 2015; p. 99.
20. Carter, S.B. City Waterworks, by Type of Ownership: 1800–1924. Table Dh236-239. In *Historical Statistics of the United States, Earliest Times to the Present: Millennial Edition*; Carter, S.B., Gartner, S.S., Haines, M.R., Olmstead, A.L., Sutch, R., Wright, G., Eds.; Cambridge University Press: New York, NY, USA, 2006.
21. Gordon, R.J. *The Rise and Fall of American Growth: The U.S. Standard of Living Since the Civil War*; Princeton University Press: Princeton, NJ, USA, 2017; p. 216.
22. Masten, S.E. Public Utility Ownership in 19th-Century America: The "Aberrant" Case of Water. *J. Law Econ. Organ.* **2011**, *27*, 604–654. [CrossRef]

23. Meeker, E. The Social Rate of Return on Investment in Public Health, 1880–1910. *J. Econ. Hist.* **1974**, *34*, 392–421. [CrossRef] [PubMed]
24. Cutler, D.; Miller, G. The Role of Public Health Improvements in Health Advances: The Twentieth-Century United States. *Demography* **2005**, *42*, 1–22. [CrossRef]
25. Hohenberg, M.; Lees, L.H. *The Making of Urban Europe, 1000–1994*; Harvard University Press: Cambridge, MA, USA, 1995; pp. 258–259.
26. Panel on Urban Population Dynamics; National Research Council. *Cities Transformed: Demographic Change and Its Implications in the Developing World*; Montgomery, M.R., Stren, R., Cohen, B., Reed, H.E., Eds.; National Academies: Washington, DC, USA, 2003; p. 271.
27. Glaeser, E.L. A World of Cities: A World of Cities: The Causes and Consequences of Urbanization in Poorer Countries. *J. Eur. Econ. Assoc.* **2014**, *12*, 1154–1199. [CrossRef]
28. Chauvin, J.P.; Glaeser, E.; Ma, Y.; Tobio, K. What Is Different About Urbanization in Rich and Poor Countries? Cities in Brazil, China, India and the United States. *J. Urban Econ.* **2017**, *98*, 17–49. [CrossRef]
29. Glaeser, E.; Henderson, J.V. Urban Economics for the Developing World: An Introduction. *J. Urban Econ.* **2017**, *98*, 1–5. [CrossRef]
30. Henderson, J.V.; Turner, M.A. Urbanization in the Developing World: Too Early or Too Slow? *J. Econ. Perspect.* **2020**, *34*, 150–173. [CrossRef]
31. Zulu, E.M.; Beguy, D.; Ezech, A.C.; Bocquier, P.; Madise, N.J.; Cleland, J.; Falkingham, J. Overview of Migration, Poverty and Health Dynamics in Nairobi City's Slum Settlements. *J. Urban Health* **2011**, *88* (Suppl. 2), S185–S199. [CrossRef]
32. Bollyky, T.J. The Future of Global Health Is Urban Health. Council on Foreign Relations. Available online: https://www.cfr.org/article/future-global-health-urban-health (accessed on 31 January 2019).
33. World Health Organization. Definitions of Indicators. Available online: https://www.who.int/water_sanitation_health/monitoring/jmp04_2.pdf (accessed on 11 March 2022).
34. Bah, E.M.; Faye, I.; Geh, Z.F. *Housing Market Dynamics in Africa*; Macmillan Publishers: London, UK, 2018.
35. United Nations. Goal 11: Make Cities and Human Settlements Inclusive, Safe, Resilient, and Sustainable. Available online: https://unstats.un.org/sdgs/report/2017/goal-11/ (accessed on 11 March 2022).
36. Institute for Health Metrics and Evaluation. Over 7 Billion People Face Unsafe Air: State of Global Air 2018. Available online: http://www.healthdata.org/news-release/over-7-billion-people-face-unsafe-air-state-global-air-2018 (accessed on 11 March 2022).
37. Ezzati, M.; Webster, C.J.; Doyle, Y.G.; Rashid, S.; Owusu, G.; Leung, G.M. Cities for Global Health. *BMJ* **2018**, *363*, k3794. [CrossRef]
38. Mberu, B.U.; Haregu, T.N.; Kyobutungi, C.; Ezeh, A.C. Health and Health-Related Indicators in Slum, Rural, and Urban Communities: A Comparative Analysis. *Glob. Health Action* **2016**, *9*, 33163. [CrossRef]
39. Bhalotra, S.R.; Diaz-Cayeros, A.; Miller, G.; Miranda, A.; Venkataramani, A.V. Urban Water Disinfection and Mortality Decline in Developing Countries. *Am. Econ. J. Econ. Policy* **2021**, *13*, 490–520. [CrossRef]
40. Ecurmen, A. Upgrading a Piped Water Supply From Intermittent to Continuous Delivery and Association with Waterborne Illness: A Matched Cohort Study in Urban India. *PLoS Med.* **2015**, *12*, e1001892. [CrossRef]
41. Danilenko, A.; van den Berg, C.; Macheve, B.; Moffit, L.J. *The IBNET Water Supply and Sanitation Performance Blue Book: The International Benchmarking Network for Water and Sanitation Utilities Databook*; World Bank: Washington, DC, USA, 2011.
42. Duflo, E.; Greenstone, M.; Guiteras, R.; Clasen, T. Toilets Can Work: Short and Medium Run Health Impacts of Addressing Complementarities and Externalities in Water and Sanitation. *NBER Work. Paper* **2015**, 21521. [CrossRef]
43. Alsan, M.; Goldin, C. Watersheds in Infant Mortality: The Role of Effective Water and Sewerage Infrastructure, 1880 to 1915. *J. Political Econ.* **2019**, *127*, 586–638. [CrossRef] [PubMed]
44. Larsen, T.A.; Hoffman, S.; Luthi, C.; Truffer, B.; Maurer, M. Emerging Solutions to the Water Challenges of an Urbanizing World. *Science* **2016**, *352*, 928–933. [CrossRef]
45. GBD Diarrhoeal Diseases Collaborators. Estimates of Global, Regional, and National Morbidity, Mortality, and Aetiologies of Diarrhoeal Diseases: A Systematic Analysis for the Global Burden of Disease Study 2015. *Lancet Infect. Dis.* **2017**, *9*, 909–948. [CrossRef]
46. Lall, S.; Wahba, S. No Urban Myth: Building Inclusive and Sustainable Cities in the Pandemic Recovery. The World Bank. Available online: https://www.worldbank.org/en/news/immersive-story/2020/06/18/no-urban-myth-building-inclusive-and-sustainable-cities-in-the-pandemic-recovery (accessed on 11 March 2022).
47. Bollyky, T.J.; Kiernan, S. From Victims to Conquerors: How Cities Can Overcome Coronavirus. *Brown J. World Aff.* **2020**, *27*, 261–272.

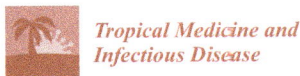

Article

An Update on Cholera Immunity and Current and Future Cholera Vaccines

Jan Holmgren

University of Gothenburg Vaccine Research Institute, Sahlgrenska Academy, University of Gothenburg, 40530 Gothenburg, Sweden; jan.holmgren@gu.se

Abstract: Individual resistance to cholera infection and disease depends on both innate host factors and adaptive immunity acquired by a previous infection or vaccination. Locally produced, intestinal-mucosal secretory IgA (SIgA) antibodies against bacterial surface lipopolysaccharide (LPS) O antigens and/or secreted cholera toxins are responsible for the protective adaptive immunity, in conjunction with an effective mucosal immunologic memory that can elicit a rapid anamnestic SIgA antibody response upon re-exposure to the antigen/pathogen even many years later. Oral cholera vaccines (OCVs), based on inactivated *Vibrio cholerae* whole-cell components, either together with the cholera toxin B subunit (Dukoral™) or administered alone (Shanchol™/Euvichol-Plus™) were shown to be consistently safe and effective in large field trials in all settings. These OCVs are recommended by the World Health Organisation (WHO) for the control of both endemic cholera and epidemic cholera outbreaks. OCVs are now a cornerstone in WHO's global strategy found in "Ending Cholera: A Global Roadmap to 2030." However, the forecasted global demands for OCV, estimated by the Global Alliance for Vaccines and Immunization (GAVI) to 1.5 billion doses for the period 2020–2029, markedly exceed the existing manufacturing capacity. This calls for an increased production capacity of existing OCVs, as well as the rapid introduction of additional and improved vaccines under development.

Keywords: cholera; oral cholera vaccine; mucosal immunity; cholera control

Citation: Holmgren, J. An Update on Cholera Immunity and Current and Future Cholera Vaccines. *TMID* **2021**, *6*, 64. https://doi.org/10.3390/tropicalmed6020064

Academic Editor: David Nalin

Received: 10 March 2021
Accepted: 17 April 2021
Published: 28 April 2021

Publisher's Note: MDPI stays neutral with regard to jurisdictional claims in published maps and institutional affiliations.

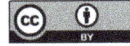

Copyright: © 2021 by the author. Licensee MDPI, Basel, Switzerland. This article is an open access article distributed under the terms and conditions of the Creative Commons Attribution (CC BY) license (https://creativecommons.org/licenses/by/4.0/).

1. Introduction

Large placebo-controlled field trials in different parts of the world in the 1960s revealed that the parenteral inactivated whole-cell cholera vaccines, which have been used widely since the early 1900s, gave little protection. This led the World Health Organisation (WHO) to remove its recommendations and most countries to abandon cholera vaccination in the 1970s [1].

It then took until 2010 before WHO was again recommending countries to use cholera vaccination in the public health control of both endemic and epidemic cholera, which was now based on oral cholera vaccines (OCVs) with much greater protective effectiveness and acceptability than the abandoned parenteral vaccines [2]. OCVs are now a cornerstone in the action plan "Ending Cholera: A Global Roadmap to 2030," which was launched in 2017 by WHO's Global Task Force on Cholera Control (GTFCC), together with 50 additional organizations. The goals are to reduce cholera deaths by at least 90% and eliminate cholera transmission in most of the currently afflicted countries by 2030 [3].

The development of the first effective OCV, namely, Dukoral™ was a result of an exceptionally successful era of international cholera research in response to the seventh cholera pandemic that began in the 1960s. Before that, most cholera research had been restricted to India. However, the rapid spread of cholera throughout Southeast Asia in the 1960s and into and across Africa in the 1970s attracted a wide range of scientists internationally. Geopolitical and military considerations of the time also mobilized increased funding to cholera research, especially in the USA and Japan. As summarized in a Nobel Symposium on cholera and related diarrheas in 1978 [4], in a "golden" research decade in the

1960s and 1970s, the pathophysiology, pathogenesis, and immune mechanisms of cholera had become better defined than any other infectious disease (see Figures 1 and 2, [5,6]). Cholera was recognized as the archetype and the "tip of the iceberg" of a whole new entity of "enterotoxic enteropathies," with enterotoxigenic *E. coli* (ETEC) as the most important additional pathogen. Practically, as had been discussed previously, the discovery and clinical introduction of life-saving oral rehydration therapy (ORT) had dramatically improved the clinical management of cholera and other diarrheal diseases, and as described below, the new knowledge about cholera pathogenesis and immunity had paved the way for the development of new, effective OCVs.

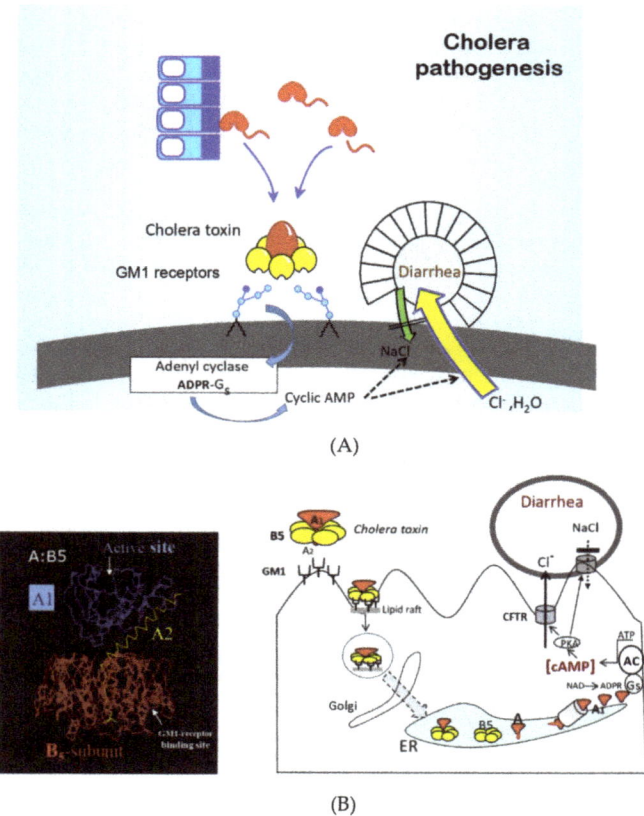

Figure 1. Pathogenesis of cholera and mode of action of the cholera toxin. (**A**) In the 1970s, the pathogenesis of cholera rapidly became better understood than any other infectious disease, as summarized in this figure from a Nobel Symposium on cholera in 1978 (A-M. Svennerholm, p.162 in [4]). After ingesting contaminated food or water, *V. cholerae* bacteria colonize the small intestine and secrete the cholera toxin, a doughnut-like protein with a central enzymatic toxic-active A ($A_1 + A_2$) subunit that is associated with a cell-binding pentamer of B subunits (B5). After binding to cell surface receptors identified as the GM1 ganglioside (the first-ever structurally defined mammalian cell receptors), the A subunit dissociates from the B subunits and its A1 entity binds to and ADP-ribosylates the GTP-binding Gs adenyl cyclase protein. This leads to the production of cyclic AMP (cAMP), which in turn induces the secretion of chloride, bicarbonate, and water from intestinal crypt cells and blocks sodium chloride and water uptake from villus cells, resulting in the watery diarrhea,

dehydration, and acidosis that is typical of severe cholera. (**B**) Subsequent crystallographic studies have confirmed the A:B5 dough-nut structure of the cholera toxin and further detailed knowledge has been gained about the way the cholera toxin induces fluid secretion. After binding to GM1 ganglioside receptors, which are mainly localized in lipid rafts on the cell surface, the toxin is endocytosed and, via a retrograde pathway, travels to the endoplasmic reticulum (ER). In the ER, the A subunit dissociates from the B subunits and, through translocation via the ER degradosome pathway, A1 is released into the cytosol. After refolding, A1 ADP-ribosylates Gs, stimulating the adenyl cyclase (AC) complex to produce increased levels of cAMP, leading to the activation of protein kinase A (PKA), phosphorylation of the major chloride channel CFTR (the cystic fibrosis transmembrane conductance regulator), and the secretion of chloride (Cl$^-$), among other effects, resulting in the often lethal cholera diarrhea and fluid loss.

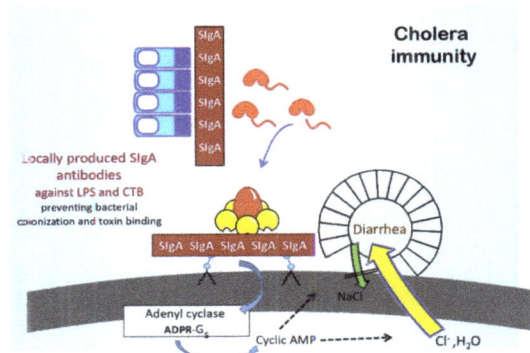

Figure 2. Protective immunity in cholera. Immune protection after infection or oral immunization is mediated mainly, if not exclusively, by locally produced SIgA antibodies that are directed against the cell surface LPS O antigen (predominantly against the A epitope defining the O1 serogroup, but also against the serotype-specific epitopes B (Ogawa) and C (Inaba) and the cholera toxin (mainly against the B subunit pentamer), and which inhibit bacterial colonization and toxin binding, respectively.

2. History of Vaccine Development

The development of cholera vaccines began almost immediately after the rediscovery and culture of *Vibrio comma (cholerae)* as the causative agent of cholera by Robert Koch in 1884 (the original discovery by Filipo Pacini in Italy in 1854 was essentially long forgotten until the international committee on nomenclature in 1965 adopted *Vibrio cholerae Pacini 1854* as the correct name of the cholera-causing organism). As reviewed by Lopez et al. [1], Ferran in Spain in the same year produced a killed bacterial vaccine, which he gave parenterally to thousands of people in an area experiencing a cholera epidemic at the time. Of those vaccinated, 1.3% got cholera compared with 7.7% of those not vaccinated. Shortly thereafter, in India, Haffkine gave a similar parenteral killed cholera vaccine to people in cholera-afflicted slums in Delhi and Calcutta (Kolkata) and noted a marked protective effect against cholera deaths. In the 1920s, Russell reported an approximately 80% protective efficacy during a 3-month follow-up period after large-scale vaccination trials in India. As a result, the parenteral cholera vaccine became widely used in Southeast Asia, especially in expatriates. In fear of cholera epidemics and with recommendations from the WHO, many countries also required cholera vaccination certificates for the entry of travelers.

However, as mentioned, several controlled studies from East Pakistan (now Bangladesh), India, the Philippines, and Indonesia during the 1960s showed that cholera vaccination gave only modest protection (approximately 50% for only a few months) and was limited to adults. Some vaccine preparations had apparent higher efficacy but were also associated with higher rates of adverse reactions, such as fever and local pain and swelling. Based on these results, in the 1970s, the WHO withdrew its previous recommendations for killed parenteral cholera vaccines.

The interest instead progressively turned to the development of orally administered cholera vaccines. The oral vaccination concept was not new. In the 1920s, a killed whole-cell OCV given together with ox bile (which had been found by Besredka to increase the immunogenicity of his killed oral *Shigella dysenterie* vaccine) was tested in India and conferred similar ($\approx$80%) protection as that provided by the injectable vaccine. However, possibly because of the bile, the vaccine also occasionally caused diarrhea; this and the "difficulty and costliness of preparing oral vaccines" led the then world experts Pollitzer and Burrows in the 1950s to conclude that "the method of cholera vaccination per os has been given up entirely" [7].

The renewed interest in oral cholera vaccination was based on new knowledge about both the mucosal immune system and the mechanisms of immune protection in cholera. In the 1960s and early 1970s, the existence of a mucosal immune system, with secretory IgA (SIgA) as its major immunoglobulin, and being preferentially activated by mucosal rather than parenteral immunization became established. In cholera, as will be discussed further below, experimental studies demonstrated that specific antibodies to either the cell wall lipopolysaccharide (LPS) O antigen or cholera toxin, when present locally in the intestine, could effectively protect against cholera infection and disease. In both animals and human volunteers, oral immunization with cholera toxin (or in humans the cholera toxin B subunit) and killed cholera bacteria could, in contrast to parenteral immunization, effectively induce protective intestinal-mucosal SIgA antitoxin and anti-LPS antibody responses. Finally, both experimental and epidemiologic studies indicated that, in contrast to the very limited and transient immune protection conferred by parenteral cholera vaccination, convalescents from cholera disease were protected against reinfection and disease for several years. These findings provided the basis for the development of the first effective OCV, the combined killed *V. cholerae* whole-cell/cholera toxin B-subunit vaccine (Dukoral™), as well as for the subsequent OCVs that are currently available.

3. Innate and Adaptive Cholera Immunity

Individual resistance to cholera infection and disease depends on a combination of innate host factors and adaptive immunity acquired by a previous infection or vaccination. The short description below focuses on those aspects that directly guided the development and/or explains the effects of current and predicted future OCVs. A comprehensive review was recently published, which is referred to for further details and supportive references [8].

Stomach acidity and ABO blood groups are the most studied innate host factors of importance for susceptibility to cholera. A low gastric acid level is associated with an increased incidence and severity of cholera disease [9]. Likewise, individuals of blood group O are at increased risk of severe cholera due to both *V. cholerae* O1 El Tor and *V. cholerae* O139 [10,11]. It was proposed that cholera might have selected for the genetically low prevalence of blood group O in the Bengal population [10].

The innate immune response is upregulated in cholera. Numerous innate immune response mediators, e.g., nitric oxide, TNF-α, and IL-1β cytokines, and several defensins and other bactericidal proteins are elevated in both blood and stool during the early stage of cholera infection [12–15]. In fact, whole-genome microarray analysis of duodenal biopsies from acutely infected cholera patients indicates that the majority of upregulated genes encode for innate response proteins [13]. Notably, the two most important protective antigens in the subsequent adaptive immune response, namely, *V. cholerae* LPS and cholera toxin, are also the predominant stimulators of innate immunity in cholera infection, including the activation of the NF-κB and IL-1 systems, which are critical for promoting mucosal IgA immune responses [13,15].

The adaptive immune response in cholera-infected or orally immunized individuals is complex. It comprises intestinal-mucosal SIgA, as well as serum IgA, IgG, and vibriocidal antibodies, and at the cellular level, e.g., antibody-secreting cells, T cells, and of special importance for long-term protection, memory B and T cells, are involved [3]. Immune protection, both in convalescents recovering from cholera disease and after oral immunization, is mediated by locally produced intestinal-mucosal SIgA antibodies [6,16]. The primary target antigens for immune protection are the LPS O antigen and cholera toxin [6,17]. The most studied correlate of adaptive immunity to *V. cholerae* is the serum vibriocidal antibody titer. Vibriocidal antibodies, which are mainly IgM directed against the LPS O antigen, increase with age in cholera endemic areas and are then associated with a reduced risk of getting cholera disease. However, these antibodies are only a surrogate marker for the intestinal-mucosal immune status and do not directly mediate or contribute to protective immunity. For instance, parenteral vaccines confer only limited and short-lived protection, even though they induce extremely high vibriocidal antibody titers.

3.1. Protective Antibodies and Mechanisms

The protective antibacterial antibodies are mainly, if not exclusively, directed against the O1 LPS [6]. The O1 LPS has a major group-specific epitope(s) "A" shared between the Inaba and Ogawa serotypes and an additional serotype-specific "B" (Ogawa) or "C" (Inaba) epitope; only a methyl group on the B epitope distinguishes Ogawa from the epitope C of Inaba [18]. Both cross-reactive and serotype-specific anti-LPS antibodies contribute to protection [6]. However, most anti-LPS antibodies after cholera infection or vaccination are directed against the shared A epitope(s) leading to predominantly serotype cross-reactive immune protection. In particular, infection with *V. cholerae* Inaba induces strong protection against subsequent cholera episodes irrespective of serotype, whereas infection with Ogawa gives rise to more serotype-specific protection [19]. Similar to the situation for *V. cholerae* O1, antibacterial protective immunity induced by *V. cholerae* O139 infection or oral immunization is mediated predominantly by antibodies to (O139) LPS, and there appears to be no cross-protection between the O1 and O139 serogroups. The protective significance, if any, of other antibacterial antibodies, including the antibodies against the toxin-coregulated pilus (TCP) and mucinase antigens that are known to contribute to intestinal colonization by *V. cholerae*, remains to be defined. The specific mechanism(s) whereby antibodies protect against *V. cholerae* LPS are also not fully understood. Their binding to LPS extending onto the flagellar sheath is known to inhibit bacterial motility in vitro, but other effects may also contribute in vivo, such as interference with bacterial biofilm formation or epithelial attachment.

There is also a clear protective role for mucosal antibodies against cholera toxin. The antitoxic antibody response is mainly directed against the B subunit pentamer and protects by blocking toxin binding to target cells. Antibodies against the A subunit induced after infection may have some, but a relatively marginal, protective effect. An important observation guiding the design of the whole-cell/B subunit OCV is the synergistic protective effect of mucosal antibacterial and antitoxic antibodies [17]. While antibodies against LPS and B subunit antigens can independently protect against disease by inhibiting bacterial colonization and toxin binding, respectively, the combined protective effect is strongly synergistic (the multiple of their individual effects).

3.2. The Intestinal-Mucosal Cholera Immune Response and Immunologic Memory

In contrast to the at best short-lasting protection that is seen after parenteral cholera vaccination, the protection found after cholera disease or oral vaccination has a duration of several years. American volunteers that were experimentally infected with virulent *V. cholerae* were protected when rechallenged 3 years after the first infection [20]. Likewise, epidemiologic studies in Bangladesh indicated that convalescents from a first episode of clinical cholera had a 90% reduced risk compared to controls to attract a new clinical reinfection during a 3-year follow-up period [21]. Similarly, immunization with an OCV conferred protection lasting for at least a 3-year period.

Even so, the gut mucosal SIgA anti-LPS and antitoxin responses after a cholera infection or oral vaccination are of much shorter duration; they peak after 1–2 weeks and then wane over a 4–9-month period (see Figure 3A,B [16,22]). Different from the generalized immune system, which meets only a few foreign antigens at a time and can then afford to respond vigorously to these antigens, the gut mucosal immune system is exposed to thousands of ingested antigens every day and has to economize on its response. By way of compensation, explaining the several-year-long protection that is seen after cholera disease or oral immunization, the mucosal response is associated with the development of a very long-lasting immunologic memory, which can mount a rapid anamnestic mucosal response upon renewed encounter with the antigen/pathogen even many years later. Thus, in Swedish volunteers who had received a standard two-dose initial immunization via an OCV, a rapid efficient recall intestinal SIgA response was elicited by a renewed single dose antigen exposure more than 10 years later (Figure 3C [23]).

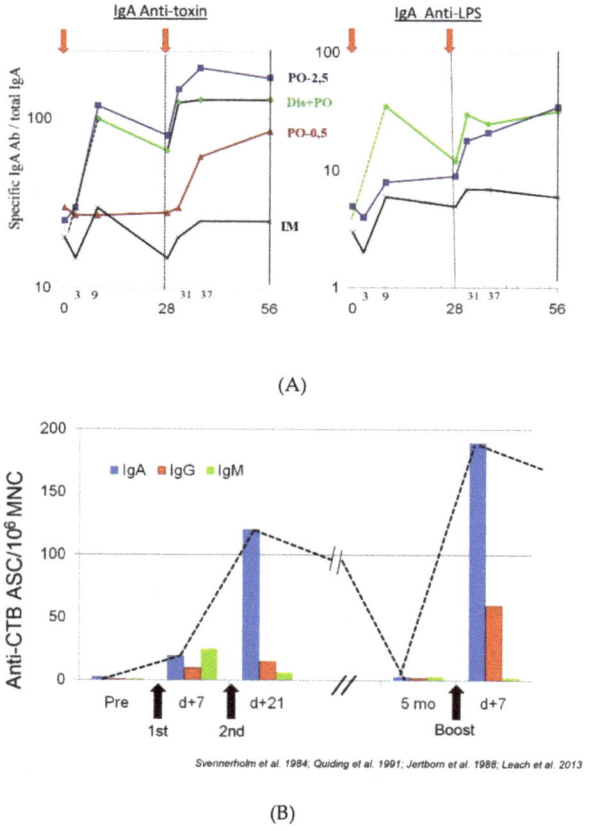

Figure 3. Cont.

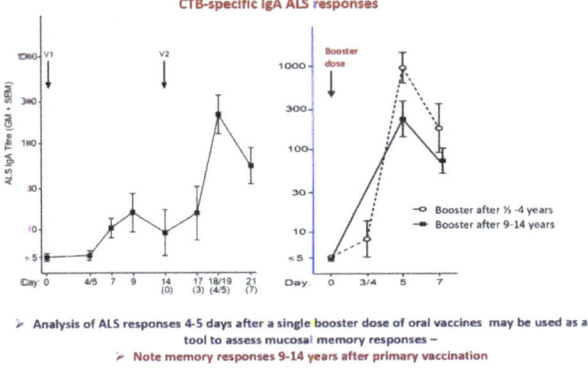

(C)

Figure 3. Intestinal IgA antibody responses and immunologic memory in cholera after oral immunization or infection. (**A**) IgA antibody responses to cholera toxin (B subunit) and LPS O antigen in intestinal lavage from adult Bangladeshi volunteers after cholera disease and/or immunizations with a B-subunit/whole-cell cholera vaccine that was administered orally (PO) or intramuscularly (IM) at an interval of 28 days. Two oral vaccine doses (in which the B subunit amounts were either 2.5 or 0.5 mg) induced antitoxin and anti-LPS intestinal IgA responses that were fully comparable to those measured after disease; in contrast, the IM route was ineffective. Adjusted from [16]. (**B**) Intestinal immune response kinetics in Swedish healthy adults after a first and second primary immunization with oral B subunit/whole-cell cholera vaccine (Dukoral) and after a single booster dose 5.5 months later; immune responses were examined as specific anti-B subunit antibody-secreting cells (ASC) in mononuclear cells (MNC) that were isolated from duodenal mucosal biopsies at various time points. Adapted from [22]. (**C**) Long-lasting immunologic memory to cholera B subunit found in Swedish adult volunteers for at least 9–14 years after an initial two-dose immunization regimen with the Dukoral OCV; this was demonstrated by giving a single booster dose at different times after the primary immunizations and finding intestine-derived IgA responses that were superior to those seen after a first dose in concomitantly first-time immunized volunteers and fully comparable in magnitude and kinetics to the second-dose responses in the latter individuals. Adapted from [23].

However, it is noteworthy that immunization by the parenteral route can also elicit a SIgA response in people whose intestinal immune system is already "primed" via previous natural exposure or oral vaccination [24]. This can explain the moderate immune protection that is observed among adults but not young children in cholera-endemic areas using the old parenteral whole-cell cholera vaccines.

4. Currently Available WHO Prequalified OCVs

The scientific findings identifying (i) intestinal-mucosal SIgA antibodies against either or both of *V. cholerae* O1 LPS and cholera toxin mediating the immune protection against cholera [25] and (ii) oral immunization as superior to parenteral immunization for eliciting this immunity [16] directly paved the way for the development of currently used OCVs. As mentioned, the first effective OCV that was developed was the inactivated whole-cell/cholera toxin B subunit vaccine Dukoral™, which was licensed in the early 1990s [26]. This has been followed by the licensure of additional inactivated and live attenuated OCVs. The inactivated OCVs have had the greatest success in achieving licensure and international acceptance.

Three such vaccines are recommended and prequalified by WHO (meaning that they can be purchased by United Nations agencies). These are Dukoral™, Shanchol™, and Euvichol™/Euvichol-Plus™, where the latter two have similar and between them identical whole-cell composition as in Dukoral but lacking the B subunit component (see Table 1). Several additional OCVs, both inactivated and live-attenuated ones, have been licensed nationally but have not received WHO prequalification. The available, licensed OCVs vaccines are briefly described below; for further details and supportive references beyond what is provided in this treatise, the reader is referred to several recent comprehensive reviews [27–29].

Table 1. Composition of WHO prequalified inactivated OCVs.

Dukoral™	Shanchol™, Euvichol™	Quantity per Dose
V. cholerae O1 Inaba classical strain Cairo 48 Heat inactivated	Same as in Dukoral	300 EU* LPS (~2.5×10^{10} bacteria)
V. cholerae O1 Ogawa classical strain Cairo 50 Heat inactivated	Same as in Dukoral	300 EU of LPS (~2.5×10^{10} bacteria)
V. cholerae O1 Ogawa classical strain Cairo 50 Formalin inactivated	Same as in Dukoral	300 EU of LPS (~2.5×10^{10} bacteria)
V. cholerae O1 Inaba El Tor strain Phil 6973 Formalin inactivated	Same as in Dukoral	600 EU of LPS (~5×10^{10} bacteria)
—	*V. cholerae* O139 strain 4260B Formalin inactivated	600 EU of LPS (~5×10^{10} bacteria)
Cholera toxin B subunit (rCTB)	—	1 mg

*EU stands for ELISA units, referring to the capacity of the vaccine to bind specific anti-LPS antibody in an internationally used Inhibition-ELISA method for quantification of LPS antigen.

Dukoral™ (Valneva, Sweden): Dukoral™ contains a mixture of formalin- and heat-killed *V. cholerae* O1 bacteria, representing both the Ogawa and Inaba serotypes and the classical and El Tor biotypes, and a recombinantly produced cholera toxin B subunit. It was internationally licensed in the early 1990s after having been shown as safe and effective in two pivotal phase III studies. The first of these trials, undertaken in 90,000 children and women in Bangladesh, showed an 85% protective efficacy against cholera during the first 4–6 months and 50–60% efficacy over a 3-year follow-up period after two or three vaccinations [30,31]. A second trial in Peruvian soldiers, all with blood group O and without any previous exposure to *V. cholerae* when given two oral doses at a 2-week interval of either Dukoral or a placebo, demonstrated 86% vaccine efficacy against a cholera epidemic 6–8 months later [32]. Several large phase IV effectiveness trials in, e.g., Mozambique and Zanzibar, later confirmed the excellent safety of this vaccine and demonstrated an 80–90% protective effectiveness of a two-dose regimen of Dukoral against cholera outbreaks occurring one or two years after vaccination. The large field trial in Bangladesh also showed that because of the extensive immunological cross-reactivity between the cholera toxin B subunit and the heat-labile toxin (LT) of *E. coli*, the whole-cell/B-subunit OCV tested there provided significant protection for 3–9 months against diarrhea caused by LT-producing ETEC bacteria; the overall protective efficacy was 67% against hospitalization due to LT ETEC and 85% against severe dehydrating disease [33]. These findings, together with observations in placebo-controlled randomized studies of 50–70% protection against LT-associated ETEC diarrhea after two doses of Dukoral in European travelers to North Africa [34] and U.S. travelers to Latin America [35], have made Dukoral widely used as a travelers' vaccine for both cholera and ETEC diarrhea.

Shanchol™ (Sanofi-Shantha Biotechnics, India): In the late 1980s, the technology for OCV manufacturing was transferred from Sweden to Vietnam for the local production of an oral killed whole-cell OCV. This vaccine contained the same *V. cholerae* O1 components as in

Dukoral but lacked the cholera toxin B subunit in order to reduce the cost and complexity of production. A two-dose vaccination was found to give 66% protection against cholera in adults and children from one year of age. In 1992, following the emergence of O139 in India and Bangladesh, the vaccine was modified to also include killed *V. cholerae* O139 cells and it was licensed nationally, first as OrcVax™ and later after modification as mOrcVax™. More than 15 million doses of OrcVax™/mOrcVax™ OCVs were used from 1998 in Vietnam's national cholera control program, mainly in the Mekong delta 1998–2006, where cholera was prevalent at that time.

A problem preventing WHO prequalification and thereby international use of the Vietnamese OCV was that the National Regulatory Agency (NRA) of Vietnam at that time was not WHO approved. To ensure that the reformulated vaccine could be made available internationally, the International Vaccine Institute (IVI) arranged a technology transfer from Vietnam to Shantha Biotechnics in India since India had a WHO-approved NRA. A large, cluster-randomized, placebo-controlled efficacy trial was undertaken in Kolkata and demonstrated that the two-dose oral immunization had an overall 65% protective efficacy over a 3–5 year follow-up period, although efficacy in children 1–5 years of age was seen for only 2 years [36,37]. In 2009, the vaccine was licensed in India as Shanchol™ and was WHO prequalified in 2011.

Euvichol™/Euvichol-Plus™ (Eubiologics, S. Korea): To address the increasing demand for OCVs, IVI also transferred the reformulated OCV technology to Eubiologics, Seoul, Republic of Korea. This has led to the successful production of Euvichol™ OCVs, which has an identical composition as Shanchol™. Based on studies in different countries demonstrating the "non-inferiority" of Euvichol™ in comparison with Shanchol with regard to both safety and vibriocidal antibody responses, Euvichol™ received both licensure and WHO prequalification in 2016. A new plastic tube presentation, Euvichol-Plus®Plus, providing easier storage, transportation, and administration, was WHO prequalified in 2017 and is currently the dominating OCV that is used in the global cholera vaccine stockpile [38].

5. Nationally Licensed but Not WHO-Prequalified OCVs

The Vietnamese mOraVax™ OCV has also been the model for a third identical OCV, Cholvax™, produced by Incepta (Dhaka, Bangladesh) and licensed in Bangladesh for use in the national cholera control program [28,29]. There are also a few other, nationally licensed OCVs on the market:

OraVacs™ (Shanghai United cell Biotechnology, China): This is a dry formulation enteric-coated capsule vaccine, which contains inactivated whole-cell (WC) *V. cholerae* O1 classical biotype or El Tor biotype and recombinant cholera B subunit and thus has a similar composition as Dukoral™. OraVacs™ is licensed in China and the Philippines for protection against cholera and traveler's diarrhea caused by ETEC. For initial immunization, three capsules are taken on days 0, 7, and 28 [28,29].

Vaxchora (PaxVax, United States): Different from the other licensed OCVs, this is a live-attenuated, single-dose vaccine developed by Levine et al. [39]. It consists of lyophilized *V. cholerae* "CVD 103-HgR" O1 bacteria that are derived from a classical Inaba strain (569B) via the deletion of the cholera toxin A subunit gene, and with its long development process since the 1980s, it has acted as a "role model" to guide essentially all the subsequent live OCVs that are currently under development (see next section). Previous efforts to generate live-attenuated cholera vaccines via random chemical mutagenesis had resulted in unacceptably reactogenic vaccine candidates. Even after modern genetic technologies were used to specifically delete the cholera toxin A subunit gene, the resulting vaccine strains continued to cause diarrhea in vaccinated volunteers, although with a much-reduced severity compared to the parent wild-type strains. It was only when this technology was applied to a *V. cholerae* strain 569B with known poor colonizing ability that an acceptably safe and yet immunogenic vaccine strain, CVD 103 HgR, could be generated. This vaccine was initially manufactured under the trade names Orochol™ and Mutacol™ (Swiss Serum and Vaccine Institute Berne), but the production was stopped for market reasons after a large field trial in Indonesia had failed to show significant efficacy [40]. Recently, the US FDA approved CVD 103-Hg under the name of Vaxchora™ for use in U.S. travelers based on human volunteer studies showing that the vaccine is well tolerated and gives up to 90% protection against a cholera challenge with either the Inaba or Ogawa *V. cholerae* O1 serotype for 3–6 months after a single dose immunization [28,29]. As of 2021, Vaxchora is also approved for use in European travelers from age 2 years.

6. Generation of Herd Protection Can Markedly Increase the Protective Impact of OCVs

A very important finding when analyzing the protective effectiveness of OCVs is that in addition to their specific vaccine efficacy, they can provide strong herd protection (previously often called herd immunity). Such herd protection is due to the ability of an OCV, which is linked to its vaccine-specific efficacy, to reduce the within-community transmission of *V. cholerae*, thus also protecting non-vaccinees who reside in vaccinated neighborhoods, as well as increased protection in vaccinees. The magnitude is proportional to the vaccination coverage of the target population. The generation of herd protection can markedly increase the overall protective impact of OCVs in vaccinated communities. This no doubt had a pivotal role in changing the public health perception of the value of OCVs in the global fight against cholera.

The herd protective effect of OCVs was first shown by Ali et al. [41] when re-examining the results from the large field trial of the whole-cell/B-subunit and whole-cell only OCVs that were undertaken in Bangladesh in 1985–1988. They found that the vaccines, in addition to their specific efficacy in vaccinated individuals, also conferred indirect "herd protection" to the unvaccinated individuals of the community. They found that the magnitude of herd protection was directly proportional to the vaccine coverage in the community and could be as high as 77% in the communities with the highest (>55%) vaccination coverage. Since in many settings, cholera cases occur with a marked clustering in space and time due to a frequent fecal–oral spread of cholera from an index case to other members of the same household and secondarily to neighboring households, with an up to 36-fold higher risk of secondary cholera observed among individuals living within 50 m of a confirmed cholera case in the first 3 days compared to the risk among individuals living elsewhere in the community, the herd protection effect is highest in a "ring" around a confirmed cholera case [42–45].

The ability of killed OCVs to confer herd protection has been repeatedly confirmed, e.g., in studies of Dukoral™ in Zanzibar and of Shanchol™ in India and Bangladesh. The combination of direct and indirect protection induced by OCVs significantly increases the overall protective impact of vaccination. The combined effect can be substantial even with relatively modest vaccination coverage. Thus, the findings from several large studies in different settings in Asia, Africa, and Hispaniola indicate that the available WHO prequalified OCVs with their 60–70% direct vaccine efficacy can confer almost complete elimination of cholera at vaccination coverages exceeding 50% [46,47]. This makes OCVs highly cost-effective by WHO measures, both in terms of numbers of lives saved and disease cases averted in relation to expense.

It is also important to note that the herd-protection effect of killed OCVs has been consistently found using various study designs. These have included individually randomized controlled clinical trials, cluster-randomized clinical trials, observational cohort studies, and observational case–control studies. Using all of these study designs, significant herd protection has been observed in unvaccinated persons, as well as in the community as a whole [45].

7. From Dismissal to Universal Acceptance of OCVs as an Important Public Health Tool for Cholera Control

As mentioned, an effective, WHO-prequalified OCV (Dukoral) has been available since the early 1990s, and was accompanied in the 1990s and 2000s with more affordable, locally produced OCVs, first from Vietnam and then from India (Shanchol). It is therefore remarkable that despite the consistent, positive results showing safety, protective efficacy, and feasibility, as well as herd protection that could further increase the overall impact, it took so long for (parts of) the WHO and the international public health community to change their negative attitude to using OCVs in cholera control programs. The positive experience from Vietnam of using an OCV in its national cholera control program since 1998 did not change the global policy.

Why Did It Take So Long before OCVs Were Accepted for Global Control of Cholera?

For many years, there were concerns among parts of the WHO that the introduction of OCVs might have a negative impact on the national implementation of oral rehydration therapy (ORT) and water, sanitation, and hygiene (WASH) activities. One concern was that people might feel safe by being protected by the vaccine and, thus, would be less compliant with WASH practices; another concern was that access to OCVs would take away the pressure on communities and governments to make needed investments toward sustainable access to clean water and adequate sanitation. These concerns are now seen as unfounded. Instead, WASH interventions and cholera vaccination should work well and probably even synergistically together, with OCVs improving the effectiveness of WASH and vice versa. Immunization will decrease the proportion of susceptible individuals in the community and reduce environmental contamination, thus helping to stop transmission of the disease and improving the effectiveness of WASH interventions. Conversely, WASH could make cholera vaccination more effective by reducing the risk of ingestion of a very high dose of *V. cholerae*.

The event that was pivotal for a rapid change in attitude to public health use of OCV was the cholera epidemic in Haiti in 2010. In the wake of a big earthquake, Haiti was hit by a devastating cholera epidemic, which in the first year caused >8000 cholera deaths. It soon became obvious how ineffective the traditional cholera control methods were for interrupting the spread of the epidemic. This and strong evidence that cholera had been brought to Haiti by UN peacekeeping staff from Nepal, and probably also the geographic proximity to the USA, created a rapidly increasing pressure on the WHO to use OCVs in the fight against cholera in Haiti. This rapidly led to strengthened recommendations from the WHO in 2010 to use OCVs both for the prevention of endemic cholera and interrupting and preventing the spread of cholera in outbreaks. It also led to the important decision to establish, with support from the GAVI, a global OCV stockpile for use primarily in settings afflicted by or at imminent risk for a cholera outbreak.

OCVs have been used in several settings in Haiti since 2012. It has shown excellent effectiveness, even when applied in the midst of the ongoing epidemic [46] and has also conferred long-lasting protection. A recently published study found the average 4-year effectiveness of two OCV doses to be 76% [47].

8. Challenges Ahead for the Elimination of Cholera

There is now great hope that the new global commitment expressed in the "Ending Cholera: A Global Road Map to 2030" program by the WHO and many partners will be revolutionary in the global war against cholera. However, there are still many challenges before its goals to reduce cholera deaths by 90% and eliminate cholera transmission in most of the currently afflicted countries will become a reality. Success will require a sustained political will at all levels, adequate sustained financing for the whole period, a motivated global health community, and an effective research and development program.

A political challenge, which is seen by many as critical for achieving the Global Roadmap's goals, will be to convince India to use OCVs in the public health control of cholera, especially in West Bengal. Cholera is still prevalent in the West Bengal region and global genomic studies have convincingly documented that each of the major waves of the global spread of cholera during the seventh pandemic did originate from the Bay of Bengal region, i.e., the West Bengal of India and Bangladesh [48]. The same is true for each of the 10–15 introductions and reintroductions of cholera into African countries in recent years [49]. It remains unknown which environmental or human conditions fueled the Bengal incubator for the seventh pandemic *V. cholerae* lineages (and probably previous ones). However, it seems clear that the implementation of all available control methods, including the extensive use of OCVs in the populations of the Bay of Bengal, should be a priority in the global elimination efforts. The government of Bangladesh has stated it will use OCVs broadly in its national cholera control program; hopefully, India will soon do the same.

Another urgent challenge is to increase the availability of OCVs to the levels required for the implementation of the Global Roadmap. The OCV global stockpile, which was started in 2013 at a level of only 2 million doses, has now increased to 20–25 million doses annually with financial support from the GAVI. More than 50 million doses have been used in more than 100 mass vaccination campaigns in 22 countries. However, this is still significantly below the OCV requests from countries, which already exceed 50 million doses annually, mainly for outbreak control use. With the projected further use of OCVs by the Global Roadmap to be focused on prevention of endemic cholera (or cholera reintroduction) in "hotspots" the annual OCV needs will exceed 100 million doses for the coming 5–10 year period. The GAVI has recently estimated that more than 1.5 billion doses will be required globally for combatting endemic cholera in 2020–2029 [50]. Even if restricted only to the GAVI-supported countries (therefore, excluding India), the OCV needs are expected to increase to approximately 64 million doses by 2021, reaching 74 million doses in 2022, and then stabilizing at about 65–70 million doses per year from 2025 onwards. The travelers and military markets are also expected to increase from about 1.3 to 2 million doses/year over the next ten years.

Besides funding, these projected needs will require a major expansion of the global OCV production capacity, including the attraction of additional manufacturers. The latter may, in itself, be a challenge given the limited commercial market for OCV. It will be important that the GAVI, UNICEF, and other purchasers can balance the lowest-possible-cost ambition against the risk of deterring manufacturers when negotiating with existing and potential new manufacturers.

Outside the OCV supply problem, operational research is needed to define and evaluate the best ways of using OCVs together with other interventions in different settings. When a broad range of cholera experts and stakeholders recently identified the most important knowledge gaps and established a priority list of key research questions for achieving the goals of the Global Roadmap [51], the top five priorities were all focused on the best use of OCVs (Table 2).

Table 2. Top Five Priorities of the Cholera Roadmap Research Agenda of January 2021 (from [51]).

1	What are the optimal oral cholera vaccine schedules (number of doses and dosing intervals) to enhance immune response and clinical effectiveness in children that are 1 to 5 years of age?
2	What are potential delivery strategies that can be used to optimize oral cholera vaccine coverage in hard-to-reach populations (including during humanitarian emergencies and areas of insecurity)?
3	Is there additional benefit to adding WASH packages, for example, household WASH kits, to an oral cholera vaccine campaign?
4	What is the optimal number of doses of oral cholera vaccine to be used for follow-up campaigns in communities previously that were vaccinated with a two-dose schedule?
5	Can the impact of an oral cholera vaccine on disease transmission, morbidity, and mortality be maximized by targeting specific populations and/or targeted delivery strategies?

One important question is whether (or when) the prescribed two-dose regimen of an OCV can be modified to a single-dose administration, which would be easier to deliver and, if working, would allow limited doses of OCVs to vaccinate twice as many people. The answer to this question is highly context dependent.

8.1. Prevention of Endemic Cholera

Large studies in Bangladesh and high-endemicity regions have shown that, while significant protection can be achieved among adults and children above 5 years of age after a single dose of an OCV, children below 5 years of age remain largely unprotected unless they receive an initial two-dose regimen. These findings are consistent with immunological studies showing that a single-dose OCV could effectively elicit ("boost") a protective immune response in individuals who were already immunologically "primed" by previous natural exposure to *V. cholerae*, whereas it takes two doses to induce an effective intestinal-mucosal immune response in immunologically "naïve" individuals, such as the whole population in previously unexposed communities and young children in endemic settings.

8.2. Use for Outbreak Control

When OCVs are used for the control of an outbreak in a known high-endemicity hotspot and/or late in an outbreak, it may be practical and cost-effective to use a single-dose OCV in order to maximize the number of individuals that can be reached with a first dose. This should also maximize the indirect herd protection among those not receiving a vaccine in the community, which will also benefit children below 5 years of age, even though this group may not get much direct protection from the vaccine. The aim should then be to give a second dose to as many young children as is practical after 1–2 weeks or later. In contrast, for an early OCV intervention in a cholera outbreak occurring in a setting that has previously not been exposed to cholera, only a two-dose regimen with an interval of at least one week between doses is likely to work, irrespective of age.

8.3. Booster Doses

Even though the available OCVs are licensed for two-dose administration with an interval of two (one to six) weeks between the doses, which is to be followed by a recommended renewed two-dose immunization at three-year intervals, it is most likely that single-dose OCV boosting at 3-year intervals would work equally well, thereby simplifying the boosting process and saving on vaccines. There is good immunological support for this recommendation. Intestinal immunologic memory was found to be effective and long-lasting, and Swedish volunteers who had received an initial two-dose immunization with Dukoral™ and then were given a single OCV boost more than 10 years later elicited a rapid, strong anamnestic mucosal IgA antibody response, which was fully comparable to that achieved by a two-dose regimen [23] (Figure 3C).

9. Future Cholera Vaccines

While the currently used OCVs are effective, they have a complex multicomponent composition, which adds to production costs. They also have a less-than-ideal formulation, which adds to transport and usage costs. Several new or improved OCVs are under development, as listed in Table 3 and briefly described below.

Table 3. Not yet licensed oral cholera vaccines under development.

Type of Vaccine	Name/Description/Stage of Development
Simplified compositions of current OCVs	• Formalin-killed Cairo 50 (Classical/Ogawa) and Phil6973 (El Tor/Inaba), which is in preclinical development in South Korea. • Hillchol™, which contains formalin-killed Hikojima El Tor strain MS1568 and is developed in India and Sweden. This OCV is in planned phase 3 testing in India. • Formalin-killed co-cultured isogenic El Tor Ogawa and Inaba, which is in preclinical development in Sweden.
Thermostable dry formulation capsule OCV	• DuoChol™, which contains lyophilized formalin-killed isogenic El Tor Ogawa and Inaba strains and recombinant cholera toxin B subunit in an enteroprotected capsule. This OCV is in preclinical development in Sweden.
Live attenuated OCVs	Genetically engineered *V. cholerae* O1 strains with deletions of ctx and other mutations: • Peru 15, which is derived from an O1 El Tor Inaba clinical isolate from 1991 in Peru, and is developed in the USA. This OCV has displayed phase 1 (also including challenge) and phase 2 immunogenicity. • El Tor Ogawa strain *638*, which is developed in Cuba. This OCV has displayed phase 1 (also including challenge) and phase 2 immunogenicity. • VA 1.4 El Tor Inaba strain, which is developed in India. This OCV has displayed phase 1 immunogenicity. • IEM 108 El Tor Ogawa strain, which is developed in China. This OCV has displayed phase 1 immunogenicity. • HaitiV, which is derived from a variant El Tor O1 Ogawa isolated in Haiti, and is in preclinical development in the USA.

9.1. Simplified Compositions of Current Types of OCVs

The three WHO prequalified OCVs are as mentioned based on (the same) three *V. cholerae* O1 strains and using both formalin and heat inactivation methods; in addition, the Shanchol and Euvichol vaccines contain a formalin-killed *V. cholerae* O139 whole-cell component. The only established protective *V. cholerae* O1 bacterial antigens are the Ogawa and Inaba LPS antigens. These antigens are exposed and preserved equally well after heat or formalin inactivation, indicating that one inactivation method is enough, with formalin being the most practical for large-scale manufacturing. *V. cholerae* O139 has almost completely disappeared as a cause of cholera since the late 1990s; therefore, the *V. cholerae* O139 component in two of the current vaccines has since been an immunologically meaningless, yet cost-adding "decoration." Based on this, it is recommended that the current whole-cell OCVs contain only formalin-killed Ogawa and Inaba bacteria from two of the current strains, preferably Cairo 50 (Classical/Ogawa) and Phil6973 (El Tor/Inaba). Efforts are underway by Eubiologics and IVI to produce and evaluate this cost-saving vaccine.

A more fundamental simplification was developed by us and further pursued in collaboration with the MSD-Wellcome Trust Hilleman Laboratories in India. A Hikojima serotype vaccine strain (El Tor biotype) stably co-expressing the Ogawa and Inaba O1 LPS antigens was generated for use as a formalin-killed single strain OCV [52,53]. The strain was constructed by introducing a partially inactivating mutation in the *wbeT* gene that is responsible for the LPS methylation differentiating the Ogawa and Inaba serotypes. This vaccine, namely, Hillchol™, was as safe and immunogenic as the comparator vaccine Shanchol when tested side-by-side in a noninferiority phase 1/phase 2 study in adults and children in Bangladesh. Bharat Biotech in India has licensed the rights to the commercialization of this easy-to-produce, low-cost Hillchol OCV, which will hopefully soon add to the global OCV supply market.

A third, recently invented, approach to simplifying and reducing the cost of vaccine production is to grow two isogenic *V. cholerae* O1 vaccine strains, one Ogawa and the other Inaba, in a mixture in the same fermentation process and then formalin-inactivating the cell mixture. Normally, one of the strains in a bacterial co-culture rapidly outgrows the companion strain, but this problem is overcome by generating and using isogenic variants with identical growth properties that only differ in that one strain expresses the *wbeT* gene resulting in serotype Ogawa and the other, by lacking this gene, has the Inaba serotype [54].

9.2. Thermostable, Dry Formulation Capsule OCV

The WHO Global Task Force on Cholera Control (GTFCC) has identified a thermostable dry formulation vaccine, ideally a tablet or capsule, as a priority for further OCV development. Such a vaccine would have significant logistical advantages over current OCVs with regard to transport, storage, and deployment. We recently described such a thermostable, low-cost OCV consisting of a lyophilized mixture of formalin-inactivated *V. cholerae* O1 bacteria and rCTB formulated in an enteroprotected capsule. We initially used the previously described Hikojima/Hillchol™ strain co-expressing the Ogawa and Inaba LPS antigens as the whole-cell vaccine component for such an experimental vaccine, namely, Hillchol-B [55]. However, we have instead now changed to use the described (cocultured and then formalin-inactivated) mixture of isogenic Ogawa and Inaba strains [54] as the preferred whole-cell component in a dry formulation whole-cell/B-subunit capsule OCV called DuoChol™. The affordable cost, practical formulation, and increased efficacy obtained by including the B subunit and also increasing the whole-cell amount/LPS O antigen content should make DuoChol™ an attractive OCV overall and an ideal vaccine for stockpiling and use in cholera outbreaks, where rapid deployment and maximal short-term efficacy are essential.

9.3. Live Attenuated OCVs

Several live oral attenuated OCVs are also under development. The oldest is Peru 15 (CholeraGarde), which was derived from an O1 El Tor Inaba strain isolated in Peru in 1991. Its multiple attenuating mutations include the deletion of the entire CT operon and flanking recombination sites; deletion of flagellar genes, making the strain non-motile; inactivating the *recA* gene by inserting the coding region for CTB under the control of a heat-shock promoter. The vaccine was safe and highly efficacious in a cholera challenge study of U.S. volunteers. A single-dose regimen was also found to be safe and immunogenic when tested in Bangladeshi adults, children, and infants [56,57].

Another live OCV is the Cuban El Tor Ogawa strain 638, which is attenuated by the deletion of the CTXPhi prophage and inactivation of the hemagglutinin/protease coding sequences (*hapA*). This vaccine was well tolerated and conferred complete protection in Cuban volunteers against a challenge with a virulent strain of El Tor *V. cholerae* O1 [58,59].

A third live OCV candidate is the VA 1.4 El Tor Inaba strain generated by Indian investigators from a clinical nontoxigenic strain that naturally lacked the CTX prophage and into which the *ctxB* gene has been inserted. The vaccine was found to be safe and immunogenic when given as a single 10^9 CFU dose to adult volunteers in India [60].

A fourth live OCV candidate strain as yet in preclinical development is IEM 108 developed in China. It is an El Tor Ogawa strain that is naturally deficient in CTXPhi and equipped with an inserted *ctxB* gene and an *rstR* gene, which blocks the reacquisition of CTXPhi [61].

Recently, yet another live attenuated vaccine strain, HaitiV, which was derived from a variant El Tor O1 Ogawa *V. cholerae* clinical isolate from the 2010 Haiti outbreak, has attracted interest by demonstrating a rapid probiotic-like protective activity, as well as more traditional longer-lasting protective immunogenicity against experimental cholera in animals [62,63]. HaitiV harbors several genetic alterations that render it avirulent and resistant to reversion. In an infant rabbit model of cholera, oral administration of HaitiV conferred protection against challenge with a lethal dose of wild-type *V. cholerae* within 24 h of vaccination, which is suggestive of a "probiotic"-like protection mechanism. In germ-free female mice, oral immunization with HaitiV elicited serum vibriocidal antibodies and protected their pups from lethal challenge with virulent *V. cholerae*. It remains to be studied whether these properties of HaitiV (or a Hikojima variant of this strain) will apply in humans after immunization and subsequent challenge with wild-type *V. cholerae* O1 and whether the rapid "probiotic" effect is specific for HaitiV or may be seen with other and possibly all live attenuated OCVs.

Despite their significant and often impressive protective efficacy against V. cholerae O1 infection and disease, even after a single dose immunization when tested in the human challenge model, live attenuated OCVs have to date met problems that have so far prevented their acceptance for use in developing countries. This is true for both the Vaxchora OCV (which, as mentioned above, has been approved for use in travelers) and for the live attenuated vaccines under development. Apart from the initial problem of residual unacceptable reactogenicity of strains even after the cholera toxin gene had been deleted, which has been overcome by developing colonization-deficient and/or multiply mutated vaccine strains, a remaining problem has been the difficulty in balancing safety against immunogenicity of the vaccine dosage in different settings. Thus, what has been both a safe and immunogenic dosage in industrialized country volunteers has often been too low dosage for inducing an adequate intestinal-mucosal immune response in developing country populations, including those living in cholera-endemic areas. For instance, a 5×10^8 CFU dose of CVD103 HgR (the predecessor of Vaxchora), which was highly immunogenic in subjects in industrialized countries, resulting in greater than 90% seroconversion of a vibriocidal antibody, elicited seroconversions in only 16% of Indonesian subjects; however, a 10-fold-higher vaccine dose resulted in seroconversion in 75–87% of vaccinated Indonesians [64].

10. Need for Novel Pathways for Licensing New Generation OCVs

Traditionally, the licensure of a new vaccine usually requires proof of clinical protection against the targeted disease in one or more pivotal, individually randomized, placebo-controlled double-blinded clinical trials (RCTs). For current OCVs, this was the path leading to the licensure of Dukoral™ and Shanchol™.

However, when an effective and safe vaccine already exists, such RCTs may be ethically problematic, which is now the case for the new and improved OCVs under development (as well as for vaccines under development for some other diseases). This problem was discussed at a recent "Expert meeting on evaluating new generation vaccines against infectious diseases for which there are licensed vaccines that are recommended for routine use" organized by the Wellcome Trust. The comments below reflect the (as yet unpublished) main observations and recommendations from this meeting.

When there is a validated immunological correlate of protection (ICP), this can be used as the primary measure of vaccine efficacy for similar or new-generation vaccines. When an established ICP is lacking, as is the case for cholera, a "surrogate" immune response may be used for comparing the new and existing vaccines. However, this approach requires that the protective antigen(s) of the compared vaccines are defined and identical, the routes of administration of the vaccines are the same, and the vaccines are identical or similar in composition. The Euvichol™ OCV, having the same composition as the already-licensed and WHO-prequalified OCV Shanchol™, and later Euvichol-Plus™, were licensed based on human studies demonstrating the noninferior safety and the same serum vibriocidal antibody responses as for Shanchol based on the vibriocidal antibodies being specific for the targeted key protective antigen, namely, the O1 LPS.

In some instances, vaccines can be licensed based on protective efficacy demonstrated in human volunteer challenge studies. This pathway was used to license the Vaxchora live OCV as a travelers' vaccine in U.S. adults, but it has not allowed for licensure in LMICs or children.

For vaccines against diseases for which there is a significant unmet medical need, the EMA pathway termed "conditional marketing authorization" may also be applied. This pathway typically requires the demonstration of an immunological endpoint after vaccination that is reasonably predictive of clinical benefit, substantial data on vaccine safety, and an overall favorable risk/benefit assessment for authorization.

Thus, for future cholera vaccines, both those described above and others yet to be developed, there are alternative ways to receive either full or conditional licensure based mainly on demonstrated safety and relevant noninferior "surrogate" immunogenicity to existing OCVs. However, in these cases, there will probably be requirements for vaccine effectiveness studies post-licensure to demonstrate vaccine protection. The operational criteria for the design, conduct, analysis, and reporting of such post-licensure studies should be defined in a dialogue between the cholera scientific community and vaccine regulators.

11. Concluding Remarks

For those of us who have been "OCV musketeers" since the 1990s, it is of course gratifying that the WHO now describes the use of OCVs as "a game-changer in the fight against cholera" in its strategy for the global control of cholera "Ending Cholera: A Global Roadmap to 2030." It underlines that by providing effective protection and being available now, OCVs can effectively bridge the time and resource gap until adequate WASH infrastructure may be universally available as a means for permanent prevention.

The development of OCVs is a good example of how basic research can be translated into a life-saving medical product. At the same time, the OCV story also illustrates how long and tedious the process even from an available product to public health use can be, especially for vaccines and drugs that are targeted against diseases for which there is no or minimal commercial market in higher-income countries. Cholera is a typical "disease of poverty" that mainly affects the poorest populations in low- or at best middle-income countries. Had it not been for the fact that Dukoral™, the first effective OCV, in addition to protecting against cholera, also protects against diarrhea caused by ETEC through its B subunit component and, thus, offered a commercial market for Dukoral as a traveler's vaccine, the licensure of an effective cholera vaccine would almost certainly have been delayed by many years.

Several challenges, both financial and political, remain to accomplish the set goals of the Global Roadmap to have decreased cholera deaths by at least 90% and largely eliminated cholera transmission by 2030. Yet, it is gratifying that the earlier question regarding whether to use OCVs has now changed to "When, how and where should OCV be used most effectively to control endemic cholera and interrupt cholera outbreaks?" and "How can we increase manufacturing of existing and new OCVs to meet current and future needs?"

Funding: The author's own cited research was funded mainly by the Swedish Research Council, the Swedish International Agency for Research Cooperation (Sida), and the Knut and Alice (KAW) and Marianne and Marcus (MMW) Wallenberg Foundations.

Institutional Review Board Statement: Not applicable.

Informed Consent Statement: Not applicable.

Acknowledgments: I wish to thank my many collaborators, both in Sweden and internationally, who over many years have contributed to both cited and uncited work that is summarized in this survey. Special thanks go to Ann-Mari Svennerholm for her support and invaluable contributions to the development of the first effective OCV, namely, Dukoral™. Further special thanks go to John Clemens for his invaluable contributions, collaboration, and friendship over soon 40 years, and for many of the perspectives of the present survey, not least those in Section 10, which as mentioned, are largely taken from the conclusions of a conference organized by John on these aspects at the Wellcome Trust in London in 2018.

Conflicts of Interest: The author has been deeply involved in the development and testing of several of the oral cholera vaccines described in the article, mainly Dukoral™, but also OrcVax™/mOrcVax™, Shanchol™, Hillchol™/Hillchol-B™, and Duochol™, and he is a co-inventor on patent applications relating to the two latter vaccines.

References

1. Lopez, A.L.; Gonzales, M.L.A.; Josephine, G.; Aldaba, J.G.; Nair, G.B. Killed oral cholera vaccines: History, development and implementation challenges. *Ther. Adv. Vaccines* **2014**, *2*, 123–136. [CrossRef] [PubMed]
2. World Health Organisation. Cholera vaccines: WHO position paper. *Weekly Epidemiol. Rec.* **2017**, *92*, 477–500. Available online: http://www.who.int/wer2 (accessed on 10 March 2021).
3. World Health Organization—Global Task Force on Cholera Control. Ending cholera—A roadmap for 2030. 2017. Available online: https://www.who.int/cholera/publications/global-roadmap/en/ (accessed on 10 March 2021).
4. *Cholera and Related Diarrheas: Molecular Aspects of a Global Health Problem 43rd Nobel Symposium 1978*; Ouchterlony, Ö.; Holmgren, J. (Eds.) S. Karger: Basel, Switzerland, 1980.
5. Holmgren, J. Actions of cholera toxin and the prevention and treatment of cholera. *Nature* **1981**, *292*, 413–417. [CrossRef] [PubMed]
6. Holmgren, J.; Svennerholm, A.M. Cholera and the immune response. *Prog. Allergy* **1983**, *33*, 106–119. [PubMed]
7. Pollitzer, R.; Burrows, W. Cholera studies. IV. Problems in immunology. *Bull. World Health Organ.* **1955**, *12*, 945–1107. [PubMed]
8. Qadri, F.; Clemens, J.D.; Holmgren, J. Cholera immunity and development and use of oral cholera vaccines for disease control. In *Mucosal Vaccines*, 2nd ed.; Kiyono, H., Pascual, D.W., Eds.; Elsevier: Amsterdam, The Netherlands, 2020; pp. 537–561.
9. Evans, C.A.; Gilman, R.H.; Rabbani, G.H.; Salazar, G.; Ali, A. Gastric acid secretion and enteric infection in Bangladesh. *Trans. R. Soc. Trop. Med. Hyg.* **1997**, *91*, 681–685. [CrossRef]
10. Glass, R.I.; Holmgren, J.; Haley, C.E.; Khan, M.R.; Svennerholm, A.M.; Stoll, B.J.; Hossain, B.K.M.; Black, R.E.; Yunus, M.; Barua, D. Predisposition for cholera of individuals with O blood group. Possible evolutionary significance. *Am. J. Epidemiol.* **1985**, *121*, 791–796. [CrossRef] [PubMed]
11. Clemens, J.D.; Sack, D.A.; Harris, J.R.; Chakraborty, J.; Khan, M.R.; Huda, S.; Ahmed, F.; Gomes, J.; Rao, M.R.; Svennerholm, A.; et al. ABO blood groups and cholera: New observations on specificity of risk and modification of vaccine efficacy. *J. Infect. Dis.* **1989**, *159*, 770–773. [CrossRef] [PubMed]
12. Qadri, F.; Bhuiyan, T.R.; Dutta, K.K.; Raqib, R.; Alam, M.S.; Alam, N.H.; Svennerholm, A.-M.; Mathan, M.M. Acute dehydrating disease caused by Vibrio cholerae serogroups O1 and O139 induce increases in innate cells and inflammatory mediators at the mucosal surface of the gut. *Gut* **2004**, *53*, 62–69. [CrossRef] [PubMed]
13. Flach, C.F.; Qadri, F.; Bhuiyan, T.R.; Alam, N.H.; Jennische, E.; Lönnroth, I.; Holmgren, J. Broad up-regulation of innate defense factors during acute cholera. *Infect. Immun.* **2007**, *75*, 2343–2350. [CrossRef]
14. Shirin, T.; Rahman, A.; Danielsson, Å.; Uddin, T.; Bhuyian, T.R.; Sheikh, A.; Qadri, S.S.; Qadri, F.; Hammarström, M.L. Antimicrobial peptides in the duodenum at the acute and convalescent stages in patients with diarrhea due to Vibrio cholerae O1 or enterotoxigenic Escherichia coli infection. *Microbes Infect.* **2011**, *13*, 1111–1120. [CrossRef]
15. Terrinoni, M.; Holmgren, J.; Lebens, M.; Larena, M. Requirement for Cyclic AMP/Protein Kinase A-Dependent Canonical NFκB Signaling in the Adjuvant Action of Cholera Toxin and Its Non-toxic Derivative mmCT. *Front. Immunol.* **2019**, *10*, 269. [CrossRef]
16. Svennerholm, A.-M.; Jertborn, M.; Gothefors, L.; Karim, A.M.M.M.; Sack, D.A.; Holmgren, J. Mucosal antitoxic and antibacterial immunity after cholera disease and after immunization with a combined B subunit-whole cell vaccine. *J. Infect. Dis.* **1984**, *149*, 884–893. [CrossRef]
17. Svennerholm, A.-M.; Holmgren, J. Synergistic protective effect in rabbits of immunization with *V. cholerae* lipopolysaccharide and toxin/toxoid. *Infect. Immun.* **1976**, *13*, 735–740. [CrossRef]
18. Chatterjee, S.N.; Chaudhuri, K. Lipopolysaccharides of Vibrio cholerae. I. Physical and chemical characterization. *Biochim. Biophys. Acta* **2003**, *1639*, 65–79. [CrossRef]
19. Ali, M.; Emch, M.; Park, J.K.; Yunus, M.; Clemens, J. Natural cholera infection-derived immunity in an endemic setting. *J. Infect. Dis.* **2011**, *204*, 912–918. [CrossRef]
20. Levine, M.M.; Black, R.E.; Clements, M.L.; Cisneros, L.; Nalin, D.R.; Young, C.R. Duration of infection-derived immunity to cholera. *J. Infect. Dis.* **1981**, *143*, 818–820. [CrossRef]

21. Glass, R.I.; Becker, S.; Huq, I.; Stoll, B.J.; Khan, M.U.; Merson, M.H.; Lee, J.V.; Black, R.E. Endemic cholera in rural Bangladesh, 1966–1980. *Am. J. Epidemiol.* **1982**, *116*, 959–970. [CrossRef]
22. Quiding, M.; Nordström, I.; Kilander, A.; Andersson, G.; Hanson, L.Å.; Holmgren, J.; Czerkinsky, C. Intestinal immune responses in humans. Oral cholera vaccination induces strong intestinal antibody responses, gamma-interferon production, and evokes local immunological memory. *J. Clin. Investig.* **1991**, *88*, 143–148. [CrossRef]
23. Leach, S.; Lundgren, A.; Svennerholm, A.M. Different kinetics of circulating antibody-secreting cell responses after primary and booster oral immunizations: A tool for assessing immunological memory. *Vaccine* **2013**, *31*, 3035–3038. [CrossRef]
24. Svennerholm, A.M.; Holmgren, J.; Hanson, L.A.; Lindblad, B.S.; Quereshi, F.; Rahimtoola, R.J. Boosting of secretory IgA antibody responses in man by parenteral cholera vaccination. *Scand. J. Immunol.* **1977**, *6*, 1345–1349. [CrossRef]
25. Holmgren, J.; Svennerholm, A.-M.; Lönnroth, I.; Fall-Persson, M.; Markman, B.; Lundbäck, H. Development of improved cholera vaccine based on subunit toxoid. *Nature* **1977**, *269*, 602–604. [CrossRef]
26. Holmgren, J.; Svennerholm, A.-M.; Jertborn, M.; Clemens, J.; Sack, D.A.; Salenstedt, R.; Wigzell, H. An oral B subunit: Whole cell vaccine against cholera. *Vaccine* **1992**, *10*, 911–914. [CrossRef]
27. Clemens, J.D.; Nair, G.B.; Ahmed, T.; Qadri, F.; Holmgren, J. Cholera. *Lancet* **2017**, *390*, 1539–1549. [CrossRef]
28. Shaikh, H.; Lynch, J.; Kim, J.; Excler, J.L. Current and future cholera vaccines. *Vaccine* **2020**, *29* (Suppl. 1), A118–A126. [CrossRef]
29. Clemens, J.D.; Desai, S.N.; Qadri, F.; Nair, G.B.; Holmgren, J. Cholera Vaccines. In *Plotkin's Vaccines*, 8th ed.; Plotkin, S.A., Offit, P.A., Orenstein, W.A., Edwards, K.M., Eds.; Elsevier: Amsterdam, The Netherlands, 2021.
30. Clemens, J.; Sack, D.A.; Harris, J.R.; Atkinson, W.; Chakraborty, J.; Khan, M.R.; Stanton, B.F.; Kay, B.A.; Khan, M.U.; Yunus, M.D.; et al. Field trial of oral cholera vaccines in Bangladesh. *Lancet* **1986**, *328*, 124–127. [CrossRef]
31. Clemens, J.D.; Sack, D.A.; Harris, J.R.; Van Loon, F.; Chakraborty, J.; Ahmed, F.; Rao, M.R.; Khan, M.R.; Yunus, M.D.; Huda, N.; et al. Field trial of oral cholera vaccines in Bangladesh: Results from three-year follow-up. *Lancet* **1990**, *335*, 270–273. [CrossRef]
32. Sanchez, J.L.; Vasquez, B.; Begue, R.E.; Meza, R.; Castellares, G.; Cabezas, C.; Watts, D.M.; Svennerholm, A.M.; Sadoff, J.C.; Taylor, D.N. Protective efficacy of oral whole-cell/recombinant-B-subunit cholera vaccine in Peruvian military recruits. *Lancet* **1994**, *344*, 1273–1276 [CrossRef]
33. Clemens, J.D.; Sack, D.A.; Harris, J.R.; Chakraborty, J.; Neogy, P.K.; Stanton, B.; Huda, N.; Khan, M.U.; Kay, B.A.; Khan, M.R.; et al. Cross-protection by B subunit-whole cell cholera vaccine against diarrhea associated with heat-labile toxin-producing enterotoxigenic *Escherichia coli*: Results of a large-scale field trial. *J. Infect. Dis.* **1988**, *158*, 372–377. [CrossRef]
34. Peltola, H.; Siitonen, A.; Kyrönseppä, H.; Simula, I.; Mattila, L.; Oksanen, P.; Kataja, M.J.; Cadoz, M. Prevention of travellers' diarrhoea by oral B-subunit/whole-cell cholera vaccine. *Lancet* **1991**, *338*, 1285–1289. [CrossRef]
35. Scerpella, E.G.; Sanchez, J.L.; Mathewson, J.J., III.; Torres-Cordero, J.V.; Sadoff, J.C.; Svennerholm, A.M.; DuPont, H.L.; Taylor, D.N.; Ericsson, C.D. Safety, Immunogenicity, and Protective Efficacy of the Whole-Cell/Recombinant B Subunit (WC/rBS) Oral Cholera Vaccine Against Travelers' Diarrhea. *J. Travel Med.* **1995**, *2*, 22–27. [CrossRef] [PubMed]
36. Sur, D.; Lopez, A.L.; Kanungo, S.; Paisley, A.; Manna, B.; Ali, M.; Niyogi, S.K.; Park, J.K.; Sarkar, B.; Puri, M.K.; et al. Efficacy and safety of a modified killed-whole-cell oral cholera vaccine in India: An interim analysis of a cluster-randomised, double-blind, placebo-controlled trial. *Lancet* **2009**, *374*, 1694–1702. [CrossRef]
37. Bhattacharya, S.K.; Sur, D.; Ali, M.; Kanungo, S.; You, Y.A.; Manna, B.; Sah, B.; Niyogi, S.K.; Park, J.K.; Sarkar, B.; et al. 5 year efficacy of a bivalent killed whole-cell oral cholera vaccine in Kolkata, India: A cluster-randomised, double-blind, placebo-controlled trial. *Lancet Infect. Dis.* **2013**, *13*, 1050–1056. [CrossRef]
38. Odevall, L.; Hong, D.; Digilio, L.; Sahastrabuddhe, S.; Mogasale, V.; Baik, Y.; Choi, S.; Kim, J.H.; Lynch, J. The Euvichol story—Development and licensure of a safe, effective and affordable oral cholera vaccine through global public private partnerships. *Vaccine* **2018**, *36*, 6606–6614. [CrossRef]
39. Levine, M.M.; Chen, W.H.; Kaper, J.B.; Lock, M.; Danzig, L.; Gurwith, M. PaxVax CVD 103-HgR single-dose live oral cholera vaccine. *Expert Rev. Vaccines* **2017**, *16*, 197–213. [CrossRef]
40. Richie, E.E.; Punjabi, N.H.; Sidharta, Y.Y.; Peetosutan, K.K.; Sukandar, M.M.; Wasserman, S.S.; Lesmana, M.M.; Wangsasaputra, F.F.; Pandam, S.S.; Levine, M.M.; et al. Efficacy trial of single-dose live oral cholera vaccine CVD 103-HgR in North Jakarta, Indonesia, a cholera-endemic area. *Vaccine* **2000**, *18*, 2399–2410. [CrossRef]
41. Ali, M.; Emch, M.; von Seidlein, L.; Yunus, M.; Sack, D.A.; Rao, M.; Holmgren, J.; Clemens, J.D. Herd immunity conferred by killed oral cholera vaccines in Bangladesh: A reanalysis. *Lancet* **2005**, *366*, 44–49. [CrossRef]
42. Ali, M.; Debes, A.K.; Luquero, F.J.; Kim, D.R.; Park, J.Y.; Digilio, L.; Manna, B.; Kanungo, S.; Dutta, S.; Sur, D.; et al. Potential for Controlling Cholera Using a Ring Vaccination Strategy: Re-analysis of Data from a Cluster-Randomized Clinical Trial. *PLoS Med.* **2016**, *13*, e1002120. [CrossRef]
43. Debes, A.K.; Ali, M.; Azman, A.S.; Yunus, M.; Sack, D.A. Cholera cases cluster in time and space in Matlab, Bangladesh: Implications for targeted preventive interventions. *Int. J. Epidemiol.* **2016**, *45*, 2134–2139. [CrossRef]
44. Roskosky, M.; Ali, M.; Upreti, S.R.; Sack, D. Spatial clustering of cholera cases in the Kathmandu Valley: Implications for a ring vaccination strategy. *Int. Health* **2021**, *13*, 170–177. [CrossRef]
45. Ali, M.; Clemens, J. Assessing Vaccine Herd Protection by Killed Whole-Cell Oral Cholera Vaccines Using Different Study Designs. *Front Public Health* **2019**, *7*, 211. [CrossRef]
46. Sévère, K.; Rouzier, V.; Anglade, S.B. Bertil, C.; Joseph, P.; Deroncelay, A.; Mabou, M.; Wright, P.F.; Guillaume, F.D.; Pape, J.W. Effectiveness of Oral Cholera Vaccine in Haiti: 37-Month Follow-Up. *Am. J. Trop. Med. Hyg.* **2016**, *94*, 1136–1142. [CrossRef]

47. Franke, M.F.; Ternier, R.; Jerome, J.G.; Matias, W.R.; Harris, J.B.; Ivers, L.C. Long-term effectiveness of one and two doses of a killed, bivalent, whole-cell oral cholera vaccine in Haiti: An extended case-control study. *Lancet Glob. Health* **2018**, *6*, e1028–e1035. [CrossRef]
48. Mutreja, A.; Kim, D.W.; Thomson, N.R.; Connor, T.R.; Lee, J.H.; Kariuki, S.; Croucher, N.J.; Choi, S.Y.; Harris, S.R.; Lebens, M.; et al. Evidence for several waves of global transmission in the seventh cholera pandemic. *Nature* **2011**, *477*, 462–465. [CrossRef]
49. Weill, F.X.; Domman DNjamkepo, E.; Tarr, C.; Rauzier, J.; Fawal, N.; Keddy, K.H.; Salje, H.; Moore, S.; Mukhopadhyay, A.K.; Bercion, R.; et al. Genomic history of the seventh pandemic of cholera in Africa. *Science* **2017**, *358*, 785–789. [CrossRef]
50. GAVI. Cholera Supply and Procurement Roadmap Update, December 2018. 2018. Available online: https://www.gavi.org/sites/default/files/document/cholera-roadmap-public-summarypdf.pdf (accessed on 10 March 2021).
51. WHO Global Task Force for Cholera Control. Cholera Roadmap Research Agenda. 2021. Available online: www.gtfcc.org (accessed on 10 March 2021).
52. Karlsson, S.L.; Ax, E.; Nygren, E.; Källgård, S.; Blomquist, M.; Ekman, A.; Benktander, J.; Holmgren, J.; Lebens, M. Development of stable Vibrio cholerae O1 Hikojima type vaccine strains co-expressing the Inaba and Ogawa lipopolysaccharide antigens. *PLoS ONE* **2014**, *9*, e108521. [CrossRef]
53. Sharma, T.; Joshi, N.; Mandyal, A.K.; Nordqvist, S.L.; Kanchan, V.; Ahasan, M.M.; Khan, I.; Muktadir, A.; Gill, D.; Holmgren, J. Development of Hillchol®, a low-cost inactivated single strain Hikojima oral cholera vaccine. *Vaccine* **2020**, *38*, 7998–8009. [CrossRef]
54. Holmgren, J.; Lebens, M. Whole Cell Vaccines and Methods of Production Thereof. In *PCT/EP/083082 25 November 2019*; WIPO: Geneva, Switzerland, 2019.
55. Holmgren, J.; Lebens, M.; Nordqvist, S.; Terrinoni, M.; Löfstrand, M.; Jeverstam, F.; Källgård, S.; Tarun Sharma, T.; Khalid Ali, K.; Gill, G. Hillchol-B™: Low-cost, thermostable dry formulation Hikojima whole-cell/B-subunit enterocoated capsule oral cholera vaccine. In Proceedings of the Vaccines for Enteric Diseases, Lausanne, Switzerland, 16–18 October 2019; 2019.
56. Sack, D.A.; Sack, R.B.; Shimko, J.; Gomes, G.; O'Sullivan, D.; Metcalfe, K.; Spriggs, D. Evaluation of Peru-15, a new live oral vaccine for cholera, in volunteers. *J. Infect. Dis.* **1997**, *176*, 201–205. [CrossRef]
57. Qadri, F.; Chowdhury, M.I.; Faruque, S.M.; Salam, M.A.; Ahmed, T.; Begum, Y.A.; Saha, A.; Alam, M.S.; Zaman, K.; Seidlein, L.V.; et al. Peru-15 Study Group. Randomized, controlled study of the safety and immunogenicity of Peru-15, a live attenuated oral vaccine candidate for cholera, in adult volunteers in Bangladesh. *J. Infect. Dis.* **2005**, *192*, 573–579. [CrossRef]
58. García, L.; Jidy, M.D.; García, H.; Rodríguez, B.L.; Fernández, R.; Año, G.; Cedré, B.; Valmaseda, T.; Suzarte, E.; Ramírez, M.; et al. The vaccine candidate Vibrio cholerae 638 is protective against cholera in healthy volunteers. *Infect. Immun.* **2005**, *73*, 3018–3024. [CrossRef]
59. Valera, R.; García, H.M.; Jidy, M.D.; Mirabal, M.; Armesto, M.I.; Fando, R.; García, L.; Fernández, R.; Año, G.; Cedré, B.; et al. Randomized, double-blind, placebo-controlled trial to evaluate the safety and immunogenicity of live oral cholera vaccine 638 in Cuban adults. *Vaccine* **2009**, *27*, 6564–6569. [CrossRef]
60. Mahalanabis, D.; Ramamurthy, T.; Nair, G.B.; Ghosh, A.; Shaikh, S.; Sen, B.; Thungapathra, M.; Ghosh, R.K.; Pazhani, G.P.; Nandy, R.K.; et al. Randomized placebo controlled human volunteer trial of a live oral cholera vaccine VA1.3 for safety and immune response. *Vaccine* **2009**, *27*, 4850–4856. [CrossRef]
61. Liang, W.; Wang, S.; Yu, F.; Zhang, L.; Qi, G.; Liu, Y.; Gao, S.; Kan, B. Construction and evaluation of a safe, live, oral Vibrio cholerae vaccine candidate, IEM108. *Infect. Immun.* **2003**, *71*, 5498–5504. [CrossRef]
62. Hubbard, T.P.; Billings, G.; Dörr, T.; Sit, B.; Warr, A.R.; Kuehl, C.J.; Kim, M.; Delgado, F.; Mekalanos, J.J.; Lewnard, J.A.; et al. A live vaccine rapidly protects against cholera in an infant rabbit model. *Sci. Transl. Med.* **2018**, *10*, eaap8423. [CrossRef]
63. Sit, B.; Zhang, T.; Fakoya, B.; Akter, A.; Biswas, R.; Ryan, E.T.; Waldor, M.K. Oral immunization with a probiotic cholera vaccine induces broad protective immunity against Vibrio cholerae colonization and disease in mice. *PLoS Negl. Trop. Dis.* **2019**, *13*, e0007417. [CrossRef]
64. Simanjuntak, C.H.; O'Hanley, P.; Punjabi, N.H.; Noriega, F.; Pazzaglia, G.; Dykstra, P.; Kay, B.; Budiarso, A.; Rifai, A.R.; Wasserman, S.S.; et al. Safety, immunogenicity, and transmissibility of single-dose live oral cholera vaccine strain CVD 103-HgR in 24- to 59-month-old Indonesian children. *J. Infect. Dis.* **1993**, *168*, 1169–1176. [CrossRef]

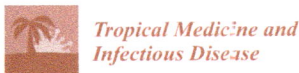

Review

Licensed and Recommended Inactivated Oral Cholera Vaccines: From Development to Innovative Deployment

Jacqueline Deen [1] and John D. Clemens [2,3,*]

1. Institute of Child Health and Human Development, National Institutes of Health, University of the Philippines, Pedro Gil Street, Ermita, Manila 1000, Philippines; jldeen@up.edu.ph
2. International Centre for Diarrhoeal Disease Research, GPO Box 128, Dhaka 1000, Bangladesh
3. UCLA Fielding School of Public Health, 550 Charles E Young Drive South, Los Angeles, CA 90095-1772, USA
* Correspondence: jclemens@icddrb.org; Tel.: +63-2-254-5205

Abstract: Cholera is a disease of poverty and occurs where there is a lack of access to clean water and adequate sanitation. Since improved water supply and sanitation infrastructure cannot be implemented immediately in many high-risk areas, vaccination against cholera is an important additional tool for prevention and control. We describe the development of licensed and recommended inactivated oral cholera vaccines (OCVs), including the results of safety, efficacy and effectiveness studies and the creation of the global OCV stockpile. Over the years, the public health strategy for oral cholera vaccination has broadened—from purely pre-emptive use to reactive deployment to help control outbreaks. Limited supplies of OCV doses continues to be an important problem. We discuss various innovative dosing and delivery approaches that have been assessed and implemented and evidence of herd protection conferred by OCVs. We expect that the demand for OCVs will continue to increase in the coming years across many countries.

Keywords: cholera; oral cholera vaccine; efficacy; effectiveness

1. Introduction

Cholera remains a threat to many impoverished populations around the world. The long-term public health strategies against cholera and other enteric diseases are the establishment of safe water sources and the improvement of sanitation and hygiene (WASH). However, these measures are years away in many areas where cholera strikes, especially when war, political upheaval or natural disasters such as earthquakes and floods occur. The oral cholera vaccine (OCV) is an important complementary tool for cholera prevention and control.

In this article we describe the history of the development of licensed oral cholera vaccines (OCVs). We discuss the accumulation of evidence on OCV safety, efficacy and effectiveness leading up to the recommendation by the World Health Organization (WHO) on mass oral cholera vaccination as both pre-emptive and reactive strategies. We discuss the initiation and expansion of the global OCV stockpile and its support by the Global Alliance for Vaccines and Immunizations (Gavi Alliance). We review various dose-sparing approaches (single-dose mass campaigns, targeting of specific high-risk groups and ring vaccination), evidence of herd protection conferred by OCVs and new delivery strategies. This article focuses on internationally licensed and recommended inactivated OCVs used during cholera outbreaks and in cholera-endemic sites.

2. Search Strategy

For this narrative review, we searched PubMed using the terms "oral cholera vaccine", "cholera outbreak response" and "cholera vaccination campaign", restricted to publications in English. We reviewed and included (a) relevant articles on the history of the development of inactivated OCVs, (b) publications during the last ten years on various innovative dosing and delivery strategies and (c) evidence of herd protection conferred by inactivated OCVs.

3. Development of Oral Cholera Vaccines and the Recommendation for Use

Injectable killed whole cell *Vibrio cholerae* O1 vaccines were widely available for many years [1]. These vaccines had poor efficacy and high reactogenicity and have not been recommended since the 1970s [2]. In the 1980s, a killed OCV consisting of inactivated whole cells of *V cholerae* O1 and the B-subunit of the cholera toxin (WC/rBS) was developed in Sweden [3]. Large scale trials of the vaccine in Bangladesh and Peru showed that the WC/rBS and the killed whole cell formulation alone were safe and conferred significant protection for up to 3 years [4,5]. An initial efficacy of 85–90% was obtained with the WC/rBS, declining to about 50% after 6 months. The oral vaccine without the B-subunit gave a somewhat lower initial level of protection but after 6 months the protection afforded by the two vaccines was similar. The WC/rBS vaccine is marketed as Dukoral (Valneva, Lyon, France) and is administered to those two years of age and older, as a two-dose regimen with a buffer (Table 1). Dukoral was the first OCV to obtain international licensure (in 1991) and WHO prequalification (in 2001). At that time, the WHO recommended inclusion of the WC/rBS vaccine among the tools to prevent cholera in populations believed to be at risk of cholera epidemic within 6 months and not experiencing a current outbreak [6].

The manufacturing technology of the Swedish vaccine was transferred to Vietnamese scientists at the National Institute of Hygiene and Epidemiology in Hanoi. A two-dose regimen of the first generation monovalent (anti-O1) OCV, containing only killed cholera whole cells and produced at USD 0.10 per dose in Vietnam, showed that it conferred 66% protection in a trial in Hue [7]. In 1997, killed *V. cholerae* O139 whole cells were added to the Vietnamese OCV due to the emergence of the new form of epidemic cholera caused by this serogroup. A bridging study found the bivalent (O1 and O139) OCV to be safe and immunogenic in adults and children one year and older [8]. The bivalent OCV was locally licensed as ORC-Vax (Vabiotech, Ha Noi, Viet Nam). The Vietnamese OCV has been used extensively in the Viet Nam public health system through mass immunization of high-risk populations. The burden of cholera in Vietnam has declined significantly in recent years, associated with widespread deployment of OCV and improvements in socioeconomic and WASH conditions [9]. The Vietnamese OCV has several distinct advantages over the original Swedish vaccine. Without a B-subunit component, the 2-dose Vietnamese OCV is easier and less expensive to manufacture, has less stringent cold chain requirements and is administered without a buffer.

The International Vaccine Institute (IVI) worked with VaBiotech to modify the strain composition of the bivalent OCV and improve the manufacturing process to conform with WHO standards [2]. The modified bivalent OCV was found to be safe and immunogenic in trials in Vietnam and India [10,11]. In 2009, the reformulated vaccine was licensed as mORC-Vax (Vabiotech, Viet Nam) but is not pre-qualified by WHO. To facilitate the international availability of mORC-Vax, manufacture of the reformulated vaccine was transferred to Shantha Biotechnics in India [12]. This led to the development of Shanchol (Shantha Biotechnics, Andhra Pradesh, India). A randomized, placebo-controlled trial in Kolkata, India showed that Shanchol is safe and confers 67% protective efficacy against cholera within two years of vaccination [12], 66% at three years [13] and 65% at five years [14] of follow-up. Shanchol, given as a 2-dose regimen to those one year of age and older, was licensed in India in 2009 and received WHO pre-qualification in 2011 (Table 1).

By then, the majority of countries reporting cholera to the WHO were in Sub-Saharan Africa [15]. A large and protracted cholera outbreak spread all over Zimbabwe from 2008 to 2009 and resulted in 98,585 cases and more than 4000 deaths [16], as well as increasing pressure by the global public health community to deploy OCVs reactively [17,18]. With amassing evidence on OCV safety and efficacy and data on field effectiveness and feasibility of OCV mass vaccination in an African setting [19–21], in October 2009, the WHO Strategic Advisory Group of Experts (SAGE) on immunization recommended that oral cholera vaccination should be considered as a reactive strategy during outbreaks, in addition to the already recommended preventive use of OCV in endemic areas [22].

The recommendation on reactive use is very important since where and when a cholera outbreak will occur is difficult or impossible to predict. Reactive mass oral cholera vaccination was documented to be feasible and effective as an outbreak response in Guinea [23,24]. Following an initial hesitation to deploy OCV in Haiti shortly after the catastrophic 2010 earthquake [25], a large reactive mass oral cholera vaccination campaign in Haiti was shown to be successful despite logistic challenges [26,27]. An increasing number of reactive mass oral cholera vaccinations has been successfully conducted in different areas around the world under diverse circumstances [28].

With the broadening of the recommendation for oral cholera vaccination, the most important concern is ensuring a sufficient and sustainable supply of OCV doses. In September 2011, the WHO convened a meeting of experts at which an OCV stockpile was affirmed as necessary and feasible [29] and an OCV stockpile was created in 2012 [30], with pivotal support from Gavi starting in 2014 [31]. From 2013 to 2017, over 25 million doses were requested from the cholera vaccine stockpile, of which only 51% could be allocated and shipped to countries for 46 deployments [32]. Due to the limited number of OCV doses available, supplies were prioritized for cholera outbreaks, making preventive OCV campaigns difficult to plan and carry-out. To expand the global OCV production capacity, Euvichol (Eubiologics, Gangwon-do, South Korea), was developed based on the same formulation as Shanchol through a technology transfer from IVI. After a Phase I trial in Korea [33] and a bridging non-inferiority immunogenicity study in the Philippines [34], Euvichol was licensed and WHO-prequalified in December 2015 [35] (Table 1). Availability of Euvichol increases the number of affordable OCV doses that can be distributed through the stockpile to affected populations [35].

Table 1. Internationally Licensed and Recommended Inactivated Oral Cholera Vaccines [28,35].

Vaccine	Dukoral	Shanchol	Euvichol
Manufacturer	Valneva, Lyon, France	Shantha Biotechnics, Andhra Pradesh, India	Eubiologics, Gangwon-do, South Korea
Description	Monovalent inactivated vaccine	Bivalent inactivated vaccine	Bivalent inactivated vaccine
Components	Killed whole-cells of *V. cholerae* O1 (Classical and El Tor biotypes) and recombinant B-subunit of cholera toxin	Killed whole cells of *V. cholerae* O1 (Classical and El Tor biotypes) and *V. cholerae* O139	Killed whole cells of *V. cholerae* O1 (Classical and El Tor biotypes) and *V. cholerae* O139
Recommended age	2 years and older	1 year and older	1 year and older
Delivery	Oral	Oral	Oral
Doses	2 doses given 1–6 weeks apart 3 doses for children aged 2–5 years	2 doses given 14 days apart	2 doses given 14 days apart
Buffer solution	Buffer dissolved in 75 mL (2–6 years old) or 150 mL (>6 years old) water	Not required	Not required

In 2018, Gavi's Board approved an additional investment for pre-emptive OCV use in high-risk areas, which will become available in 2021, while continuing its support for OCV emergency use [31]. The current objectives of the GAVI investment include ongoing prevention of an OCV low demand–low supply cycle, reduction in cholera outbreaks in Gavi-supported countries and strengthening of the evidence base for periodic, pre-emptive campaigns [31]. Currently, the International Coordinating Group (comprising representatives from Médecins Sans Frontières, the International Federation of Red Cross/Crescent, Unicef, and the WHO) manage the allocation of OCV doses for outbreak response during emergency situations or humanitarian crisis. The Global Task Force on Cholera Control, a WHO coordinated network of partners, manages the allocation of OCV doses for vaccination in cholera endemic hotspots [36].

4. Dose-Sparing Approaches

Most of the OCV doses produced since 2013 enter the stockpile, which has increased from about two million doses per year in 2013–2014 to more than 17 million doses in 2018 [31]. Despite this increase, the availability of OCV doses remains limited compared with the population in need. Innovative OCV dose-sparing approaches have been evaluated.

4.1. Single-Dose Strategy

A single dose regimen could mitigate against insufficient supplies and would also address the difficulties associated with delivery of two doses particularly during humanitarian emergencies, including accessing the same population twice, maintaining vaccine storage and retaining vaccination staff during the inter-dose period. A modeling study showed that reactive vaccination campaigns using a single dose of OCV may prevent more cases and deaths than a two-dose campaign when vaccine supplies are limited, while at the same time reducing logistical complexity [37]. Field evidence on OCV single-dose protection is available from one randomized controlled trial in Bangladesh [38,39] and several observational studies [24,27,40–44]. The protection conferred by a single dose was shown to be 89% at 7 weeks [43], waning to 39% at 2 years of follow-up [39] (Figure 1). Estimates of single-dose protection were generally lower in the randomized controlled trial than in the observational studies. Importantly, a subgroup analysis of the Bangladesh single-dose randomized trial found no significant protection in children younger than five years of age [38,39], which has been attributed to the lower pre-existing natural immunity in this age group.

Although the level of protection from a single OCV dose two years following vaccination is lower than the two-dose efficacy of 67% during the Kolkata trial [12], this may be sufficient to reduce the immediate short-term risk during outbreaks or in high-risk settings. A one-dose campaign, where more people receive a dose may be better in some circumstances than a two-dose strategy, where half as many people are vaccinated. In emergency situations, short-term protection is most critical and most of the public health benefit of reactive vaccination campaigns likely comes from the first dose, regardless of whether or not the second dose is administered [37]. However, the finding from the Bangladesh trial of no protective efficacy in young children suggests that the single-dose strategy may be beneficial only in populations with pre-existing natural immunity. Ideally, a second dose should be given as soon as circumstances allow to ensure longer and more robust protection, but this may not be possible due to inadequate OCV supplies or field logistics.

In 2016, during a resurgence of cholera cases after Hurricane Matthew, Haiti launched a large emergency campaign when more than 700,000 people received a single dose of OCV [45]. During mass oral cholera vaccinations of Rohingya refugees in Bangladesh when only 900,000 doses were available, one dose was given to more than 700,000 people in October 2017, while a second dose was given in November 2017 to children between the ages of one to four years [46].

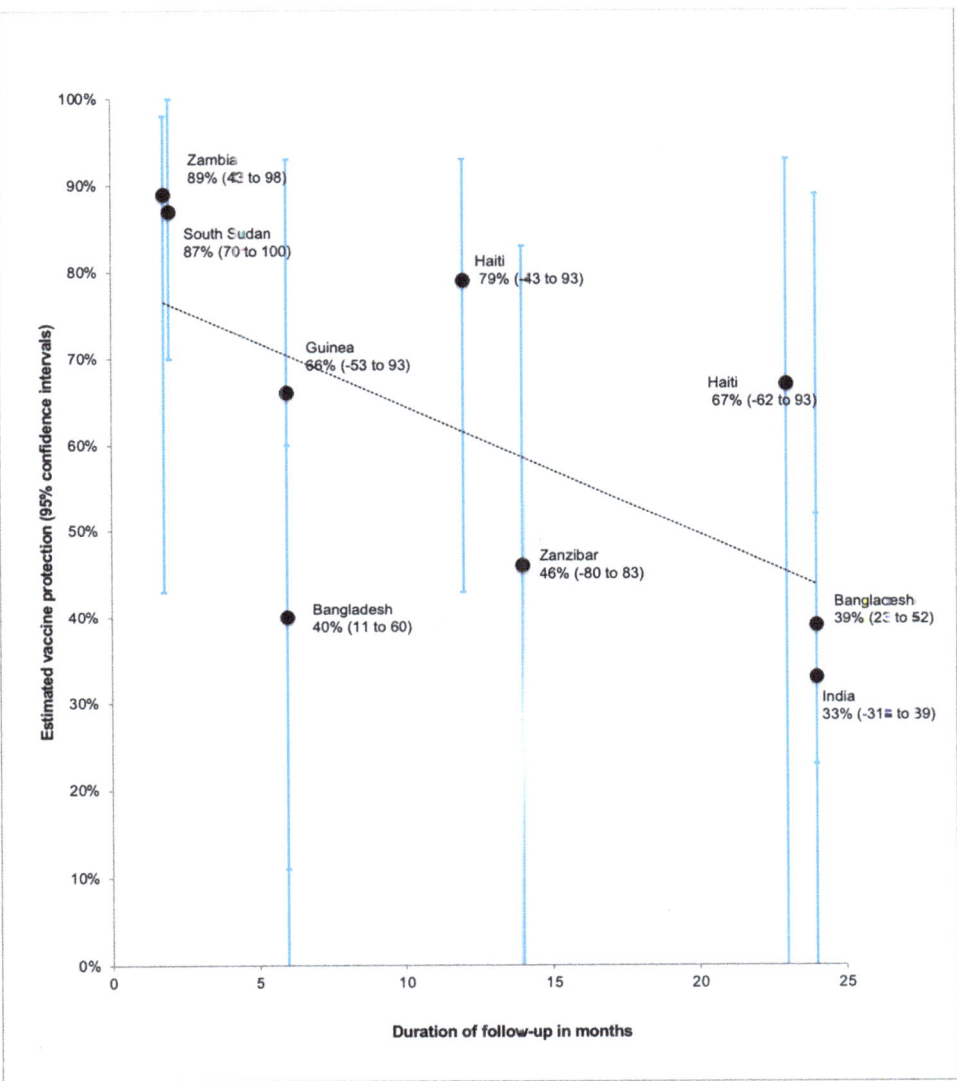

Figure 1. Estimated single-dose oral cholera vaccine protection (95% confidence intervals) with trendline, by month of follow-up. (Modified and updated from Lopez, A.L.; Deen, J.; Azman, A.S.; Luquero, F.J.; Kanungo, S.; Dutta, S.; von Seidlein, L.; Sack, D.A. Immunogenicity and Protection From a Single Dose of Internationally Available Killed Oral Cholera Vaccine: A Systematic Review and Meta-analysis. *Clinical Infectious Diseases*: 2018, 66, 1960–1971, doi:10.1093/cid/cix1039.)

4.2. Targeted Deployment of OCVs

Another dose-sparing approach is the targeted deployment of OCVs, both as a pre-emptive or reactive strategy. Targeting discrete areas within a larger population at risk for cholera is usually necessary since the number of doses approved for allocation from the global stockpile is often less than the number requested. Criteria for the selection of targeted areas include the population size in an area in relation to the number of doses available, logistics required, historical attack rates of cholera and recent reported cases of cholera [47]. The concept of "source drying" may also be used when considering where to deploy limited number of OCV doses. For example, the two-dose mass vaccination campaign in Guinea targeted the Boffa and Forecariah coastal and island populations, which are highly mobile, have limited access to health care, safe water and basic sanitation and from whom cholera cases are often first reported during an outbreak [23,24].

In 2014, a two-dose OCV campaign was successfully conducted in selected areas of Kalemie, an urbanized and highly cholera-endemic area in the Democratic Republic of Congo [48] The targeted areas covered a population of around 120,000 people and had the highest historical attack rates in Kalemie. In 2015, a two-dose OCV campaign was carried out in ten selected villages of Shashemenae, a rural district of Ethiopia [49]. In 2015, 140,249 individuals in selected neighborhoods in Juba, South Sudan received a single dose of OCV in response to a cholera outbreak [50]. Targeting high-risk neighborhoods in Juba was done since authorities were unable to secure sufficient doses to vaccinate the entire at-risk population of about one million.

4.3. Ring Vaccination

When cholera outbreaks occur, there is usually broad agreement on the need for mass vaccination campaigns. In contrast, during smaller outbreaks or when sporadic cases occur in endemic areas, public health officials may be reluctant to allocate substantial resources for mass vaccination campaigns. Since cholera cases tend to cluster in time and place, particularly among household contacts of a cholera case [51,52], ring vaccination around cases could be considered. Ring vaccination may be used as a preliminary control strategy, which could be followed by a wider mass vaccination campaign if needed [53]. Data from the OCV efficacy trial in Kolkata [14] were used to model a potential OCV ring strategy and found that high-level protection can be achieved for those living close to cholera cases [54]. More recently, simulations of case-area targeted interventions, which can include improved water quality and supply, sanitation, hand washing, oral cholera vaccine, and prophylactic antibiotics, showed that vaccinating people within 100 m around index case households and improving their water source early in epidemics could reduce the number of cases by 82% compared to uncontrolled epidemics [55]. The addition of antibiotic treatment of neighbors within a 30-m to 45-m radius around the index case was helpful, but only in the short term.

Ring vaccination using OCV may be less resource intensive than mass oral cholera vaccination but to be successful, cholera cases have to be detected quickly, sufficient OCV doses must be available on site within a short time from detection of the first cases, and the logistics for contact tracing and vaccination have to be set up immediately. A feasibility study in Nepal showed that cholera cases could be investigated within two days of a positive culture result [56]. The actual real-life feasibility and cost of integrating a sustainable cholera surveillance and ring OCV response system into a government's health infrastructure has yet to be assessed.

5. Evidence of Vaccine Herd Protection

The term vaccine herd protection is widely used but carries a variety of meanings [57]. In this discussion, we define vaccine herd protection as the extension of the defense conferred by immunization beyond the vaccinated to unvaccinated persons in a population, as well as the enhancement of the protection among the vaccinated. Vaccine herd protection results from a decline in transmission of the pathogen within the community. Included in vaccine herd protection is the reduction in disease risk among the unvaccinated in the population (indirect protection) due to decreased exposure to the pathogen, as well as enhanced protection of vaccinees due to their proximity to other vaccinees (total protection). Unlike vaccinated individuals protected through direct immunity, individuals with indirect protection remain fully susceptible to infection, should they be exposed [57].

Aside from direct vaccine protective effects, there is increasing evidence of herd protection conferred by OCV. A reanalysis of a field trial in Matlab, Bangladesh demonstrated that OCV induces indirect protection of non-vaccinees, as well as enhanced protection of vaccinees [58]. A model of cholera transmission using information from the same trial showed that if about half the population was vaccinated, this would reduce the number of cholera cases among unvaccinated people by 89% and among the entire population by 93% [59]. For children too young to be vaccinated or to mount an adequate response to OCV (particularly to a single dose), based on principles of cocooning [60], oral cholera vaccination of older children and adults would be beneficial. There is evidence for substantial indirect protection of young children when a large proportion of older persons in the community are vaccinated [61].

More recently in Zanzibar, mass oral cholera vaccination was also found to confer indirect protection, as indicated by the lower risk of cholera in non-vaccinated individuals residing in areas with high vaccine coverage than in those residing in areas with low vaccine coverage [41]. Population-level effects of OCV was inferred from a study during the cholera epidemic in South Sudan in 2014 [62] The daily cholera reproductive number among internally displaced persons living in settlements that had received OCV vaccination was <1 for most of the epidemic, compared to >1 in unvaccinated areas even though conditions were less suitable for transmission in these unvaccinated areas.

The degree of population level effectiveness induced by a vaccine is driven by several factors, including vaccine-induced direct protection, vaccine coverage and population mixing and mobility [63]. A mathematical model of a simulated displaced-persons camp indicated that the duration of OCV-derived herd protection can be short in settings with high population mobility [64].

6. New Delivery Strategies

Mass oral cholera vaccination campaigns have generally utilized fixed posts for distribution [28], but other deployment methods may be used for various reasons. In the 2014 OCV campaign in Kalemie (described above), the vaccinations were administered door-to-door as it was feared that the targeted approach would generate tensions in the area, especially among those not selected for vaccination [48]. In October 2016, a two-dose pre-emptive mass vaccination campaign was given door-to-door in Nampula, Mozambique, which targeted 193,403 people [65]. The door-to-door method was used since this is the routine local distribution strategy for polio vaccination campaigns.

OCV has been recommended to be stored at 2–8 °C but a study in Bangladesh showed that Shanchol has a good safety and immunogenic profile when stored under ambient temperature or even as high as 42 °C for up to 14 days [66]. Using OCV out of strict cold chain allows various possibilities for vaccine delivery and distribution. During the Guinea mass vaccination campaign, OCV doses were stored in cold chain but transported and used at ambient temperature during the vaccination days [23,24]. During a reactive two-dose OCV campaign in Lake Chilwa, Malawi, innovative strategies for the second vaccine dose (delivery by a community leader and self-administration) were used to facilitate vaccine access in hard-to-reach communities [67]. In another study in Dhaka, Bangladesh 41,694 people received a first OCV dose from fixed sites and the second dose was provided in a plastic zip-lock bag for the participant to take two weeks later at home [68]. Compliance for the second dose was estimated at 93% [68].

Cholera can cause serious complications in pregnant women and their fetuses if the disease is not treated promptly. Safety of the OCV during pregnancy has been demonstrated in several studies [69–73]. Pregnant women are no longer excluded during OCV mass campaigns [74].

7. Discussion

Since the availability of an effective OCV vaccine stockpile, more countries are open to acknowledging outbreaks and requesting OCV doses. The demand for OCVs will likely continue to outstrip supply in the near future. The constraints in supplies, complex logistics of administering the vaccine under difficult conditions and ensuring coverage of high-risk groups have resulted in alternative vaccination strategies, including single-dose regimens, targeted campaigns and locally adapted ways in administering OCVs. More recent campaigns have utilized a combination of these strategies. Although there is growing experience with the feasibility and acceptability of these methods, there is a need to continue documenting the protective effectiveness of OCVs when deployed using these methods.

In October 2017, the Global Task Force on Cholera Control launched an initiative to reduce cholera deaths by 90% worldwide, and eliminate cholera in at least 20 countries by 2030 [75]. A Global Roadmap to 2030 outlines three main axes for cholera prevention and control: early detection and rapid response to contain outbreaks; a multisectoral approach to prevent cholera in endemic countries (strengthening of surveillance, health care systems, water, sanitation and hygiene, and community mobilization and mass vaccination campaigns for communities at risk), targeting hotspots; and effective technical support, resource mobilization and partnership at local and international levels [76]. OCVs will play an important role to reach this ambitious goal but long-term improvements in WASH should be the ultimate aim.

Author Contributions: Conceptualization, J.D.C.; literature search and review, J.D.; original draft preparation, J.D.; review and editing, J.D.C. Both authors have read and agreed to the published version of the manuscript.

Funding: This research received no external funding.

Institutional Review Board Statement: Not applicable.

Informed Consent Statement: Not applicable.

Conflicts of Interest: The authors declare no conflict of interest.

References

1. Ryan, E.T.; Calderwood, S.B. Cholera vaccines. *Clin. Infect. Dis.* **2000**, *31*, 561–565. [CrossRef]
2. World Health Organization. *Guidelines for the Production and Control of Inactivated Oral Cholera Vaccines*; WHO Technical Report, Series No. 924; World Health Organization: Geneva, Switzerland, 2004. Available online: https://www.who.int/biologicals/publications/trs/areas/vaccines/cholera/129-149.pdf?ua=1 (accessed on 15 January 2021).
3. Holmgren, J.; Svennerholm, A.M.; Clemens, J.; Sack, D.; Black, R.; Levine, M. An oral B subunit-whole cell vaccine against cholera: From concept to successful field trial. *Adv. Exp. Med. Biol.* **1987**, *216B*, 1649–1660.
4. Clemens, J.D.; Sack, D.A.; Harris, J.R.; Van Loon, F.; Chakraborty, J.; Ahmed, F.; Rao, M.R.; Khan, M.R.; Yunus, M.; Huda, N.; et al. Field trial of oral cholera vaccines in Bangladesh: Results from three-year follow-up. *Lancet* **1990**, *335*, 270–273. [CrossRef]
5. Sanchez, J.L.; Vasquez, B.; Begue, R.E.; Meza, R.; Castellares, G.; Cabezas, C.; Watts, D.M.; Svennerholm, A.M.; Sadoff, J.C.; Taylor, D.N. Protective efficacy of oral whole-cell/recombinant-B-subunit cholera vaccine in Peruvian military recruits. *Lancet* **1994**, *344*, 1273–1276. [CrossRef]
6. World Health Organization. Cholera vaccines. *Wkl. Epidemiol. Rec.* **2001**, *76*, 117–124.
7. Trach, D.D.; Clemens, J.D.; Ke, N.T.; Thuy, H.T.; Son, N.D.; Canh, D.G.; Hang, P.V.; Rao, M.R. Field trial of a locally produced, killed, oral cholera vaccine in Vietnam. *Lancet* **1997**, *349*, 231–235. [CrossRef]
8. Trach, D.D.; Cam, P.D.; Ke, N.T.; Rao, M.R.; Dinh, D.; Hang, P.V.; Hung, N.V.; Canh, D.G.; Thiem, V.D.; Naficy, A.; et al. Investigations into the safety and immunogenicity of a killed oral cholera vaccine developed in Viet Nam. *Bull. World Health Organ.* **2002**, *80*, 2–8. [PubMed]
9. Anh, D.D.; Lopez, A.L.; Tran, H.T.; Cuong, N.V.; Thiem, V.D.; Ali, M.; Deen, J.L.; von Seidlein, L.; Sack, D.A. Oral cholera vaccine development and use in Vietnam. *PLoS Med.* **2014**, *11*, e1001712. [CrossRef]
10. Anh, D.D.; Canh, D.G.; Lopez, A.L.; Thiem, V.D.; Long, P.T.; Son, N.H.; Deen, J.; von Seidlein, L.; Carbis, R.; Han, S.H.; et al. Safety and immunogenicity of a reformulated Vietnamese bivalent killed, whole-cell, oral cholera vaccine in adults. *Vaccine* **2007**, *25*, 1149–1155. [CrossRef]
11. Mahalanabis, D.; Lopez, A.L.; Sur, D.; Deen, J.; Manna, B.; Kanungo, S.; von Seidlein, L.; Carbis, R.; Han, S.H.; Shin, S.H.; et al. A randomized, placebo-controlled trial of the bivalent killed, whole-cell, oral cholera vaccine in adults and children in a cholera endemic area in Kolkata, India. *PLoS ONE* **2008**, *3*, e2323. [CrossRef] [PubMed]
12. Sur, D.; Lopez, A.L.; Kanungo, S.; Paisley, A.; Manna, B.; Ali, M.; Niyogi, S.K.; Park, J.K.; Sarkar, B.; Puri, M.K.; et al. Efficacy and safety of a modified killed-whole-cell oral cholera vaccine in India: An interim analysis of a cluster-randomised, double-blind, placebo-controlled trial. *Lancet* **2009**, *374*, 1694–1702. [CrossRef]
13. Sur, D.; Kanungo, S.; Sah, B.; Manna, B.; Ali, M.; Paisley, A.M.; Niyogi, S.K.; Park, J.K.; Sarkar, B.; Puri, M.K.; et al. Efficacy of a low-cost, inactivated whole-cell oral cholera vaccine: Results from 3 years of follow-up of a randomized, controlled trial. *PLoS Negl. Trop. Dis.* **2011**, *5*, e1289. [CrossRef] [PubMed]

14. Bhattacharya, S.K.; Sur, D.; Ali, M.; Kanungo, S.; You, Y.A.; Manna, B.; Sah, B.; Niyogi, S.K.; Park, J.K.; Sarkar, B.; et al. 5 year efficacy of a bivalent killed whole-cell oral cholera vaccine in Kolkata, India: A cluster-randomised, double-blind, placebo-controlled trial. *Lancet Infect. Dis.* **2013**, *13*, 1050–1056. [CrossRef]
15. Gaffga, N.H.; Tauxe, R.V.; Mintz, E.D. Cholera: A new homeland in Africa? *Am. J. Trop. Med. Hyg.* **2007**, *77*, 705–713. [CrossRef]
16. Cuneo, C.N.; Sollom, R.; Beyrer, C. The Cholera Epidemic in Zimbabwe, 2008–2009: A Review and Critique of the Evidence. *Health Hum. Rights* **2017**, *19*, 249–264.
17. Bhattacharya, S.; Black, R.; Bourgeois, L.; Clemens, J.; Cravioto, A.; Deen, J.L.; Dougan, G.; Glass, R.; Grais, R.F.; Greco, M.; et al. Public health. The cholera crisis in Africa. *Science* **2009**, *324*, 885. [CrossRef] [PubMed]
18. Reyburn, R.; Deen, J.L.; Grais, R.F. Bhattacharya, S.K.; Sur, D.; Lopez, A.L.; Jiddawi, M.S.; Clemens, J.D.; von Seidlein, L. The case for reactive mass oral cholera vaccinations. *PLoS Negl. Trop. Dis.* **2011**, *5*, e952. [CrossRef] [PubMed]
19. Legros, D.; Paquet, C.; Perea, W.; Marty, I.; Mugisha, N.K.; Royer, H. Neira, M.; Ivanoff, B. Mass vaccination with a two-dose oral cholera vaccine in a refugee camp. *Bull. World Health Organ.* **1999**, *77*, 837–842.
20. Lucas, M.E.; Deen, J.L.; von Seidlein, L.; Wang, X.Y.; Ampuero, J.; Puri, M.; Ali, M.; Ansaruzzaman, M.; Amos, J.; Macuamule, A.; et al. Effectiveness of mass oral cholera vaccination in Beira, Mozambique. *N. Engl. J. Med.* **2005**, *352*, 757–767. [CrossRef]
21. Cavailler, P.; Lucas, M.; Perroud, V.; McChesney, M.; Ampuero, S.; Guerin, P.J.; Legros, D.; Nierle, T.; Mahoudeau, C.; Lab, B.; et al. Feasibility of a mass vaccination campaign using a two-dose oral cholera vaccine in an urban cholera-endemic setting in Mozambique. *Vaccine* **2006**, *24*, 4890–4895. [CrossRef]
22. Meeting of the Strategic Advisory Group of Experts on immunization, October 2009—Conclusions and recommendations. *Wkl. Epidemiol. Rec.* **2009**, *84*, 517–532
23. Ciglenecki, I.; Sakoba, K.; Luquero, F.J.; Heile, M.; Itama, C.; Mengel, M.; Grais, R.F.; Verhoustraeten, F.; Legros, D. Feasibility of mass vaccination campaign with oral cholera vaccines in response to an outbreak in Guinea. *PLoS Med.* **2013**, *10*, e1001512. [CrossRef]
24. Luquero, F.J.; Grout, L.; Ciglenecki, I.; Sakoba, K.; Traore, B.; Heile, M.; Diallo, A.A.; Itama, C.; Page, A.L.; Quilici, M.L.; et al. Use of Vibrio cholerae vaccine in an outbreak in Guinea. *N. Engl. J. Med.* **2014**, *370*, 2111–2120. [CrossRef]
25. Date, K.A.; Vicari, A.; Hyde, T.B.; Mintz, E.; Danovaro-Holliday, M.C.; Henry, A.; Tappero, J.W.; Roels, T.H.; Abrams, J.; Burkholder, B.T.; et al. Considerations for oral cholera vaccine use during outbreak after earthquake in Haiti, 2010–2011. *Emerg. Infect. Dis.* **2011**, *17*, 2105–2112. [CrossRef] [PubMed]
26. Ivers, L.C.; Teng, J.E. Lascher, J.; Raymond, M.; Weigel, J.; Victor, N.; Jerome, J.G.; Hilaire, I.J.; Almazor, C.P.; Ternier, R.; et al. Use of oral cholera vaccine in Haiti: A rural demonstration project. *Am. J. Trop. Med. Hyg.* **2013**, *89*, 617–624. [CrossRef] [PubMed]
27. Ivers, L.C.; Hilaire, I.J.; Teng, J.E.; Almazor, C.P.; Jerome, J.G.; Ternier, R.; Boncy, J.; Buteau, J.; Murray, M.B.; Harris, J.B.; et al. Effectiveness of reactive oral cholera vaccination in rural Haiti: A case-control study and bias-indicator analysis. *Lancet Glob. Health* **2015**, *3*, e162–e168. [CrossRef]
28. Martin, S.; Lopez, A.L.; Bellos, A.; Deen, J.; Ali, M.; Alberti, K.; Arth, D.D.; Costa, A.; Grais, R.F.; Legros, D.; et al. Post-licensure deployment of oral cholera vaccines: A systematic review. *Bull. World Health Organ.* **2014**, *92*, 881–893. [CrossRef]
29. WHO—World Health Organization. Consultation on Oral Cholera Vaccine (OCV) Stockpile Strategic Framework: Potential Objectives and Possible Policy Options Geneva: Department of Immunization, Vaccines and Biologicals, World Health Organization. (WHO/IVB/12.05). 2012. Available online: http://www.who.int/immunization/documents/innovation/WHO_IVB_12.05/en/ (accessed on 27 November 2020).
30. Martin, S.; Costa, A.; Perea, W. Stockpiling oral cholera vaccine. *Bull. World Health Organ.* **2012**, *90*, 714. [CrossRef] [PubMed]
31. GAVI. Oral Cholera Vaccine Support. Available online: https://www.gavi.org/types-support/vaccine-support/oral-cholera (accessed on 16 January 2020).
32. World Health Organization. Deployments from the oral cholera vaccine stockpile, 2013–2017. *Wkl. Epidemiol. Rec.* **2017**, *92*, 437–442.
33. Baik, Y.O.; Choi, S.K.; Kim, J.W.; Yang, J.S.; Kim, I.Y.; Kim, C.W.; Hong, J.H. Safety and immunogenicity assessment of an oral cholera vaccine through phase I clinical trial in Korea. *J. Korean Med. Sci.* **2014**, *29*, 494–501. [CrossRef]
34. Baik, Y.O.; Choi, S.K.; Olveda, R.M.; Espos, R.A.; Ligsay, A.D.; Montellano, M.B.; Yeam, J.S.; Yang, J.S.; Park, J.Y.; Kim, D.R.; et al. A randomized, non-inferiority trial comparing two bivalent killed, whole cell, oral cholera vaccines (Euvichol versus. Shanchol) in the Philippines. *Vaccine* **2015**, *33*, 6360–6365. [CrossRef] [PubMed]
35. Desai, S.N.; Pezzoli, L.; Martin, S.; Costa, A.; Rodriguez, C.; Legros, D.; Perea, W. A second affordable oral cholera vaccine: Implications for the global vaccine stockpile. *Lancet Glob. Health* **2016**, *4*, e223–e224. [CrossRef]
36. Desai, S.N.; Pezzoli, L.; Alberti, K.P.; Martin, S.; Costa, A.; Perea, W.; Legros, D. Achievements and challenges for the use of killed oral cholera vaccines in the global stockpile era. *Hum. Vaccines Immunother.* **2017**, *13*, 579–587. [CrossRef] [PubMed]
37. Azman, A.S.; Luquero, F.J.; Ciglenecki, I.; Grais, R.F.; Sack, D.A.; Lessler, J. The Impact of a One-Dose versus Two-Dose Oral Cholera Vaccine Regimen in Outbreak Settings: A Modeling Study. *PLoS Med.* **2015**, *12*, e1001867. [CrossRef]
38. Qadri, F.; Wierzba, T.F.; Ali, M.; Chowdhury, F.; Khan, A.I.; Saha, A.; Khan, I.A.; Asaduzzaman, M.; Akter, A.; Khan, A.; et al. Efficacy of a Single-Dose, Inactivated Oral Cholera Vaccine in Bangladesh. *N. Engl. J. Med.* **2016**, *374*, 1723–1732. [CrossRef]
39. Qadri, F.; Ali, M.; Lynch, J.; Chowdhury, F.; Khan, A.I.; Wierzba, T.F.; Excler, J.L.; Saha, A.; Islam, M.T.; Begum, Y.A.; et al. Efficacy of a single-dose regimen of inactivated whole-cell oral cholera vaccine: Results from 2 years of follow-up of a randomised trial. *Lancet Infect. Dis.* **2018**, *18*, 666–674. [CrossRef]

40. Azman, A.S.; Parker, L.A.; Rumunu, J.; Tadesse, F.; Grandesso, F.; Deng, L.L.; Lino, R.L.; Bior, B.K.; Lasuba, M.; Page, A.L.; et al. Effectiveness of one dose of oral cholera vaccine in response to an outbreak: A case-cohort study. *Lancet Glob. Health* **2016**, *4*, e856–e863. [CrossRef]
41. Khatib, A.M.; Ali, M.; von Seidlein, L.; Kim, D.R.; Hashim, R.; Reyburn, R.; Ley, B.; Thriemer, K.; Enwere, G.; Hutubessy, R.; et al. Effectiveness of an oral cholera vaccine in Zanzibar: Findings from a mass vaccination campaign and observational cohort study. *Lancet Infect. Dis.* **2012**, *12*, 837–844. [CrossRef]
42. Wierzba, T.F.; Kar, S.K.; Mogasale, V.V.; Kerketta, A.S.; You, Y.A.; Baral, P.; Khuntia, H.K.; Ali, M.; Kim, Y.H.; Rath, S.B.; et al. Effectiveness of an oral cholera vaccine campaign to prevent clinically-significant cholera in Odisha State, India. *Vaccine* **2015**, *33*, 2463–2469. [CrossRef] [PubMed]
43. Ferreras, E.; Chizema-Kawesha, E.; Blake, A.; Chewe, O.; Mwaba, J.; Zulu, G.; Poncin, M.; Rakesh, A.; Page, A.L.; Stoitsova, S.; et al. Single-Dose Cholera Vaccine in Response to an Outbreak in Zambia. *N. Engl. J. Med.* **2018**, *378*, 577–579. [CrossRef] [PubMed]
44. Franke, M.F.; Ternier, R.; Jerome, J.G.; Matias, W.R.; Harris, J.B.; Ivers, L.C. Long-term effectiveness of one and two doses of a killed, bivalent, whole-cell oral cholera vaccine in Haiti: An extended case-control study. *Lancet Glob. Health* **2018**, *6*, e1028–e1035. [CrossRef]
45. WHO. Cholera Vaccination Campaign for Haitians Hardest hit by Hurricane Matthew, 28 November 2016. Available online: http://www.who.int/en/news-room/feature-stories/detail/cholera-vaccination-campaign-for-haitians-hardest-hit-by-hurricane-matthew (accessed on 8 January 2020).
46. Qadri, F.; Azad, A.K.; Flora, M.S.; Khan, A.I.; Islam, M.T.; Nair, G.B.; Singh, P.K.; Clemens, J.D. Emergency deployment of oral cholera vaccine for the Rohingya in Bangladesh. *Lancet* **2018**, *391*, 1877–1879. [CrossRef]
47. Luquero, F.J.; Banga, C.N.; Remartinez, D.; Palma, P.P.; Baron, E.; Grais, R.F. Cholera epidemic in Guinea-Bissau (2008): The importance of "place". *PLoS ONE* **2011**, *6*, e19005. [CrossRef]
48. Massing, L.A.; Aboubakar, S.; Blake, A.; Page, A.L.; Cohuet, S.; Ngandwe, A.; Mukomena Sompwe, E.; Ramazani, R.; Allheimen, M.; Levaillant, P.; et al. Highly targeted cholera vaccination campaigns in urban setting are feasible: The experience in Kalemie, Democratic Republic of Congo. *PLoS Negl. Trop. Dis.* **2018**, *12*, e0006369. [CrossRef]
49. Teshome, S.; Desai, S.; Kim, J.H.; Belay, D.; Mogasale, V. Feasibility and costs of a targeted cholera vaccination campaign in Ethiopia. *Hum. Vaccines Immunother.* **2018**, *14*, 2427–2433. [CrossRef]
50. Parker, L.A.; Rumunu, J.; Jamet, C.; Kenyi, Y.; Lino, R.L.; Wamala, J.F.; Mpairwe, A.M.; Ciglenecki, I.; Luquero, F.J.; Azman, A.S.; et al. Adapting to the global shortage of cholera vaccines: Targeted single dose cholera vaccine in response to an outbreak in South Sudan. *Lancet Infect. Dis.* **2017**, *17*, e123–e127. [CrossRef]
51. Weil, A.A.; Khan, A.I.; Chowdhury, F.; Larocque, R.C.; Faruque, A.S.; Ryan, E.T.; Calderwood, S.B.; Qadri, F.; Harris, J.B. Clinical outcomes in household contacts of patients with cholera in Bangladesh. *Clin. Infect. Dis.* **2009**, *49*, 1473–1479. [CrossRef] [PubMed]
52. Sugimoto, J.D.; Koepke, A.A.; Kenah, E.E.; Halloran, M.E.; Chowdhury, F.; Khan, A.I.; LaRocque, R.C.; Yang, Y.; Ryan, E.T.; Qadri, F.; et al. Household Transmission of Vibrio cholerae in Bangladesh. *PLoS Negl. Trop. Dis.* **2014**, *8*, e3314. [CrossRef] [PubMed]
53. Deen, J.; von Seidlein, L. The case for ring vaccinations with special consideration of oral cholera vaccines. *Hum. Vaccines Immunother.* **2018**, *14*, 2069–2074. [CrossRef] [PubMed]
54. Ali, M.; Debes, A.K.; Luquero, F.J.; Kim, D.R.; Park, J.Y.; Digilio, L.; Manna, B.; Kanungo, S.; Dutta, S.; Sur, D.; et al. Potential for Controlling Cholera Using a Ring Vaccination Strategy: Re-analysis of Data from a Cluster-Randomized Clinical Trial. *PLoS Med.* **2016**, *13*, e1002120. [CrossRef]
55. Finger, F.; Bertuzzo, E.; Luquero, F.J.; Naibei, N.; Touré, B.; Allan, M.; Porten, K.; Lessler, J.; Rinaldo, A.; Azman, A.S. The potential impact of case-area targeted interventions in response to cholera outbreaks: A modeling study. *PLoS Med.* **2018**, *15*, e1002509. [CrossRef]
56. Roskosky, M.; Acharya, B.; Shakya, G.; Karki, K.; Sekine, K.; Bajracharya, D.; von Seidlein, L.; Devaux, I.; Lopez, A.L.; Deen, J.; et al. Feasibility of a Comprehensive Targeted Cholera Intervention in The Kathmandu Valley, Nepal. *Am. J. Trop. Med. Hyg.* **2019**, *100*, 1088–1097. [CrossRef] [PubMed]
57. Clemens, J.; Shin, S.; Ali, M. New approaches to the assessment of vaccine herd protection in clinical trials. *Lancet Infect Dis.* **2011**, *11*, 482–487. [CrossRef]
58. Ali, M.; Emch, M.; von Seidlein, L.; Yunus, M.; Sack, D.A.; Rao, M.; Holmgren, J.; Clemens, J.D. Herd immunity conferred by killed oral cholera vaccines in Bangladesh: A reanalysis. *Lancet* **2005**, *366*, 44–49. [CrossRef]
59. Longini, I.M., Jr.; Nizam, A.; Ali, M.; Yunus, M.; Shenvi, N.; Clemens, J.D. Controlling endemic cholera with oral vaccines. *PLoS Med.* **2007**, *4*, e336. [CrossRef] [PubMed]
60. Healy, C.M.; Rench, M.A.; Baker, C.J. Implementation of cocooning against pertussis in a high-risk population. *Clin. Infect. Dis.* **2011**, *52*, 157–162. [CrossRef]
61. Ali, M.; Emch, M.; Yunus, M.; Sack, D.; Lopez, A.L.; Holmgren, J.; Clemens, J. Vaccine Protection of Bangladeshi infants and young children against cholera: Implications for vaccine deployment and person-to-person transmission. *Pediatr. Infect. Dis. J.* **2008**, *27*, 33–37. [CrossRef]

62. Azman, A.S.; Rumunu, J.; Abubakar, A.; West, H.; Ciglenecki, I.; Helderman, T.; Wamala, J.F.; Vazquez Ode, L.; Perea, W.; Sack, D.A.; et al. Population-Level Effect of Cholera Vaccine on Displaced Populations, South Sudan, 2014. *Emerg. Infect. Dis.* **2016**, *22*, 1067–1070. [CrossRef]
63. Ali, M.; Clemens, J. Assessing Vaccine Herd Protection by Killed Whole-Cell Oral Cholera Vaccines Using Different Study Designs. *Front. Public Health* **2019**, *7*, 211. [CrossRef]
64. Peak, C.M.; Reilly, A.L.; Azman, A.S.; Buckee, C.O. Prolonging herd immunity to cholera via vaccination: Accounting for human mobility and waning vaccine effects. *PLoS Negl. Trop. Dis.* **2018**, *12*, e0006257. [CrossRef]
65. Semá Baltazar, C.; Rafael, F.; Langa, J.P.M.; Chicumbe, S.; Cavailler, P.; Gessner, B.D.; Pezzoli, L.; Barata, A.; Zaina, D.; Inguane, D.L.; et al. Oral cholera vaccine coverage during a preventive door-to-door mass vaccination campaign in Nampula, Mozambique. *PLoS ONE* **2018**, *13*, e0198592. [CrossRef] [PubMed]
66. Saha, A.; Khan, A.; Salma, U.; Jahan, N.; Bhuiyan, T.R.; Chowdhury, F.; Khan, A.I.; Khanam, F.; Muruganandham, S.; Reddy Kandukuri, S.; et al. The oral cholera vaccine Shanchol when stored at elevated temperatures maintains the safety and immunogenicity profile in Bangladeshi participants. *Vaccine* **2016**, *34*, 1551–1558. [CrossRef] [PubMed]
67. Sauvageot, D.; Saussier, C.; Gobeze, A.; Chipeta, S.; Mhango, L.; Kawalazira, G.; Mengel, M.A.; Legros, D.; Cavailler, P.; M'Bang'ombe, M. Oral cholera vaccine coverage in hard-to-reach fishermen communities after two mass Campaigns, Malawi, 2016. *Vaccine* **2017**, *35*, 5194–5200. [CrossRef] [PubMed]
68. Khan, A.I.; Islam, M.S.; Islam, M.T.; Ahmed, A.; Chowdhury, M.I.; Chowdhury, F.; Siddik, M.A.U.; Clemens, J.D.; Qadri, F. Oral cholera vaccination strategy: Self-administration of the second dose in urban Dhaka, Bangladesh. *Vaccine* **2019**, *37*, 827–832. [CrossRef]
69. Ali, M.; Nelson, A.; Luquero, F.J.; Azman, A.S.; Debes, A.K.; M'Bang'ombe, M.; Seyama, L.; Kachale, E.; Zuze, K.; Malichi, D.; et al. Safety of a killed oral cholera vaccine (Shanchol) in pregnant women in Malawi: An observational cohort study. *Lancet Infect. Dis.* **2017**, *17*, 538–544. [CrossRef]
70. Khan, A.I.; Ali, M.; Chowdhury, F.; Saha, A.; Khan, I.A.; Khan, A.; Akter, A.; Asaduzzaman, M.; Islam, M.T.; Kabir, A.; et al. Safety of the oral cholera vaccine in pregnancy: Retrospective findings from a subgroup following mass vaccination campaign in Dhaka, Bangladesh. *Vaccine* **2017**, *35*, 1538–1543. [CrossRef] [PubMed]
71. Khan, A.I.; Ali, M.; Lynch, J.; Kabir, A.; Excler, J.L.; Khan, M.A.; Islam, M.T.; Akter, A.; Chowdhury, F.; Saha, A.; et al. Safety of a bivalent, killed, whole-cell oral cholera vaccine in pregnant women in Bangladesh: Evidence from a randomized placebo-controlled trial. *BMC Infect. Dis.* **2019**, *19*, 422. [CrossRef] [PubMed]
72. Hashim, R.; Khatib, A.M.; Enwere, G.; Park, J.K.; Reyburn, R.; Ali, M.; Chang, N.Y.; Kim, D.R.; Ley, B.; Thriemer, K.; et al. Safety of the recombinant cholera toxin B subunit, killed whole-cell (rBS-WC) oral cholera vaccine in pregnancy. *PLoS Negl. Trop. Dis.* **2012**, *6*, e1743. [CrossRef]
73. Grout, L.; Martinez-Pino, I.; Ciglenecki, I.; Keita, S.; Diallo, A.A.; Traore, B.; Delamou, D.; Toure, O.; Nicholas, S.; Rusch, B.; et al. Pregnancy Outcomes after a Mass Vaccination Campaign with an Oral Cholera Vaccine in Guinea: A Retrospective Cohort Study. *PLoS Negl. Trop. Dis.* **2015**, *9*, e0004274. [CrossRef] [PubMed]
74. Friedrich, M.J. Cholera Vaccine Safe During Pregnancy. *JAMA* **2017**, *317*, 2362. [CrossRef]
75. Legros, D.; Partners of the Global Task Force on Cholera Control. Global Cholera Epidemiology: Opportunities to Reduce the Burden of Cholera by 2030. *J. Infect. Dis.* **2018**, *218*, S137–S140. [CrossRef] [PubMed]
76. World Health Organization. *Ending Cholera: A Global Roadmap to 2030 Strategy*; World Health Organization: Geneva, Switzerland, 2017. Available online: https://www.who.int/cholera/publications/global-roadmap.pdf?ua=1 (accessed on 9 January 2021).

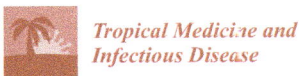

Review

Systemic, Mucosal, and Memory Immune Responses following Cholera

Edward T. Ryan [1,2,3], Daniel T. Leung [4], Owen Jensen [4], Ana A. Weil [5], Taufiqur Rahman Bhuiyan [6], Ashraful Islam Khan [6], Fahima Chowdhury [6], Regina C. LaRocque [1,2], Jason B. Harris [1,7,8,9], Stephen B. Calderwood [1,2,10], Firdausi Qadri [6] and Richelle C. Charles [1,2,3,*]

1. Division of Infectious Diseases, Massachusetts General Hospital, Boston, MA 02114, USA; etryan@mgh.harvard.edu (E.T.R.); rclarocque@mgh.harvard.edu (R.C.L.); jbharris@mgh.harvard.edu (J.B.H.); scalderwood@mgh.harvard.edu (S.B.C.)
2. Department of Medicine, Harvard Medical School, Boston, MA 02115, USA
3. Department of Immunology and Infectious Diseases, Harvard T.H. Chan School of Public Health, Boston, MA 02115, USA
4. Division of Infectious Diseases, Department of Internal Medicine, University of Utah School of Medicine, Salt Lake City, UT 84132, USA; daniel.leung@utah.edu (D.T.L.); owen.jensen@path.utah.edu (O.J.)
5. Division of Allergy and Infectious Diseases, University of Washington, Seattle, WA 98109, USA; anaweil@uw.edu
6. International Centre for Diarrhoeal Disease Research, Bangladesh (icddr,b), Dhaka 1212, Bangladesh; taufiqur@icddrb.org (T.R.B.); ashrafk@icddrb.org (A.I.K.); fchowdhury@icddrb.org (F.C.); fqadri@icddrb.org (F.Q.)
7. Department of Pediatrics, MassGeneral Hospital for Children, Boston, MA 02114, USA
8. Mucosal Immunology and Biology Research Center, Division of Pediatric Gastroenterology and Nutrition, Massachusetts General Hospital, Boston MA 02115, USA
9. Division of Pediatric Global Health, Massachusetts General Hospital, Boston, MA 02115, USA
10. Department of Microbiology, Harvard Medical School, Boston, MA 02115, USA
* Correspondence: rcharles@mgh.harvard.edu

Citation: Ryan, E.T.; Leung, D.T.; Jensen, O.; Weil, A.A.; Bhuiyan, T.R.; Khan, A.I.; Chowdhury, F.; LaRocque, R.C.; Harris, J.B.; Calderwood, S.B.; et al. Systemic, Mucosal, and Memory Immune Responses following Cholera. *TMID* **2021**, *6*, 192. https://doi.org/10.3390/tropicalmed6040192

Academic Editor: David Nalin

Received: 28 September 2021
Accepted: 23 October 2021
Published: 27 October 2021

Publisher's Note: MDPI stays neutral with regard to jurisdictional claims in published maps and institutional affiliations.

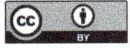

Copyright: © 2021 by the authors. Licensee MDPI, Basel, Switzerland. This article is an open access article distributed under the terms and conditions of the Creative Commons Attribution (CC BY) license (https://creativecommons.org/licenses/by/4.0/).

Abstract: *Vibrio cholerae* O1, the major causative agent of cholera, remains a significant public health threat. Although there are available vaccines for cholera, the protection provided by killed whole-cell cholera vaccines in young children is poor. An obstacle to the development of improved cholera vaccines is the need for a better understanding of the primary mechanisms of cholera immunity and identification of improved correlates of protection. Considerable progress has been made over the last decade in understanding the adaptive and innate immune responses to cholera disease as well as *V. cholerae* infection. This review will assess what is currently known about the systemic, mucosal, memory, and innate immune responses to clinical cholera, as well as recent advances in our understanding of the mechanisms and correlates of protection against *V. cholerae* O1 infection.

Keywords: cholera; *Vibrio cholerae*; immunity; innate; adaptive; antibody; cellular; mucosal; systemic; memory; vaccine

1. Introduction

Cholera is a severe dehydrating disease of humans caused by *Vibrio cholerae* serogroup O1 and O139. Over one billion people remain at risk for cholera in 51 endemic countries, and there are an estimated three million cases and 95,000 deaths from the disease each year [1]. The current global cholera pandemic began in 1961 with El Tor *V. cholerae* O1 and shows no signs of abating, as evidenced by recent large outbreaks in Haiti, Yemen, and South Sudan and annual epidemics in countries in Asia and Africa. This reality has led to enhanced commitments to cholera control strategies [2]. Such strategies now include vaccination against cholera, as well as improved water and sanitation efforts [2]. Currently available oral killed-cholera vaccines (kOCVs) have been a transformative addition to these control efforts; however, these vaccines may provide limited durable protection, especially in immunologically naïve individuals, including children under five years of age who bear a large proportion of the global cholera burden [3]. In comparison, survivors of clinical cholera, including young children, have high-level protective immunity that persists for years [4]. An improved understanding of immune responses associated with protection against cholera could lead to next-generation vaccines or prevention strategies. This review will assess what is currently known about the systemic, mucosal, memory, and innate immune responses to clinical cholera, as well as recent advances in our understanding of the mechanisms and correlates of protection against *V. cholerae* O1 infection

2. *V. cholerae*-Antigen Repertoire
V. cholerae O-Specific Polysaccharide (Lipopolysaccharide)

Protection against cholera is serogroup-specific, and serogroup specificity is dictated by the O-specific polysaccharide (OSP) component of *V. cholerae* lipopolysaccharide (LPS). Because of this, there is no cross-protection between infection with *V. cholerae* O1 and O139, even though these organisms can both cause epidemic cholera and are essentially genetically identical except for differences in the *rfb* genes encoding the OSP of these two serogroups [5–7]. Antibodies that bind externally to *V. cholerae* are binding to surface displayed antigens, either outer membrane proteins or LPS. Previous work has shown that the vibriocidal response is mediated by antibodies that bind to LPS, and specifically OSP [8,9]. Following clinical cholera, over a third of all induced antibodies target *V. cholerae* OSP [10,11]. These data would suggest that anti-LPS and specifically OSP-specific immune antibody responses are the actual mediators of protection against cholera.

Before OSP became available as a reagent for use in immunologic assays, a body of evidence showed that LPS responses (plasma, mucosal and memory) occur following cholera and vaccination in both children and adults, and that these responses correlated with protection against cholera, including in young children [12–15]. These findings were confirmed with OSP, once it became available for study [9,16–19]. Anti-OSP/LPS IgG, IgA and IgM responses following immunization of children in Bangladesh with killed oral cholera vaccines are significantly lower than those induced following clinical disease in age-matched patients, including the absence of anti-LPS memory responses in vaccinees despite induction of vibriocidal responses [15,16,18]. Specifically, infants and young children receiving kOCVs did not mount IgG, IgA, or IgM antibody responses to *V. cholerae* OSP or LPS, whereas older children showed significant responses.

In comparison to the vaccinees, young children with wild-type *V. cholerae* O1 infection showed significant antibody responses against OSP/LPS. OSP responses correlated with age in vaccinees, but not in cholera patients, reflecting the ability of even young children with wild-type cholera to develop OSP responses. These differences might contribute to the lower efficacy of protection rendered by kOCV than by wild-type disease in young children and suggest that efforts to improve OSP-specific responses might be critical for achieving optimal cholera vaccine efficacy in this younger age group [15,16]. In addition, avidity of anti-LPS IgG and IgA antibodies following wild-type disease is high and prolonged, despite a decrease in vibriocidal titers by day 180; and anti-LPS avidity correlates with induction of memory B-cell responses [20]. Anti-LPS avidity falls rapidly to baseline by day 30 following oral vaccination, suggesting a possible explanation for lower and shorter-term immunity afforded by kOCVs [20]. These data suggest that LPS/OSP specific responses may be better markers of long-term protection against cholera in endemic zones than other immune responses.

Much effort is now being made to assess how OSP-specific antibodies might protect against cholera, with a growing body of evidence suggesting that protection against infection may involve the ability of OSP-specific antibodies to impede the motility of *V. cholerae* organisms in the human intestine. This effect requires at least two-point binding of OSP-specific antibodies [21–26].

3. Protein Antigens

In addition to OSP, well-characterized *V. cholerae* antigens include the following proteins: cholera toxin B subunit (CTB), the toxin co-regulated pilus (TCP) subunit A (TcpA), and *V. cholerae* cytolysin (VCC), also referred to as hemolysin A (HlyA). Cholera toxin is a major virulence factor for all toxigenic strains of *V. cholerae* and consists of five B (CTB) subunits associated non-covalently with a single, enzymatically active A subunit [27]. TcpA is a major structural component of TCP, a colonizing factor essential for virulence in humans [28]. VCC generates membrane pores in eukaryotic cells and has been shown to induce fluid accumulation in ligated rabbit ileal loops and induce chloride secretion in intact human intestinal mucosa [29,30]. CTB, TcpA, and VCC have been shown to induce systemic, mucosal, and memory B-cell responses after *V. cholerae* infection [17,31–33].

Additional antigenic targets of the immune response to *V. cholerae* have recently been identified. The antigenic repertoire recognized by the cholera-induced plasmablast population was assessed through generation of a panel of monoclonal antibodies (mAbs) isolated following single-cell expression of day 7 plasmablasts from *V. cholerae*-infected patients [11]. Plasmablasts are activated antibody-secreting cells that are transiently found in the circulation after either infection or vaccination. Both cholera and cholera vaccines induce a potent mucosal homing plasmablast response that peaks seven days after infection and is strongly predictive of the presence of specific duodenal plasma cells for up to six months after cholera [10,34], suggesting that a proportion of these cells ultimately take up residence in the intestine as plasma cells. Of the 138 mAbs that were generated from a total of seven participants, 24 were OSP-specific, 37 were CtxB-specific, 12 were CtxA-specific, and none were TcpA-specific [11]. Using a *V. cholerae*-antigen array containing 95% of the *V. cholerae* proteome, nine additional antigenic targets were identified, most notably *V. cholerae* sialidase/mucinase (NanH), which was the target of 6 mAbs (or 5% of all circulating plasmablasts). Flagellin protein A and ToxR-regulated mucinase tagA were also identified.

This work was further supported by an immunoscreen using the *V. cholerae* antigen array above with plasma and antibodies recovered from culture supernatants of activated plasmablasts [35]. Fifty-nine antigens were demonstrated to have higher immunoreactivity at the early convalescent stage of infection compared to the acute stage or healthy controls [17]. These included the known antigens OSP, CTB, TcpA, VCC as well as several novel antigens, including NanH, cholera toxin A subunit (CtxA), an outer membrane protein (OmpV), a protein phosphotransferase (PtsP), and flagellar proteins (FlaC, FlaD).

Systemic, mucosal, and memory B-cells responses to NanH occur after clinical cholera, with NanH found to be the third most common antigenic target of a mucosal homing plasmablast response [11,17,36]. NanH is a virulence factor that catalyzes the cleavage of terminal sialic acid residues from gangliosides on the membrane of intestinal epithelial cells to generate monogangliosides (GM1), the binding site for CT [37]. NanH-neutralizing antibodies have been shown to block the toxin-potentiating effect of NanH in vitro [11]. These findings together suggest a possible functional role for NanH in protective immunity to cholera and antibody responses to NanH have been found to correlate with protection [36].

4. Correlates of Protection

4.1. Vibriocidal Response-Pros/cons

The vibriocidal response has historically been used to assess protection against cholera, but antibody-based bacterial killing of *V. cholerae* in the intestinal lumen is unlikely. There is no evidence that enhanced opsonophagocytosis or antibody-dependent cytotoxic activity in the intestinal lumen plays a role in mediating protection against cholera. Although cell-free antibody-based killing via complement lysis might be considered possible in the intestinal lumen, viability studies in animals have shown that bactericidal activity is not required for protection from disease [22,25,26]. In addition, although C3 and earlier components of the complement cascade have been detected in the intestinal lumen/epithelium, the terminal components of the complement cascade have not been detected in the lumen in the absence of epithelial breakdown and intestinal inflammation [38–40]. The primary antibody secreted at mucosal surfaces is IgA; however, IgA lacks the Fc regions of IgG and IgM that bind C1q, and consequently does not activate complement via the classical complement pathway; moreover, IgA complexed to antigen actually inhibits complement activation by IgM and IgG [41–43]. These data suggest that IgA plays a minimal, if any, role in complement activation in the intestine. The vibriocidal antibody assay, however, assesses complement activation [12,44,45].

While the vibriocidal response is associated with protection against cholera [46] and is an important biomarker of recent infection [47], there is no absolute value above which protection is assured [44]; and cholera vaccines that have been equivalent to wild type infection in inducing vibriocidal antibody responses have failed in clinical field trials in humans [48]. Similarly, although vibriocidal antibody titers increase sharply within 10 days of symptomatic cholera, they then fall rapidly within 30 days of infection, returning to baseline within 6–12 months, despite the fact that an episode of symptomatic cholera induces long-term immunity against cholera that exists for at least three to 10 years [4,49,50]. In addition, individuals can be protected against cholera with no increase of vibriocidal antibody responses following challenge and exposure, suggesting that other immune responses mediate protection against cholera [50–53]. Importantly, OSP responses differ substantially in naïve North Americans and low-to-middle-income country residents infected with *V. cholerae*, despite induction of comparable vibriocidal responses [54]. These data strongly suggest that the vibriocidal antibody is at best an imperfect non-mechanistic correlate of protection against cholera.

The majority of the vibriocidal response consists of IgM antibodies that specifically target OSP, giving the vibriocidal its serogroup specificity [9]. Interestingly, IgM antibodies, just like IgA antibodies, are actively transported across intact intestinal epithelium into the intestinal lumen, so it is quite possible that anti-vibrio OSP IgM antibodies may play a role in mediating at least short-term protection against cholera (for instance, following vaccination). Still, there are no data that this protection is mediated by complement-dependent membrane attack complex (MAC)-based lysis at a mechanistic level. If the vibriocidal antibody response is only a surrogate/correlate of protection against cholera, is there a related mechanistic antibody response that might actually mediate protection, especially long-term protection not afforded by IgM? Mucosal IgA and IgM antibodies may protect against pathogens at mucosal surfaces by inhibiting bacterial-epithelial cell interactions ("immune exclusion"), and/or via bacterial "clumping" either via agglutination at high bacterial concentrations ($\geq 10^8$ non-motile bacteria per gram), or "enchaining growth" (antibody-mediated cross-linking preventing bacterial separation after bacterial division) at lower bacterial concentrations, with facilitated mucosal clearance of clumped bacteria [55]. Recent data also suggest that inhibition of motility of *V. cholerae* in the intestinal lumen may contribute mechanistically to protection against cholera [25,26].

4.2. Memory B-Cells

Individuals with cholera are protected for a period well beyond when the serum vibriocidal antibody, circulating antigen-specific plasmablasts, and serum antibody to specific cholera antigens have disappeared or waned in the circulation, suggesting that longer-term protection may depend on anamnestic responses mediated by immunologic memory following primary infection. During primary infection, naïve B-cells traffic through secondary lymphoid tissues, where the B-cell receptor may recognize an antigen presented on an antigen-presenting cell, priming that B-cell to internalize, process, and present that antigen on MHC class II molecules. Primed B-cells interact with primed T follicular helper cells, a subset of CD4-positive T-cells that have been similarly primed from a naïve T-cell by interaction with the same specific antigen presented on an antigen-presenting cell. The interaction of the primed B and T follicular helper cells activate the B-cell to undergo further proliferation, somatic hypermutation, and isotype switching, and subsequently to differentiate into memory B-cells and long-lived plasma cells specific for that antigen, which mediate immunologic memory [56].

Both adults and children with cholera develop memory B-cells of the IgG and IgA isotypes specific to protein antigens, such as CTB and TcpA, which persist in the circulation out to at least one year following infection. Sialidase-specific IgA memory B-cells have also been demonstrated after cholera [36]. Similarly, memory B-cells also develop that recognize both LPS and the OSP of *V. cholerae* O1, which persist in the circulation out to at least 90–180 days following infection [15,32,33,47,57]. The mechanisms by which isotype-switched memory B-cells develop to the T-cell-independent antigens LPS and OSP are currently unknown.

Individuals receiving kOCVs develop memory B-cells to CTB and OSP, but at substantially lower levels than seen with natural infection and are shorter-lived [15,57,58]. These differences might contribute to the lower efficacy of protection rendered by these vaccines. The live-attenuated cholera vaccine, CVD 103-HgR (approved in the United States as a traveler's vaccine), has been shown in clinical trials in developed countries to induce vibriocidal responses that persist beyond two years in older children [59] and beyond one year in adults [60]. In addition, induction of memory B-cells to LPS and CTB has also been demonstrated in a US population [60,61]. However, oral vaccines (including CVD 103-HgR) induce lower immune responses and efficacy in resource-poor countries compared to developed countries [62]. More studies of live attenuated vaccines are needed in endemic countries as several host factors are suspected to impact responses in different geographic populations including nutritional status, intestinal epithelial barrier integrity, enteric enteropathy, concurrent infection, and diet [62–66].

Using a household contact study approach, OSP responses were found to correlate with protection in cholera endemic populations, including in young children [57]; and OSP and LPS responses were found to correlate with protection against cholera in an experimental infection model in humans [67,68]. However, no protection was mediated by the presence of circulating memory B-cells recognizing CTB [14,57]. There is currently inadequate data on the presence and persistence of antigen-specific memory B-cells or long-lived plasma cells in gastrointestinal mucosa and whether these might mediate more direct local protection from infection or disease.

5. Innate Immune Responses to Cholera

Microscopic characterization of intestinal mucosal tissue obtained by endoscopic biopsy shows that *V. cholerae* disrupts components of the epithelium and is associated with an influx of inflammatory cells, including neutrophils, lymphocytes and macrophages, into the lamina propria [69,70]. At a molecular level, early changes include the increased expression of a wide array of antibacterial effector proteins such as lactoferrin (LTF), lipocalin2 (LCN2) and Bactericidal/Permeability-increasing-fold-containing family B member 1 (BPIFB1; also known as LPLUNC1), as well as oxidases including nitric oxide synthase (NOS2) and dual oxidase 2 (DUOX2) [71–73]. *V. cholerae* infection also results in the upregulation of key cytokine signaling hubs. Several of these activated signaling pathways, such as the NLR family pyrin domain containing 3 (NLRP3) inflammasome and interferon regulatory factor 7 (IRF7)/type I interferon, are not typical of the innate immune response to pyogenic bacterial infections and are instead more typical of the response seen with viral infection [73].

The functional significance of the innate immune responses to *V. cholerae* infection is not fully understood. While the innate immune system does not entirely prevent infection—since most immunologically naïve individuals who ingest enough organisms will become infected—it nonetheless plays an essential role in directing the adaptive immune response. For example, the innate immune response to live pathogenic *V. cholerae* results in the expression of key cytokines such as IL-23 that promote B- and T-cell differentiation [74].

The innate immune system may also impact disease severity. For example, human biopsy-derived enteroids (an in vitro model for the intestinal epithelium) engineered to express the human blood group O-antigen are more susceptible to the effects of cholera toxin than enteroids expressing the A-type antigen [75]. This provides a molecular basis for the link between the blood group O phenotype and increased disease severity, and also may explain why the lowest prevalence of the O blood group phenotype in the world is observed the Bengal region of South Asia, where cholera is historically endemic [76]. Similarly, a genome-wide association study found that variations in both the type I interferon and NLRP3 inflammasome signaling pathways have been under strong selective pressure in Bangladesh, suggesting that these cholera-linked innate immune responses have played an important role in human survival historically in this region [77].

6. Interaction between Microbiota and Cholera Immunity

The composition of the gut microbiota may also impact susceptibility to *V. cholerae* infection, the clinical severity of disease, and subsequent immune responses. For the identification of microbial markers associated with susceptibility to infection, a recent study characterized the microbiota of close contacts of cholera patients in Bangladesh [78] by measuring the gut microbiota at the time of a shared exposure to the household case or common water source. The study assessed the microbial composition before and after exposure and found that the gut microbiota predicted susceptibility to infection at least as well as the clinical risk factors known to contribute to susceptibility, such as age, baseline vibriocidal titer, and blood group O-status.

Several taxonomic groups, such as *Enterobacteriaceae* and *Streptococcus*, were correlated with the stool of individuals who developed infection. At the same time, the genera *Prevotella, Bacteroides,* and *Lactobacillus* were more dominant among contacts who did not develop infection during the follow-up period. Using the same cohort of household contacts, a metagenomic study was conducted that identified specific gene groups that correlated with the development of infection [79]. For example, iron metabolism and regulation genes were more common in the gut microbiota of persons who did not develop infection after exposure. Like most bacteria, *V. cholerae* has several mechanisms of scavenging iron in the gut, and defects in iron metabolism have been shown to be critical to *V. cholerae* virulence in animal studies [80–82]. Bile acids are also metabolized by the gut microbiota and may impact susceptibility to *V. cholerae* infection. The bacterium *Blautia obeum* has been found to impact the ability of *V. cholerae* to colonize an animal host by degrading taurocholate, a conjugated bile acid [83]. *V. cholerae* senses taurocholate in the small intestinal environment and this triggers virulence factor expression; however, in the presence of *B. obeum*, this effect is reduced [83,84]. These studies demonstrate that commensal microbes in the human gut microbiota may potentially impact susceptibility to *V. cholerae* infection, through signaling molecules or other mechanisms. They may also impact responses to oral cholera vaccination. This remains an area of active study.

7. Mucosal-Associated Invariant T (MAIT) Cells

Mucosal-associated invariant T (MAIT) cells are innate-like T-cells defined by the expression of an invariant T-cell receptor (TCR) alpha chain, Vα7.2 (TRAV1-2) in humans, with a limited diversity of TCR beta chains [85–87]. The MAIT TCR recognizes microbial-derived metabolites of the riboflavin biosynthetic pathway presented on the MHC Class 1-related protein, MR1 [88]. MAIT cells make up approximately 1-10% of T-cells in healthy human blood, and are enriched in the liver, skin, lymph nodes and intestinal and respiratory mucosa [86,89–93]. MAIT cells are potent producers of pro-inflammatory cytokines and cytotoxic molecules and have been shown to provide protection against mucosal bacterial pathogens in murine challenge models [94–97]. Given their potential to participate in both innate and adaptive immunity, MAIT cells have been postulated to play key roles in mucosal infections. Observational studies have shown that MAIT cell frequency is reduced in the blood of humans with mucosal infections [98–101]. This finding, along with an increase in activation and gut homing markers [98,102,103] suggests that MAIT cells may traffic to the mucosa during infection. Despite their enrichment in the human gastrointestinal (GI) tract, knowledge about MAIT cells in the context of GI bacterial infections remains limited.

V. cholerae is capable of de novo riboflavin biosynthesis using the riboflavin biosynthetic pathway [104]), the intermediates of which can activate MAIT cells [105]. Flow cytometric analysis of MAIT cells in Bangladeshi adult and pediatric patients presenting with severe culture-confirmed cholera showed that at seven days post-cholera onset, peripheral blood MAIT cells had increased expression of activation markers, and MAIT frequency was significantly decreased in pediatric but not adult patients, suggesting potential trafficking to the mucosa [106]. In support, analysis of duodenal biopsies and peripheral blood MAIT cells from another cohort of adult Bangladeshi cholera patients revealed increases in duodenal lamina propria MAIT cell frequency and expression of gut homing markers in peripheral blood MAIT cells [107]. Changes in frequency of peripheral blood MAIT cells were also found to correlate with LPS IgA and IgG responses, suggesting that MAIT cells may be associated with class switching for T-cell-independent antigens [106]. Furthermore, in a murine model of *V. cholerae* intranasal vaccination in T-cell deficient mice, adoptive transfer of MAIT cells rescued *V. cholerae*-specific IgA responses and promoted B-cell differentiation [108]. Although these data highlight that MAIT cells, especially those in the duodenal mucosa, are activated in response to *V. cholerae* infection, further investigation into their function and phenotype is necessary to understand the role that MAIT cells play in cholera immunity.

8. Conclusions

Our understanding of cholera immunity has greatly increased over the last two decades. However, gaps remain in our understanding of the primary mechanisms of protective immunity to cholera, specifically whether antigen-specific memory B-cells or long-lived plasma cells are present and persist in gastrointestinal mucosa and the various physiologic mechanisms of an effective antibody-mediated response against cholera. In addition, further assessment of how the gut microbiome and innate immune response modulate the adaptive immune response to infection and vaccination will be important for a full understanding cholera immunity. These insights into the variation in immune responses between natural infection and vaccination will lead to improved vaccination strategies.

Author Contributions: All authors contributed to this summary of their investigative work on immune responses targeting *V. cholerae*, including performing the original investigative work, and in writing and editing this review. All authors have read and agreed to the published version of the manuscript.

Funding: This work was supported in part through programs funded by the National Institutes of Health, including the National Institute of Allergy and Infectious Diseases (AI106878 [ETR and FQ], AI130378 [DTL and TRB], AI135115 [DTL and FQ], and AI137164 [RCC, JBH]), the Fogarty International Center, Training Grant in Vaccine Development and Public Health (TW005572 [TRB, FQ], and the Emerging Global Fellowship Award TW010362 [TRB]. The work was also supported by icddr,b in part by core and unrestricted funds provided by the Government of Bangladesh, Canada, Sweden and the United Kingdom.

Conflicts of Interest: The authors declare no conflict of interest. The funders had no role in the interpretation of prior studies, the writing of the manuscript, or in the decision of which manuscripts to include in this review.

References

1. Ali, M.; Nelson, A.R.; Lopez, A.L.; Sack, D.A. Updated global burden of cholera in endemic countries. *PLoS Negl. Trop. Dis.* **2015**, *9*, e0003832. [CrossRef]
2. World Health Organization. Cholera vaccines: WHO position paper—August 2017. *Wkly. Epidemiol. Rec.* **2017**, *92*, 477–498.
3. Bi, Q.; Ferreras, E.; Pezzoli, L.; Legros, D.; Ivers, L.C.; Date, K.; Qadri, F.; Digilio, L.; Sack, D.A.; Ali, M.; et al. Protection against cholera from killed whole-cell oral cholera vaccines: A systematic review and meta-analysis. *Lancet Infect. Dis.* **2017**, *17*, 1080–1088. [CrossRef]

4. Koelle, K.; Rodo, X.; Pascual, M.; Yunus, M.; Mostafa, G. Refractory periods and climate forcing in cholera dynamics. *Nature* **2005**, *436*, 696–700. [CrossRef]
5. Albert, M.J.; Alam, K.; Rahman, A.S.; Huda, S.; Sack, R.B. Lack of cross-protection against diarrhea due to Vibrio cholerae O1 after oral immunization of rabbits with V. cholerae O139 Bengal. *J. Infect. Dis.* **1994**, *169*, 709–710. [CrossRef] [PubMed]
6. Waldor, M.K.; Colwell, R.; Mekalanos, J.J. The Vibrio cholerae O139 serogroup antigen includes an O-antigen capsule and lipopolysaccharide virulence determinants. *Proc. Natl. Acad. Sci. USA* **1994**, *91*, 11388–11392. [CrossRef]
7. Qadri, F.; Wenneras, C.; Albert, M.J.; Hossain, J.; Mannoor, K.; Begum, Y.A.; Mohi, G.; Salam, M.A.; Sack, R.B.; Svennerholm, A.M. Comparison of immune responses in patients infected with Vibrio cholerae O139 and O1. *Infect. Immun.* **1997**, *65*, 3571–3576. [CrossRef]
8. Losonsky, G.A.; Yunyongying, J.; Lim, V.; Reymann, M.; Lim, Y.L.; Wasserman, S.S.; Levine, M.M. Factors influencing secondary vibriocidal immune responses: Relevance for understanding immunity to cholera. *Infect. Immun.* **1996**, *64*, 10–15. [CrossRef]
9. Johnson, R.A.; Uddin, T.; Aktar, A.; Mohasin, M.; Alam, M.M.; Chowdhury, F.; Harris, J.B.; LaRocque, R.C.; Bufano, M.K.; Yu, Y.; et al. Comparison of immune responses to the O-specific polysaccharide and lipopolysaccharide of Vibrio cholerae O1 in Bangladeshi adult patients with cholera. *Clin. Vaccine Immunol.* **2012**, *19*, 1712–1721. [CrossRef]
10. Rahman, A.; Rashu, R.; Bhuiyan, T.R.; Chowdhury, F.; Khan, A.I.; Islam, K.; LaRocque, R.C.; Ryan, E.T.; Wrammert, J.; Calderwood, S.B.; et al. Antibody-secreting cell responses after Vibrio cholerae O1 infection and oral cholera vaccination in adults in Bangladesh. *Clin. Vaccine Immunol. CVI* **2013**, *20*, 1592–1598. [CrossRef]
11. Kauffman, R.C.; Bhuiyan, T.R.; Nakajima, R.; Mayo-Smith, L.M.; Rashu, R.; Hoq, M.R.; Chowdhury, F.; Khan, A.I.; Rahman, A.; Bhaumik, S.K.; et al. Single-cell analysis of the plasmablast response to Vibrio cholerae demonstrates expansion of cross-reactive memory B cells. *mBio* **2016**, *7*, e02021-16. [CrossRef] [PubMed]
12. Harris, J.B.; Larocque, R.C.; Chowdhury, F.; Khan, A.I.; Logvinenko, T.; Faruque, A.S.; Ryan, E.T.; Qadri, F.; Calderwood, S.B. Susceptibility to Vibrio cholerae infection in a cohort of household contacts of patients with cholera in Bangladesh. *PLoS Negl. Trop. Dis.* **2008**, *2*, e221. [CrossRef] [PubMed]
13. Leung, D.T.; Rahman, M.A.; Mohasin, M.; Riyadh, M.A.; Patel, S.M.; Alam, M.M.; Chowdhury, F.; Khan, A.I.; Kalivoda, E.J.; Aktar, A.; et al. Comparison of memory B cell, antibody-secreting cell, and plasma antibody responses in young children, older children, and adults with infection caused by Vibrio cholerae O1 El Tor Ogawa in Bangladesh. *Clin. Vaccine Immunol. CVI* **2011**, *18*, 1317–1325. [CrossRef] [PubMed]
14. Patel, S.M.; Rahman, M.A.; Mohasin, M.; Riyadh, M.A.; Leung, D.T.; Alam, M.M.; Chowdhury, F.; Khan, A.I.; Weil, A.A.; Aktar, A.; et al. Memory B cell responses to Vibrio cholerae O1 lipopolysaccharide are associated with protection against infection from household contacts of patients with cholera in Bangladesh. *Clin. Vaccine Immunol. CVI* **2012**, *19*, 842–848. [CrossRef]
15. Leung, D.T.; Rahman, M.A.; Mohasin, M.; Patel, S.M.; Aktar, A.; Khanam, F.; Uddin, T.; Riyadh, M.A.; Saha, A.; Alam, M.M.; et al. Memory B cell and other immune responses in children receiving two doses of an oral killed cholera vaccine compared to responses following natural cholera infection in Bangladesh. *Clin. Vaccine Immunol. CVI* **2012**, *19*, 690–698. [CrossRef] [PubMed]
16. Leung, D.T.; Uddin, T.; Xu, P.; Aktar, A.; Johnson, R.A.; Rahman, M.A.; Alam, M.M.; Bufano, M.K.; Eckhoff, G.; Wu-Freeman, Y.; et al. Immune responses to the O-specific polysaccharide antigen in children who received a killed oral cholera vaccine compared to responses following natural cholera infection in Bangladesh. *Clin. Vaccine Immunol. CVI* **2013**, *20*, 780–788. [CrossRef]
17. Charles, R.C.; Nakajima, R.; Liang, L.; Jasinskas, A.; Berger, A.; Leung, D.T.; Kelly, M.; Xu, P.; Kovac, P.; Giffen, S.R.; et al. The plasma and mucosal IgM, IgA, and IgG responses to the Vibrio cholerae O1 protein immunome in adults with cholera in Bangladesh. *J. Infect. Dis.* **2017**, *216*, 125–134. [CrossRef] [PubMed]
18. Uddin, T.; Aktar, A.; Xu, P.; Johnson, R.A.; Rahman, M.A.; Leung, D.T.; Afrin, S.; Akter, A.; Alam, M.M.; Rahman, A.; et al. Immune responses to O-specific polysaccharide and lipopolysaccharide of Vibrio cholerae O1 Ogawa in adult Bangladeshi recipients of an oral killed cholera vaccine and comparison to responses in patients with cholera. *Am. J. Trop. Med. Hyg.* **2014**, *90*, 873–881. [CrossRef] [PubMed]
19. Aktar, A.; Rahman, M.A.; Afrin, S.; Faruk, M.O.; Uddin, T.; Akter, A.; Sami, M.I.; Yasmin, T.; Chowdhury, F.; Khan, A.I.; et al. O-specific polysaccharide-specific memory B cell responses in young children, older children, and adults infected with *Vibrio cholerae* O1 Ogawa in Bangladesh. *Clin. Vaccine Immunol. CVI* **2016**, *23*, 427–435. [CrossRef] [PubMed]
20. Alam, M.M.; Leung, D.T.; Akhtar, M.; Nazim, M.; Akter, S.; Uddin, T.; Khanam, F.; Mahbuba, D.A.; Ahmad, S.M.; Bhuiyan, T.R.; et al. Antibody avidity in humoral immune responses in Bangladeshi children and adults following administration of an oral killed cholera vaccine. *Clin. Vaccine Immunol. CVI* **2013**, *20*, 1541–1548. [CrossRef] [PubMed]
21. Wang, Z.; Lazinski, D.W.; Camilli, A. Immunity provided by an outer membrane vesicle cholera vaccine is due to O-antigen-specific antibodies inhibiting bacterial motility. *Infect. Immun.* **2016**, *85*, e00626-16. [CrossRef]
22. Bishop, A.L.; Schild, S.; Patimalla, B.; Klein, B.; Camilli, A. Mucosal immunization with *Vibrio cholerae* outer membrane vesicles provides maternal protection mediated by antilipopolysaccharide antibodies that inhibit bacterial motility. *Infect. Immun.* **2010**, *78*, 4402–4420. [CrossRef]
23. Levinson, K.J.; De Jesus, M.; Mantis, N.J. Rapid effects of a protective O-polysaccharide-specific monoclonal IgA on *Vibrio cholerae* agglutination, motility, and surface morphology. *Infect. Immun.* **2015**, *83*, 1674–1683. [CrossRef]

24. Levinson, K.J.; Baranova, D.E.; Mantis, N.J. A monoclonal antibody that targets the conserved core/lipid A region of lipopolysaccharide affects motility and reduces intestinal colonization of both classical and El Tor *Vibrio cholerae* biotypes. *Vaccine* **2016**, *34*, 5833–5836. [CrossRef]
25. Charles, R.C.; Kelly, M.; Tam, J.M.; Akter, A.; Hossain, M.; Islam, K.; Biswas, R.; Kamruzzaman, M.; Chowdhury, F.; Khan, A.I.; et al. Humans surviving cholera develop antibodies against *Vibrio cholerae* O-specific polysaccharide that inhibit pathogen motility. *mBio* **2020**, *11*, e02847-20. [CrossRef]
26. Kauffman, R.C.; Adekunle, O.; Yu, H.; Cho, A.; Nyhoff, L.E.; Kelly, M.; Harris, J.B.; Bhuiyan, T.R.; Qadri, F.; Calderwood, S.B.; et al. Impact of immunoglobulin isotype and epitope on the functional properties of *Vibrio cholerae* O-specific polysaccharide-specific monoclonal antibodies. *mBio* **2021**, *12*, e03679-20. [CrossRef]
27. Gill, D.M. The arrangement of subunits in cholera toxin. *Biochemistry* **1976**, *15*, 1242–1248. [CrossRef]
28. Herrington, D.A.; Hall, R.H.; Losonsky, G.; Mekalanos, J.J.; Taylor, R.K.; Levine, M.M. Toxin, toxin-coregulated pili, and the toxR regulon are essential for *Vibrio cholerae* pathogenesis in humans. *J. Exp. Med.* **1988**, *168*, 1487–1492. [CrossRef]
29. Debellis, L.; Diana, A.; Arcidiacono, D.; Fiorotto, R.; Portincasa, P.; Altomare, D.F.; Spirli, C.; de Bernard, M. The Vibrio cholerae cytolysin promotes chloride secretion from intact human intestinal mucosa. *PLoS ONE* **2009**, *4*, e5074. [CrossRef]
30. Saka, H.A.; Bidinost, C.; Sola, C.; Carranza, P.; Collino, C.; Ortiz, S.; Echenique, J.R.; Bocco, J.L. Vibrio cholerae cytolysin is essential for high enterotoxicity and apoptosis induction produced by a cholera toxin gene-negative V. cholerae non-O1, non-O139 strain. *Microb. Pathog.* **2008**, *44*, 118–128. [CrossRef]
31. Weil, A.A.; Arifuzzaman, M.; Bhuiyan, T.R.; Larocque, R.C.; Harris, A.M.; Kendall, E.A.; Hossain, A.; Tarique, A.A.; Sheikh, A.; Chowdhury, F.; et al. Memory T cell responses to Vibrio cholerae O1 infection. *Infect. Immun.* **2009**, *77*, 5090–5096. [CrossRef]
32. Jayasekera, C.R.; Harris, J.B.; Bhuiyan, S.; Chowdhury, F.; Khan, A.I.; Faruque, A.S.; Larocque, R.C.; Ryan, E.T.; Ahmed, R.; Qadri, F.; et al. Cholera toxin-specific memory B cell responses are induced in patients with dehydrating diarrhea caused by Vibrio cholerae O1. *J. Infect. Dis.* **2008**, *198*, 1055–1061. [CrossRef]
33. Harris, A.M.; Bhuiyan, M.S.; Chowdhury, F.; Khan, A.I.; Hossain, A.; Kendall, E.A.; Rahman, A.; LaRocque, R.C. Wrammert, J.; Ryan, E.T.; et al. Antigen-specific memory B-cell responses to Vibrio cholerae O1 infection in Bangladesh. *Infect. Immun.* **2009**, *77*, 3850–3856. [CrossRef]
34. Uddin, T.; Harris, J.B.; Bhuiyan, T.R.; Shirin, T.; Uddin, M.I.; Khan, A.I.; Chowdhury, F.; Larocque, R.C.; Alam, N.H.; Ryan, E.T.; et al. Mucosal immunologic responses in cholera patients in Bangladesh. *Clin. Vaccine Immunol. CVI* **2011**, *18*, 506–512. [CrossRef]
35. Qadri, F.; Ryan, E.T.; Faruque, A.S.; Ahmed, F.; Khan, A.I.; Islam, M.M.; Akramuzzaman, S.M.; Sack, D.A.; Calderwood, S.B. Antigen-specific immunoglobulin A antibodies secreted from circulating B cells are an effective marker for recent local immune responses in patients with cholera: Comparison to antibody-secreting cell responses and other immunological markers. *Infect. Immun.* **2003**, *71*, 4808–4814. [CrossRef]
36. Kaisar, M.H.; Bhuiyan, M.S.; Akter, A.; Saleem, D.; Iyer, A.S.; Dash, P.; Hakim, A.; Chowdhury, F.; Khan, A.I.; Calderwood, S.B.; et al. Vibrio cholerae sialidase-specific immune responses are associated with protection against cholera. *mSphere* **2021**, *6*, e01232-20. [CrossRef]
37. Galen, J.E.; Ketley, J.M.; Fasano, A.; Richardson, S.H.; Wasserman, S.S.; Kaper, J.B. Role of Vibrio cholerae neuraminidase in the function of cholera toxin. *Infect. Immun.* **1992**, *60*, 406–415. [CrossRef]
38. Halstensen, T.S.; Hvatum, M.; Scott, H.; Fausa, O.; Brandtzaeg, P. Association of subepithelial deposition of activated complement and immunoglobulin G and M response to gluten in celiac disease. *Gastroenterology* **1992**, *102*, 751–759. [CrossRef]
39. Halstensen, T.S.; Mollnes, T.E.; Garred, P.; Fausa, O.; Brandtzaeg, P. Epithelial deposition of immunoglobulin G1 and activated complement (C3b and terminal complement complex) in ulcerative colitis. *Gastroenterology* **1990**, *98*, 1264–1271. [CrossRef]
40. Halstensen, T.S.; Mollnes, T.E.; Fausa, O.; Brandtzaeg, P. Deposits of terminal complement complex (TCC) in muscularis mucosae and submucosal vessels in ulcerative colitis and Crohn's disease of the colon. *Gut* **1989**, *30*, 361–366. [CrossRef]
41. Griffiss, J.M.; Goroff, D.K. IgA blocks IgM and IgG-initiated immune lysis by separate molecular mechanisms. *J. Immunol.* **1983**, *130*, 2882–2885. [PubMed]
42. Hiemstra, P.S.; Biewenga, J.; Gorter, A.; Stuurman, M.E.; Faber, A.; van Es, L.A.; Daha, M.R. Activation of complement by human serum IgA, secretory IgA and IgA1 fragments. *Mol. Immunol.* **1988**, *25*, 527–533. [CrossRef]
43. Woof, J.M.; Russell, M.W. Structure and function relationships in IgA. *Mucosal Immunol.* **2011**, *4*, 590–597. [CrossRef]
44. Saha, D.; LaRocque, R.C.; Khan, A.I.; Harris, J.B.; Begum, Y.A.; Akramuzzaman, S.M.; Faruque, A.S.; Ryan, E.T.; Qadri, F.; Calderwood, S.B. Incomplete correlation of serum vibriocidal antibody titer with protection from Vibrio cholerae infection in urban Bangladesh. *J. Infect. Dis.* **2004**, *189*, 2318–2322. [CrossRef] [PubMed]
45. Qadri, F.; Mohi, G.; Hossain, J.; Azim, T.; Khan, A.M.; Salam, M.A.; Sack, R.B.; Albert, M.J.; Svennerholm, A.M. Comparison of the vibriocidal antibody response in cholera due to *Vibrio cholerae* O139 Bengal with the response in cholera due to *Vibrio cholerae* O1. *Clin. Diagn. Lab. Immunol.* **1995**, *2*, 685–688. [CrossRef]
46. Glass, R.I.; Svennerholm, A.M.; Khan, M.R.; Huda, S.; Huq, M.I.; Holmgren, J. Seroepidemiological studies of El Tor cholera in Bangladesh: Association of serum antibody levels with protection. *J. Infect. Dis.* **1985**, *151*, 236–242. [CrossRef]
47. Azman, A.S.; Lessler, J.; Luquero, F.J.; Bhuiyan, T.R.; Khan, A.I.; Chowdhury, F.; Kabir, A.; Gurwith, M.; Weil, A.A.; Harris, J.B.; et al. Estimating cholera incidence with cross-sectional serology. *Sci. Transl. Med.* **2019**, *11*, 6242. [CrossRef]

48. Richie, E.E.; Punjabi, N.H.; Sidharta, Y.Y.; Peetosutan, K.K.; Sukandar, M.M.; Wasserman, S.S.; Lesmana, M.M.; Wangsasaputra, F.F.; Pandam, S.S.; Levine, M.M.; et al. Efficacy trial of single-dose live oral cholera vaccine CVD 103-HgR in North Jakarta, Indonesia, a cholera-endemic area. *Vaccine* **2000**, *18*, 2399–2410. [CrossRef]
49. Ali, M.; Emch, M.; Park, J.K.; Yunus, M.; Clemens, J. Natural cholera infection-derived immunity in an endemic setting. *J. Infect. Dis.* **2011**, *204*, 912–918. [CrossRef]
50. Levine, M.M.; Black, R.E.; Clements, M.L.; Cisneros, L.; Nalin, D.R.; Young, C.R. Duration of infection-derived immunity to cholera. *J. Infect. Dis.* **1981**, *143*, 818–820. [CrossRef]
51. Clements, M.L.; Levine, M.M.; Young, C.R.; Black, R.E.; Lim, Y.L.; Robins-Browne, R.M.; Craig, J.P. Magnitude, kinetics, and duration of vibriocidal antibody responses in North Americans after ingestion of Vibrio cholerae. *J. Infect. Dis.* **1982**, *145*, 465–473. [CrossRef]
52. Tacket, C.O.; Losonsky, G.; Nataro, J.P.; Cryz, S.J.; Edelman, R.; Kaper, J.B.; Levine, M.M. Onset and duration of protective immunity in challenged volunteers after vaccination with live oral cholera vaccine CVD 103-HgR. *J. Infect. Dis.* **1992**, *166*, 837–841. [CrossRef]
53. Clemens, J.D.; van Loon, F.; Sack, D.A.; Chakraborty, J.; Rao, M.R.; Ahmed, F.; Harris, J.R.; Khan, M.R.; Yunus, M.; Huda, S. Field trial of oral cholera vaccines in Bangladesh: Serum vibriocidal and antitoxic antibodies as markers of the risk of cholera. *J. Infect. Dis.* **1991**, *163*, 1235–1242. [CrossRef]
54. Hossain, M.; Islam, K.; Kelly, M.; Mayo Smith, L.M.; Charles, R.C.; Weil, A.A.; Bhuiyan, T.R.; Kovac, P.; Xu, P.; Calderwood, S.B.; et al. Immune responses to O-specific polysaccharide (OSP) in North American adults infected with Vibrio cholerae O1 Inaba. *PLoS Negl. Trop. Dis.* **2019**, *13*, e0007874. [CrossRef] [PubMed]
55. Moor, K.; Diard, M.; Sellin, M.E.; Felmy, B.; Wotzka, S.Y.; Toska, A.; Bakkeren, E.; Arnoldini, M.; Bansept, F.; Co, A.D.; et al. High-avidity IgA protects the intestine by enchaining growing bacteria. *Nature* **2017**, *544*, 498–502. [CrossRef]
56. Akkaya, M.; Kwak, K.; Pierce, S.K. B cell memory: Building two walls of protection against pathogens. *Nat. Rev. Immunol.* **2020**, *20*, 229–238. [CrossRef] [PubMed]
57. Aktar, A.; Rahman, M.A.; Afrin, S.; Akter, A.; Uddin, T.; Yasmin, T.; Sami, M.I.N.; Dash, P.; Jahan, S.R.; Chowdhury, F.; et al. Plasma and memory B cell responses targeting O-specific polysaccharide (OSP) are associated with protection against Vibrio cholerae O1 infection among household contacts of cholera patients in Bangladesh. *PLoS Negl. Trop. Dis.* **2018**, *12*, e0006399. [CrossRef]
58. Alam, M.M.; Riyadh, M.A.; Fatema, K.; Rahman, M.A.; Akhtar, N.; Ahmed, T.; Chowdhury, M.I.; Chowdhury, F.; Calderwood, S.B.; Harris, J.B.; et al. Antigen-specific memory B-cell responses in bangladeshi adults after one- or two-dose oral killed cholera vaccination and comparison with responses in patients with naturally acquired cholera. *Clin. Vaccine Immunol. CVI* **2011**, *18*, 844–850. [CrossRef]
59. McCarty, J.M.; Cassie, D.; Bedell, L.; Lock, M.D.; Bennett, S. Long-term immunogenicity of live oral cholera vaccine CVD 103-HgR in adolescents aged 12–17 years in the United States. *Am. J. Trop. Med. Hyg.* **2021**, *104*, 1758–1760. [CrossRef]
60. Adekunle, O.; Dretler, A.; Kauffman, R.C.; Cho, A.; Rouphael, N.; Wrammert, J. Longitudinal analysis of human humoral responses after vaccination with a live attenuated *V. cholerae* vaccine. *PLoS Negl. Trop. Dis.* **2021**, *15*, e0009743. [CrossRef] [PubMed]
61. Haney, D.J.; Lock, M.D.; Gurwith, M.; Simon, J.K.; Ishioka, G.; Cohen, M.B.; Kirkpatrick, B.D.; Lyon, C.E.; Chen, W.H.; Sztein, M.B.; et al. Lipopolysaccharide-specific memory B cell responses to an attenuated live cholera vaccine are associated with protection against *Vibrio cholerae* infection. *Vaccine* **2018**, *36*, 2768–2773. [CrossRef] [PubMed]
62. Levine, M.M. Immunogenicity and efficacy of oral vaccines in developing countries: Lessons from a live cholera vaccine. *BMC Biol.* **2010**, *8*, 129. [CrossRef] [PubMed]
63. Zimmermann, P.; Curtis, N. Factors that influence the immune response to vaccination. *Clin. Microbiol. Rev.* **2019**, *32*, e00084–18. [CrossRef]
64. Uddin, M.I.; Islam, S.; Nishat, N.S.; Hossain, M.; Rafique, T.A.; Rashu, R.; Hoq, M.R.; Zhang, Y.; Saha, A.; Harris, J.B.; et al. Biomarkers of environmental enteropathy are positively associated with immune responses to an oral cholera vaccine in Bangladeshi children. *PLoS Negl. Trop. Dis.* **2016**, *10*, e0005039. [CrossRef]
65. Savy, M.; Edmond, K.; Fine, P.E.; Hall, A.; Hennig, B.J.; Moore, S.E.; Mulholland, K.; Schaible, U.; Prentice, A.M. Landscape analysis of interactions between nutrition and vaccine responses in children. *J. Nutr.* **2009**, *139*, 2154S–2218S. [CrossRef]
66. Weil, A.A.; Becker, R.L.; Harris, J.B. Vibrio cholerae at the intersection of immunity and the microbiome. *mSphere* **2019**, *4*, e00597–19. [CrossRef] [PubMed]
67. Islam, K.; Hossain, M.; Kelly, M.; Mayo Smith, L.M.; Charles, R.C.; Bhuiyan, T.R.; Kovac, P.; Xu, P.; LaRocque, R.C.; Calderwood, S.B.; et al. Anti-O-specific polysaccharide (OSP) immune responses following vaccination with oral cholera vaccine CVD 103-HgR correlate with protection against cholera after infection with wild-type *Vibrio cholerae* O1 El Tor Inaba in North American volunteers. *PLoS Negl. Trop. Dis.* **2018**, *12*, e0006376. [CrossRef]
68. Haney, D.J.; Lock, M.D.; Simon, J.K.; Harris, J.; Gurwith, M. Antibody-based correlates of protection against cholera analysis of a challenge study in a cholera-naive population. *Clin. Vaccine Immunol. CVI* **2017**, *24*, e00098-17. [CrossRef]
69. Mathan, M.M.; Chandy, G.; Mathan, V.I. Ultrastructural changes in the upper small intestinal mucosa in patients with cholera. *Gastroenterology* **1995**, *109*, 422–430. [CrossRef]

70. Qadri, F.; Raqib, R.; Ahmed, F.; Rahman, T.; Wenneras, C.; Das, S.K.; Alam, N.H.; Mathan, M.M.; Svennerholm, A.M. Increased levels of inflammatory mediators in children and adults infected with Vibrio cholerae O1 and O139. *Clin. Diagn. Lab. Immunol.* **2002**, *9*, 221–229. [CrossRef]
71. Flach, C.F.; Qadri, F.; Bhuiyan, T.R.; Alam, N.H.; Jennische, E.; Lonnroth, I.; Holmgren, J. Broad up-regulation of innate defense factors during acute cholera. *Infect. Immun.* **2007**, *75*, 2343–2350. [CrossRef]
72. Ellis, C.N.; LaRocque, R.C.; Uddin, T.; Krastins, B.; Mayo-Smith, L.M.; Sarracino, D.; Karlsson, E.K.; Rahman, A.; Shirin, T.; Bhuiyan, T.R.; et al. Comparative proteomic analysis reveals activation of mucosal innate immune signaling pathways during cholera. *Infect. Immun.* **2015**, *83*, 1089–1103. [CrossRef]
73. Bourque, D.L.; Bhuiyan, T.R.; Genereux, D.P.; Rashu, R.; Ellis, C.N.; Chowdhury, F.; Khan, A.I.; Alam, N.H.; Paul, A.; Hossain, L.; et al. Analysis of the Human Mucosal Response to Cholera Reveals Sustained Activation of Innate Immune Signaling Pathways. *Infect. Immun.* **2018**, *86*, e00594-17. [CrossRef] [PubMed]
74. Weil, A.A.; Ellis, C.N.; Debela, M.D.; Bhuiyan, T.R.; Rashu, R.; Bourque, D.L.; Khan, A.I.; Chowdhury, F.; LaRocque, R.C.; Charles, R.C.; et al. Posttranslational Regulation of IL-23 Production Distinguishes the Innate Immune Responses to Live Toxigenic versus Heat-Inactivated Vibrio cholerae. *mSphere* **2019**, *4*, e00206-19. [CrossRef] [PubMed]
75. Kuhlmann, F.M.; Santhanam, S.; Kumar, P.; Luo, Q.; Ciorba, M.A.; Fleckenstein, J.M. Blood Group O-Dependent Cellular Responses to Cholera Toxin: Parallel Clinical and Epidemiological Links to Severe Cholera. *Am. J. Trop. Med. Hyg.* **2016**, *95*, 440–443. [CrossRef]
76. Harris, J.B.; LaRocque, R.C. Cholera and ABO Blood Group: Understanding an Ancient Association. *Am. J. Trop. Med. Hyg.* **2016**, *95*, 263–264. [CrossRef]
77. Karlsson, E.K.; Harris, J.B.; Tabrizi, S.; Rahman, A.; Shlyakhter, I.; Patterson, N.; O'Dushlaine, C.; Schaffner, S.F.; Gupta, S.; Chowdhury, F.; et al. Natural selection in a bangladeshi population from the cholera-endemic ganges river delta. *Sci. Transl. Med.* **2013**, *5*, 192ra186. [CrossRef]
78. Midani, F.S.; Weil, A.A.; Chowdhury, F.; Begum, Y.A.; Khan, A.I.; Debela, M.D.; Durand, H.K.; Reese, A.T.; Nimmagadda, S.N.; Silverman, J.D.; et al. Human gut microbiota predicts susceptibility to Vibrio cholerae infection. *J. Infect. Dis.* **2018**, *218*, 645–653. [CrossRef] [PubMed]
79. Levade, I.; Saber, M.M.; Midani, F.S.; Chowdhury, F.; Khan, A.I.; Begum, Y.A.; Ryan, E.T.; David, L.A.; Calderwood, S.B.; Harris, J.B.; et al. Predicting Vibrio cholerae infection and disease severity using metagenomics in a prospective cohort study. *J. Infect. Dis.* **2021**, *223*, 342–351. [CrossRef]
80. Payne, S.M.; Mey, A.R.; Wyckoff, E.E. Vibrio iron transport: Evolutionary adaptation to life in multiple environments. *Microbiol. Mol. Biol. Rev.* **2016**, *80*, 69–90. [CrossRef]
81. Mey, A.R.; Wyckoff, E.E.; Kanukurthy, V.; Fisher, C.R.; Payne, S.M. Iron and *fur* regulation in Vibrio cholerae and the role of *fur* in virulence. *Infect. Immun.* **2005**, *73*, 8167–8178. [CrossRef] [PubMed]
82. Wyckoff, E.E.; Mey, A.R.; Payne, S.M. Iron acquisition in Vibrio cholerae. *Biometals* **2007**, *20*, 405–416. [CrossRef]
83. Alavi, S.; Mitchell, J.D.; Cho, J.Y.; Liu, R.; Macbeth, J.C.; Hsiao, A. Interpersonal gut microbiome variation drives susceptibility and resistance to cholera infection. *Cell* **2020**, *181*, 1533–1546.e3. [CrossRef]
84. Yang, M.; Liu, Z.; Hughes, C.; Stern, A.M.; Wang, H.; Zhong, Z.; Kan, B.; Fenical, W.; Zhu, J. Bile salt-induced intermolecular disulfide bond formation activates Vibrio cholerae virulence. *Proc. Natl. Acad. Sci. USA* **2013**, *110*, 2348–2353. [CrossRef]
85. Tilloy, F.; Treiner, E.; Park, S.H.; Garcia, C.; Lemonnier, F.; de la Salle, H.; Bendelac, A.; Bonneville, M.; Lantz, O. An invariant T cell receptor alpha chain defines a novel TAP-independent major histocompatibility complex class Ib-restricted alpha/beta T cell subpopulation in mammals. *J. Exp. Med.* **1999**, *189*, 1907–1921. [CrossRef]
86. Reantragoon, R.; Corbett, A.J.; Sakala, I.G.; Gherardin, N.A.; Furness, J.B.; Chen, Z.; Eckle, S.B.; Uldrich, A.P.; Birkinshaw, R.W.; Patel, O.; et al. Antigen-loaded MR1 tetramers define T cell receptor heterogeneity in mucosal-associated invariant T cells. *J. Exp. Med.* **2013**, *210*, 2305–2320. [CrossRef]
87. Lepore, M.; Kalinichenko, A.; Colone, A.; Paleja, B.; Singhal, A.; Tschumi, A.; Lee, B.; Poidinger, M.; Zolezzi, F.; Quagliata, L.; et al. Parallel T-cell cloning and deep sequencing of human MAIT cells reveal stable oligoclonal TCRbeta repertoire. *Nat. Commun.* **2014**, *5*, 3866. [CrossRef]
88. Kjer-Nielsen, L.; Patel, O.; Corbett, A.J.; Le Nours, J.; Meehan, B.; Liu, L.; Bhati, M.; Chen, Z.; Kostenko, L.; Reantragoon, R.; et al. MR1 presents microbial vitamin B metabolites to MAIT cells. *Nature* **2012**, *491*, 717–723. [CrossRef] [PubMed]
89. Dusseaux, M.; Martin, E.; Serriari, N.; Peguillet, I.; Premel, V.; Louis, D.; Milder, M.; Le Bourhis, L.; Soudais, C.; Treiner, E.; et al. Human MAIT cells are xenobiotic-resistant, tissue-targeted, CD161hi IL-17-secreting T cells. *Blood* **2011**, *117*, 1250–1259. [CrossRef] [PubMed]
90. Sobkowiak, M.J.; Davanian, H.; Heymann, R.; Gibbs, A.; Emgard, J.; Dias, J.; Aleman, S.; Kruger-Weiner, C.; Moll, M.; Tjernlund, A.; et al. Tissue-resident MAIT cell populations in human oral mucosa exhibit an activated profile and produce IL-17. *Eur. J. Immunol.* **2019**, *49*, 133–143. [CrossRef]
91. Booth, J.S.; Salerno-Goncalves, R.; Blanchard, T.G.; Patil, S.A.; Kader, H.A.; Safta, A.M.; Morningstar, L.M.; Czinn, S.J.; Greenwald, B.D.; Sztein, M.B. Mucosal-Associated Invariant T Cells in the Human Gastric Mucosa and Blood: Role in Helicobacter pylori Infection. *Front. Immunol.* **2015**, *6*, 466. [CrossRef] [PubMed]

92. Gibbs, A.; Leeansyah, E.; Introini, A.; Paquin-Proulx, D.; Hasselrot, K.; Andersson, E.; Broliden, K.; Sandberg, J.K.; Tjernlund, A. MAIT cells reside in the female genital mucosa and are biased towards IL-17 and IL-22 production in response to bacterial stimulation. *Mucosal. Immunol.* **2017**, *10*, 35–45. [CrossRef]
93. Li, J.; Reantragoon, R.; Kostenko, L.; Corbett, A.J.; Varigos, G.; Carbone, F.R. The frequency of mucosal-associated invariant T cells is selectively increased in dermatitis herpetiformis. *Australas. J. Derm.* **2017**, *58*, 200–204. [CrossRef]
94. Meierovics, A.; Yankelevich, W.J.; Cowley, S.C. MAIT cells are critical for optimal mucosal immune responses during in vivo pulmonary bacterial infection. *Proc. Natl. Acad. Sci. USA* **2013**, *110*, E3119–E3128. [CrossRef] [PubMed]
95. Georgel, P.; Radosavljevic, M.; Macquin, C.; Bahram, S. The non-conventional MHC class I MR1 molecule controls infection by Klebsiella pneumoniae in mice. *Mol. Immunol.* **2011**, *48*, 769–775. [CrossRef] [PubMed]
96. Chen, Z.; Wang, H.; D'Souza, C.; Sun, S.; Kostenko, L.; Eckle, S.B.; Meehan, B.S.; Jackson, D.C.; Strugnell, R.A.; Cao, H.; et al. Mucosal-associated invariant T-cell activation and accumulation after in vivo infection depends on microbial riboflavin synthesis and co-stimulatory signals. *Mucosal. Immunol.* **2017**, *10*, 58–68. [CrossRef]
97. Wang, H.; D'Souza, C.; Lim, X.Y.; Kostenko, L.; Pediongco, T.J.; Eckle, S.B.G.; Meehan, B.S.; Shi, M.; Wang, N.; Li, S.; et al. MAIT cells protect against pulmonary Legionella longbeachae infection. *Nat. Commun.* **2018**, *9*, 3350. [CrossRef]
98. Salerno-Goncalves, R.; Luo, D.; Fresnay, S.; Magder, L.; Darton, T.C.; Jones, C.; Waddington, C.S.; Blohmke, C.J.; Angus, B.; Levine, M.M.; et al. Challenge of Humans with Wild-type Salmonella enterica Serovar Typhi Elicits Changes in the Activation and Homing Characteristics of Mucosal-Associated Invariant T Cells. *Front. Immunol.* **2017**, *8*, 398. [CrossRef] [PubMed]
99. Kwon, Y.S.; Cho, Y.N.; Kim, M.J.; Jin, H.M.; Jung, H.J.; Kang, J.H.; Park, K.J.; Kim, T.J.; Kee, H.J.; Kim, N.; et al. Mucosal-associated invariant T cells are numerically and functionally deficient in patients with mycobacterial infection and reflect disease activity. *Tuberculosis* **2015**, *95*, 267–274. [CrossRef] [PubMed]
100. Lu, B.; Liu, M.; Wang, J.; Fan, H.; Yang, D.; Zhang, L.; Gu, X.; Nie, J.; Chen, Z.; Corbett, A.J.; et al. IL-17 production by tissue-resident MAIT cells is locally induced in children with pneumonia. *Mucosal. Immunol.* **2020**, *13*, 824–835. [CrossRef]
101. Cosgrove, C.; Ussher, J.E.; Rauch, A.; Gartner, K.; Kurioka, A.; Huhn, M.H.; Adelmann, K.; Kang, Y.H.; Fergusson, J.R.; Simmonds, P.; et al. Early and nonreversible decrease of CD161++ /MAIT cells in HIV infection. *Blood* **2013**, *121*, 951–961. [CrossRef]
102. Le Bourhis, L.; Dusseaux, M.; Bohineust, A.; Bessoles, S.; Martin, E.; Premel, V.; Core, M.; Sleurs, D.; Serriari, N.E.; Treiner, E.; et al. MAIT cells detect and efficiently lyse bacterially-infected epithelial cells. *PLoS Pathog.* **2013**, *9*, e1003681. [CrossRef] [PubMed]
103. Vorkas, C.K.; Wipperman, M.F.; Li, K.; Bean, J.; Bhattarai, S.K.; Adamow, M.; Wong, P.; Aube, J.; Juste, M.A.J.; Bucci, V.; et al. Mucosal-associated invariant and gammadelta T cell subsets respond to initial Mycobacterium tuberculosis infection. *JCI Insight* **2018**, *3*, e121899. [CrossRef] [PubMed]
104. Cisternas, I.S.; Torres, A.; Flores, A.F.; Angulo, V.A.G. Differential regulation of riboflavin supply genes in Vibrio cholerae. *Gut Pathog.* **2017**, *9*, 10. [CrossRef] [PubMed]
105. Corbett, A.J.; Eckle, S.B.; Birkinshaw, R.W.; Liu, L.; Patel, O.; Mahony, J.; Chen, Z.; Reantragoon, R.; Meehan, B.; Cao, H.; et al. T-cell activation by transitory neo-antigens derived from distinct microbial pathways. *Nature* **2014**, *509*, 361–365. [CrossRef]
106. Leung, D.T.; Bhuiyan, T.R.; Nishat, N.S.; Hoq, M.R.; Aktar, A.; Rahman, M.A.; Uddin, T.; Khan, A.I.; Chowdhury, F.; Charles, R.C.; et al. Circulating mucosal associated invariant T cells are activated in Vibrio cholerae O1 infection and associated with lipopolysaccharide antibody responses. *PLoS Negl. Trop. Dis.* **2014**, *8*, e3076. [CrossRef] [PubMed]
107. Bhuiyan, T.R.; Rahman, M.A.; Trivedi, S.; Afroz, T.; Banna, H.A.; Hoq, M.R.; Pop, I.; Jensen, O.; Rashu, R.; Uddin, M.I.; et al. Mucosal-associated invariant T (MAIT) cells are highly activated in duodenal tissue of humans with *Vibrio cholerae* O1 infection. *medRxiv* **2021**. [CrossRef]
108. Jensen, O.; Trivedi, S.; Meier, J.D.; Fairfax, K.; Scott Hale, J.; Leung, D.T. A novel subset of follicular helper-like MAIT cells has capacity for B cell help and antibody production in the mucosa. *bioRxiv* **2020**. [CrossRef]

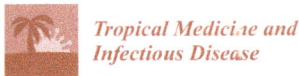 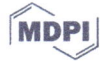

Review

The History of Intravenous and Oral Rehydration and Maintenance Therapy of Cholera and Non-Cholera Dehydrating Diarrheas: A Deconstruction of Translational Medicine: From Bench to Bedside?

David R. Nalin

Center for Immunology and Microbial Diseases, Albany Medical College, Albany, NY 12208, USA; nalindavid@gmail.com

Abstract: The "bench to bedside" (BTB) paradigm of translational medicine (TM) assumes that medical progress emanates from basic science discoveries transforming clinical therapeutic models. However, a recent report found that most published medical research is false due, among other factors, to small samples, inherent bias and inappropriate statistical applications. Translation-blocking factors include the validity (or lack thereof) of the underlying pathophysiological constructs and related therapeutic paradigms and adherence to faulty traditional beliefs. Empirical discoveries have also led to major therapeutic advances, but scientific dogma has retrospectively retranslated these into the BTB paradigm. A review of the history of intravenous (I.V.) and oral therapy for cholera and NDDs illustrates some fallacies of the BTB model and highlights pitfalls blocking translational and transformative progress, and retro-translational factors, including programmatic modifications of therapeutic advances contradicting therapeutic paradigms and medical economic factors promoting more expensive and profitable medical applications inaccessible to resource-limited environments.

Keywords: cholera; non-cholera dehydrating diarrheas; translational medicine; history

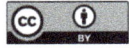

1. Introduction

The intravenous (I.V.) and oral treatment of cholera and non-cholera dehydrating diarrheas (NDDs) provide insights into translational medicine, spanning the period from the birth of clinical laboratory science (the "bench") in 1831 [1] to the development of modern oral rehydration and maintenance therapy (ORT) in 1967–1968 (the "bedside") [2], which, in terms of saving lives, has been hailed as perhaps the most important translational advance of the last century [3].

A translational medical advance rests upon three foundations: a valid *causative* paradigm derived from a correct understanding of disease pathophysiology, a valid *therapeutic* paradigm for correcting the pathophysiologic disorder, and a clinically effective (and safe) *methodology* for delivering the treatment to provide a therapeutically beneficial or life-saving outcome. The 'bench to bedside" slogan overlooks the fact that between bench and bedside are many factors which ultimately determine whether the therapy will be life saving, useless, impracticable, regressive or deadly. The notion that the bench to bedside concept of translational medicine proceeds in a linear manner is erroneous. Discoveries at the bench can take years and even decades to translate to widespread adoption and acceptance. In the case of intravenous (I.V.) and oral therapy (ORT) for cholera, the gap of 127 years from the first correct pathophysiologic and partial therapeutic paradigms for cholera (1831) to the 1960's development of effective and safe treatment methods, and its application to NDD therapy, implies that a more nuanced understanding of transitional medicine is needed, based on historical review of the phases of translation.

2. Material and Methods

Cholera and the NDDs share major aspects of pathophysiology, and methods of rehydration and maintenance therapy for cholera are adaptable for treatment of NDDs. This review will examine the causes of the lethally slow progress toward an effective and safe cholera and NDD treatment regimen, including the pathophysiologic and therapeutic paradigms underlying NDD treatment from ancient times until the arrival of the first documented European cholera epidemic in 1830 (the apocryphal period); the years 1831–1947 (the transitional period); and 1948–1968 (the translational period). Numerous contextual translation-blocking factors and retro-translational factors delayed for 127 years translation to a safe and consistently effective treatment, factors which continue even today to play a negative role.

The key indicator of translational progress for cholera and NDD treatments is the case fatality rate (CFR). Historically, persistent high CFRs indicated translational paralysis. Treatments converging towards the modern CFR of less than 1% provide a key marker of translational progress, achieved by the timely replacement of diarrheal water and electrolyte losses with matching volumes of I.V. or absorbable oral solutions of similar electrolyte composition.

3. The Apocryphal Period

Before 1831, the true extent of cholera and its epidemic frequency remain unknown, due to lack of population-based clinical reports from the endemic areas in South Asia. Microbiology did not yet exist, and *Vibrio cholerae* Pacini was as yet unknown, as was cholera itself as we define it today [4]. Even clear, accurate, virtually pathognomonic clinical case descriptions such as Latta's in 1831–1832 (vide infra) are not found in surviving documents before 1831.

In contrast, records of treatment recommendations for diarrhea go back several millennia [5]. The causes are today known to include a range from cholera and non-vibrio cholera (caused chiefly by various types of *Vibrio* sp. and *Escherichia coli*), and other potentially lethal NDDs of infants and children caused by rotavirus and other bacterial and viral pathogens.

While no quantitative or accurate CFR data exist before 1831, cholera CFRs of 40–60% or higher continued long after 1831 during a prolonged period of quantitative reporting up to the mid-20th century. Many preventable deaths still occur in cholera-affected areas lacking access to modern treatment. NDDs outnumber cholera in incidence and, before the development of modern therapeutic methods, took the lives of over five million under-5-year-olds annually [6,7].

During the "apocryphal" period from ancient times up to 1830, the main causative and pathophysiologic paradigms for diarrhea were (1) an imbalance of "humors" (bile, phlegm, blood, wind) attributed to Galen and Greek predecessors and (2) a poison in the blood, supposed to spread chiefly through the air [5]. Therapeutic recommendations were aimed at correcting imbalances of the humors or removing the poison by bloodletting and purging. Specific dietary or medicinal recommendations were not anchored in accurate therapeutic paradigms or proof of efficacy, but on alleged dietary or preventive practices of ancient hallowed authorities and/their modern interpreters, ranging from cereals or farinaceous gruels (Galen [8], p. 666) to raw oysters ([8], p. 677) (also Galen [8]). The treatments allegedly espoused by Galen and others over those centuries, including enemas to clean the intestinal surface and remove noxious intestinal contents ([8], p. 663), were as imaginative as the false theory of imbalanced "humors". Though some of these reported recommendations such as gruel or soups of chicken or beef appear to echo modern clinical trial-based rice-, other cereal- or amino acid-based oral rehydration therapy [9], there is no more evidence for efficacy for raw oyster therapy than there is that gruels or soups of chicken or beef were tested in balance studies or administered in amounts sufficient to match voluminous fluid losses in accordance with any effective therapeutic method. Isolated uncontrolled case reports remain anecdotal, not translational.

Apocryphal claims of different foods, dietary and medicinal treatments for cholera became part of the material medica based on no quantitative evidence of clinical trials or objectively documented reports of reproducible successful clinical outcomes. Claims that recommendations for sugars, porridges, chicken soup and such represent early use of oral therapy for cholera or severe NDDs overlook the lack of any evidence that such dietary advice included any reproducible methods or reduced CFRs. A brief survey of such recommendations and linked therapeutic methods illustrates that many dietary recommendations are not equivalent to effective therapeutic methods. Use of a given food or solution without a linked effective methodology or proof of net absorption and concurrent reduction in CFRs is no translational breakthrough.

4. The Post-Apocryphal Transitional Period (1830–1959): Development of I.V. Therapy

Over more than a century after 1831, there is no mention of measuring and quantitatively replacing the diarrheal losses of water and electrolytes in a timely manner so as to avoid recurrent shock, renal failure and death. The method of bolus I.V. infusions given when shock recurred could not avoid decade after decade of 40 to 60% CFRs. Accurate pathophysiologic and therapeutic paradigms existed by 1831–1832, but in the absence of an effective and safe clinical methodology, the void was filled with a lethal array of irrational and often counterintuitive and contraindicated "remedies".

Howard-Jones [10] has thoroughly reviewed the 19th c. advances in cholera pathophysiology and therapy and the numerous, mostly lethal traditional "treatments" of the time, most derived from ancient pathophysiologic paradigms based on irrational medical traditions supported by the medical hierarchy. Continued high CFRs confirm that successive treatment modalities failed to achieve life-saving outcomes during most of the 127 year evolution from bench to graveside rather than to bedside. Current misunderstandings of the progress, or lack thereof, in this period merit review of selected historical details.

By 1831, cholera had spread from Asia across Russia, Europe and into England, bringing mass panic and innumerable old and new "treatments", often including contradictory modalities. The commonest remained bloodletting, the archaic causative and therapeutic paradigm being removal of an unknown toxic element in the blood. To this end, bloodletting and replacement with transfusion of human and even animal blood was attempted in the 1830s [11].

The arrival of cholera in Europe occurred at a time when the advances in chemistry and physics of the 18th century were first being applied to biomedical phenomena. Serum-specific gravity (sp.gr.) and chemical analyses of serum, clotted blood, cholera diarrhea fluid and vomitus were introduced, but the analytic skill of the pioneer clinical biochemists varied widely, and some specimens were analyzed fresh and others after long periods at room temperature.

The correct pathophysiologic and therapeutic cholera paradigms evolved from pathophysiological and therapeutic errors of William Stevens [12,13], who claimed cures using various salts to convert the color of blood of terminal cholera patients from cyanotic into a bright red color. In Moscow, Hermann published largely incorrect serum analyses but partially correct inference of loss of blood water (and, incorrectly, acetic acid [14]) in 1830. This led Jaehnichen to give a minute amount of I.V. water with acetic acid, apparently, from his published remarks, to lubricate the thickened and inspissated blood rather than to quantitatively replace the fluid losses of cholera. Then, the more accurate analyses, pathophysiologic and therapeutic paradigms of O'Shaughnessy inspired the daring clinical application of those findings of Latta (1831–1832 [15]), who advanced rational treatment as afar as possible in the absence of sterile solutions and a valid therapeutic method.

5. William Stevens' "Saline Treatment"

The observations leading to the correct pathophysiologic and therapeutic paradigms for cholera were published in 1831–1832 during the European onslaught of cholera.

Stevens' reported in 1830 [12] and again retrospectively in 1853 [13] that yellow fever patients had dark blood, indicating to him a lack of oxygen, and a bright red color returned on adding salt in vitro. This "saline method" was extended to the dark color of cholera patients' blood as well, by giving small amounts of salt powder, saline solutions and saline and other laxatives by rectal enema, by steam bath, by mouth or injection (a word which in his texts is variably used to signify delivery not only parenterally in small amounts, but also by orointestinal or other routes). As noted by Howard-Jones [10], he had no concept of rehydration, only of inducing color change of the blood. He had no quantitative concept of cholera patients' salt and water losses or of their quantitative I.V. replacement.

Modern balance studies have proven that oral plain saline is not absorbed by cholera patients and aggravates cholera diarrhea in the absence of glucose or other substrate in the solution to enhance active sodium transport and thereby also promote concurrent water absorption [16,17]. There is also evidence indicating the non-absorbability of colonic saline enemas during diarrhea [18,19].

A review of William Stevens' claims in his book titled "Observations On the Nature and the Treatment of the Asiatic Cholera" [13] is warranted by the fact that despite his erroneous pathophysiologic and therapeutic paradigms and the non-absorbability in cholera patients of orally or rectally administered plain salt or saline solutions (or saline baths), several unwary authors [20–22] have in recent years mistakenly reported that Stevens was a pioneer in oral and I.V. rehydration therapy for cholera. This he was not, as critical reading of his publications demonstrates.

Stevens' second book is a belated attempt to rescue his reputation and defend his claims of, in his words, "miraculous" cures of cholera patients using his "saline method". However, Steven's book gives no single clear or succinct description of his "saline method". Several variants appear in different sections. In one, he states that "even at the eleventh hour, if a warm saline fluid be thrown into the intestinal canal, this vital fluid is even then rapidly absorbed by the absorbent vessels and the moment that this living fluid enters the circulation it gives new electric life to the blood." ([13], p. lvii).

In contrast, Latta correctly reported that oral or rectal saline brought no benefit to cholera patients [15]. Stevens' description of patients "throwing up" the oral salines are consistent with the lack of benefit of non-absorbable saline powders and laxatives. The latter promoted forceful evacuation along with the cholera stool, aggravating patients discomfort. Anal corks prevented expulsion of intestinal contents after laxatives and enemas [10].

Stevens held that "the non-purgative saline medicines were the most likely to be useful, for they not only redden the colour of the blood, but by increasing its fluidity they render it better fitted to serve its [intended].functions." Applying this in Coldbath-Fields prison in 1832 to patients with presumed cholera with "premonitory symptoms of diarrhea and vomiting", the treatment included a Seidlitz powder laxative, more active purgatives (e.g., sodium tartrate), Epsom salts added to the Seidlitz powder, and then, "on the bowels being moved, plenty of thin beef-tea, well seasoned with salt." "If much irritability of the stomach prevailed, a sinapism (mustard plaster) was applied to the gastric region, and thirst was relieved with seltzer, soda or pure water ad libitum." When the collapse stage was reached, a strong solution of the same salts, at a temperature of 100 degrees, was "thrown" into the bowels. Stevens claimed that the latter method succeeded far better than "injection of the vital electric salts into the veins" and patients "were generally dismissed cured in a few days." [12,13]. Of these patients, none were entered as cholera cases in the prison journal, but Stevens attributed this to an aberration of prison recordkeeping.

There was no standard case definition of cholera, which was regarded as a fatal disease often, but not always accompanied with profuse diarrhea and vomiting, with stages based on the patient's appearance and general condition: "premonitory", later "collapse", and (assuming survival after collapse) "reaction". Case reports frequently included symptoms and signs not at all characteristic of cholera as we know it (some were even said to have constipation ([13], p. 39)). Stevens' critics found his results unreproducible; many patients had mild diarrheas, or other non-diarrheal illnesses terminating in fatal "collapse" [23].

Stevens' claims of "magical" cures were challenged by the medical authorities of the day, leading to the vituperations pervading much of Stevens' 1853 book. These critics, including Sir David Barry, Mr. Wakefield and W.B. O'Shaughnessy, reported that examination of Steven's reported cholera patients revealed that none of them had cholera. Stevens retorted that his critics "were the mere instruments in the hands of the higher human serpents, or the so-called physiologists, who are the leaders of the medical profession; for ever to this day they are the false teachers that come in the garb of sheep's clothing, but inwardly they are ravening wolves." ([13], pp. 258–259).

An *enema (italics mine)* "composed of a large tablespoonful of muriate of soda dissolved in warm water, sometimes with the addition of sugar or starch" administered "at as high a temperature as the patient could well bear" was recommended, with additional "sinapisms ... frictions..., warm towels" and "a pure air for the patient to breathe."([13], p. 40).

Another patient received a Seidlitz powder laxative and mustard poultices with an "injection" (evidently per os, quotation marks mine) of four salines in a pint and a half of warm water, repeated until followed by a "copious motion" and then the saline powders were repeated every hour and saline injections used every three hours with warm flannel frictions and the third of a Seidlitz laxative given every half hour, and soda and seltzer-water ... from time to time" ([13], p. 243). Then, "a saline injection attempted to be infused into the blood, but the veins were so completely collapsed it did not succeed. The patient ... could not swallow, but a warm saline fluid was from time to time thrown slowly into the intestinal canal" ([13], p. 244]. The patient reportedly survived ([13], pp. 242–245).

In his 1832 book ([12], p.33), Stevens reported that 29 of 30 cholera patients survived after drinking 2 tablespoons of salt in 6 ounces of water hourly and one tablespoonful of a similar mixture cold every hour afterwards. Another iteration of the "saline method" as noted by Jones ([10], p. 386) included oral administration of "strong solutions of non-purgative neutral salts in half a tumbler of water" (see also ([13], p. 41)). Steven's report has sufficient detail to establish that his "saline method" could not have had any therapeutic benefit due to the non-absorbability of plain oral saline or saline mixtures given by rectal or dermal routes. The variable components and unspecified quantities of other oral fluids and the tiny amounts given I.V., typically as a last desperate measure, could not avoid fatal outcomes. There was no awareness of the need, nor any method used to match volume of saline infusion by any route to volume of fluid losses.

In summary, there is no basis for considering Stevens an I.V. or oral rehydration or maintenance pioneer, as his salines, whether powder or liquid, oral drink, enema or bath, were non-absorbable in cholera and intended only to turn cyanotic blood red. He did not conceive of rehydration and conducted no measures of intake and output. The oral plain saline and saline laxatives that he recommended would have aggravated cholera patients' diarrhea and dehydration. Use of oral salines in patients he claimed had cholera but who actually had other diseases may have been harmless or even beneficial in isolated cases, but provides no basis for considering Stevens as a rehydration pioneer. His "magical" cholera cures were evidently delusional and he confused matters further by hailing others' correct concepts of intravenous saline replacement of the large volumes of fluid losses of cholera as if they represented proof and acceptance of his color change therapeutic paradigm ([13], p. 488–491). The controversies arising over the rejection of his claims by his contemporaries and his virulent condemnations of O'Shaughnessy and others who debunked his claims make it clear that his saline method falls into the category of ineffective cholera remedies of the period, lacking valid case definitions, correct pathophysiologic or therapeutic paradigms or effective clinical methods. The concept of controlled trials did not yet exist.

6. Rudolf Hermann and Friedrich Jaehnichen

Cholera's progress through Russia led to medical commissions tasked with formulating quarantine and other supposed control measures. In Moscow, the German expatriate Hermann, a chemist, reported among the earliest measurements of serum sp.gr. in cholera and of other substances [14] which his faulty analyses convinced him were present in dehydrated cholera patients.

Hermann correctly interpreted the elevated serum sp.gr. as indicating loss of blood water, but his erroneous acetic acid measurements on cholera stools led Jaehnichen to conclude that I.V. water with added acetic acid might correct the inspissation of blood into clotted material blocking circulatory function along with the alkaline blood and acid stool erroneously identified by Hermann in cholera patients. Hermann performed no serum sodium, chloride or bicarbonate analyses, reporting only his erroneous finding of acetic acid, so Jaehnichen gave only 33 cc of dilute acetic acid (not saline or water) I.V. to relieve the thickening of the blood. The patient died soon after [24].

As Howard-Jones noted [10], Hermann and Jaehnichen had no concept of volumetric replacement of the diarrheal or emesis fluid losses. Hermann concluded that "the liquids evacuated in cholera both by the stools and by vomiting form constituent parts of the blood, which is deconstituted by their disappearance ... the immediate cause of death is consequently the thickening of the blood, which prevents its circulation." ([10], pp. 385–386). He continued that this "decomposition" was due to the "separation of the acid and aqueous liquids that are evacuated in the diarrhea and vomitus of cholera patients." ([14], p. 29).

Hermann surmised that intestinal absorption was blocked in cholera based on an alkaline diarrhea fluid of a cholera patient fed a sodium hydroxide solution and speculated that the diarrhea fluid originated as a transudate across the intestinal wall (later disproven).

Hermann ([14], pp. 29–30) agreed with Jaehnichen and others that cholera was an affliction of the symphatique or "pneumo-gastrique nerve". Here again is an ironic and seemingly prescient but totally unrelated idea which in modern times has emerged as a role for the nervous system and gut hormones in choleragenesis [25]. The chance use of seemingly prescient but actually unrelated descriptive phrases often suggests ideas that the authors could not have understood as we do today.

All Hermann's reported analyses except the elevated serum sp.gr. were erroneous, including absence of urea in anuric cholera patients. His finding of blood and stool acetic acid may have resulted from detecting indole-3-acetic acid, a product of bacterial metabolism found in contaminated blood and intestinal fecal matter [26]. Hermann noted that others had in ten cases found the stools to be alkaline, not acidic. This he attributed to "national differences" He also noted that other investigators at the time had reported highly elevated serum sp.gr. values in terminal cholera patients (e.g., Thompson: 1.057; Rose and Willstoch (Berlin): 1.0447 ([14], pp. 36,40). He believed that cholera blood had lost its normal anatomical shape and was "decomposed."

Hermann and Jaehnichen may have been first to connect the pathophysiologic dots between raised serum sp.gr. and loss of water from blood via diarrhea and vomitus. However, their therapeutic paradigm focused on the idea that the desiccated thickened blood was decomposing into woody and polypoid masses which caused death by blocking the circulation, compromising the heart. Their therapeutic paradigm was inappropriately focused on eliminating the inspissation of the blood rather than replacement of the large fluid losses, the true composition and volume of which they had failed to identify.

Hermann was not a physician and uncritically recorded the many irrational medical practices then prevailing ([14], p. 33) and not rejected by him or Jaehnichen, such as venesection and commonly used ineffective and often lethal medicinals, herbal preparations, plasters, baths and enemas. These were essentially placed on a par with the idea of replacing cholera's fluid losses with small intravenous injections. Hermann's incorrect analyses and his omission of sodium and bicarbonate analyses led to Jaehnichen omitting the crucial electrolytes lost in cholera diarrhea. Had Jaehnichen realized the volumes that were needed, and had he administered them as dilute acetic acid, fatal massive hemolysis would have occurred.

7. O'Shaughnessy

In London, O'Shaughnessy at first pursued Stevens' red color theory and advocated giving salts with more oxygen than sodium chloride to redden the blood ([27], p. 31, line 434). He read Hermann's reports and, having performed his own remarkably accurate determinations of sp.gr., sodium, chloride and bicarbonate levels in cholera patients' serum and diarrhea fluid, he published a critical report (10, p. 387 [28]) indicating correctly that all but Hermann's finding of an elevated serum sp.gr. were in error, including the findings of acetic acid in the cholera diarrheal fluid, an alkaline serum and absence of urea in anuric cholera patients' serum.

O'Shaughnessy noted that Hermann's specimens were mishandled, resulting in decomposition with erroneous high levels of alkali in cholera patients' blood and acetic acid in cholera diarrhea. Modern analyses confirm the opposite: acidosis in the blood and highly alkaline diarrheal fluid [29].

O'Shaughnessy's new pathophysiologic paradigm, whether guided by (or in opposition to) Hermann's and Jaehnichen's reports or not, led him to the essentially different and correct pathophysiologic paradigm of loss of water, salt and bicarbonate causing the cholera syndrome, with the logical therapeutic paradigm being replacement of the water and salt losses with I.V. solutions. The need for aseptic technique and sterile infusions remained undiscovered translation-blocking factors.

O'Shaughnessy's analyses led to these conclusions [28]:

1. The blood drawn in the worst cases of the cholera is unchanged in its anatomical or globular structure.
2. It has lost a large proportion of its water, 1000 parts of cholera serum having but the average of 860 parts of water.
3. It has lost also a great proportion of its neutral saline ingredients.
4. Of the free alkali contained in healthy serum, not a particle is present in some cholera cases, and barely a trace in others.
5. Urea exists in cases where suppression of urine has been a marked symptom.
6. All the salts deficient in the blood, especially the carbonate of soda, are present in large quantities in the peculiar white dejected matters.

As Howard-Jones noted [10], p. 387] O'Shaughnessy's therapeutic recommendations were "(1st) To restore the blood to its natural specific gravity and (2nd) To restore its deficient saline matters. The first of these can only be effected by absorption, by imbibition, or by the injection of aqueous fluid into the veins. The same remarks, with sufficiently obvious modification apply to the second." Absorption and imbibition were soon found blocked in cholera.

However, O'Shaughnessy continued to recommend "other remedies: such as stimulants, opioids, external warmth, etc., "which may be calculated to re-excite the circulation and promote the required absorption . . . and "tepid water enemas containing a certain proportion of the neutral salts" ([10], op cit; [28], p. 53). Unaware of the absorptive defects in cholera, he stated: *"I would expect much benefit from the frequently repeated use of the neutral salts by the mouth or by enemata."* ([10], op cit, p.-54) while noting that the salts in most cases "pre-exist in the intestinal canal." His crucial correct inference was that "In the severe cases in which absorption is totally suspended, and when stimulants . . . fail to re-excite the circulation, I would not hesitate to inject some ounces of warm water into the veins . . . and 'dissolve in that water the mild innocuous salts . . . which in cholera are deficient." His conjecture would have been more accurate had he said "pounds" instead of "ounces"

He proposed a formulation with 6 ounces of water, to be repeated every 2 h, containing sodium phosphate, sodium chloride, sodium carbonate and sodium sulphate, then covering his bets by "also obey[ing] every local indications and use cold applications, leeches, etc.".

8. Latta

Inspired by O'Shaughnessy's publications, Latta decided to replace the losses orally, rectally or I.V. with significant volumes of saline solutions and noted for the first time the failure of oral or rectal plain saline solutions to provide any benefit [15]. Treating cholera patients at an advanced stage of their dehydration, or "collapse", he infused up to ten pounds of his saline solution using the Reid's syringe used to bleed patients, and his vivid and accurate descriptions noted the immediate striking improvement in moribund cholera patients given such treatment. His solutions were hypotonic, containing less sodium than in cholera diarrhea ([15], pp. 208–213) but capable of reviving patients without inducing hemolysis.

Latta wrote ([15], pp. 275–277), "As soon as I learnt the result of Dr. O'Shaughnessy's analysis, I attempted to restore the blood to its natural state, by injecting copiously into the larger intestine warm water, holding in solution the requisite salts, and also administered quantities from time to time by the mouth, treating that the power of absorption might not be altogether lost, but by these means produced, in no case, any permanent benefit, but, on the contrary, I though the tormina, vomiting and purging were much aggravated thereby, to the further reduction of the little remaining strength of the patient; finding thus, that such, in common with all the ordinary means in use, was either useless or hurtful, I at length resorted to throw the fluid immediately into the circulation . . . .. The first subject of experiment was an aged female, on whom all the usual remedies had been fully tried, without producing one good symptom; the disease, uninterrupted, holding steadily on its course, had apparently reached the last moments of her earthly existence, and now nothing could injure her—indeed, so entirely was she reduced, that I feared I would be unable to get my apparatus ready ere she expired. Having inserted a tube in the basilic vein, cautiously—anxiously, I watched the effects; ounce after ounce was injected, but no visible change was produced. Still persevering, I thought she began to breathe less laboriously, soon her sharpened features, and sunken eye, and fallen jaw, pale and cold, bearing the manifest impress of death's signet, began to glow with returning animation; the pulse, which had long ceased, returned to the wrist; at first small and weak, by degrees it became more and more distinct, fuller, slower and firmer, and in the short space of half an hour, when six pints had been injected, she expressed in a firm voice that she was free from all uneasiness, actually became jocular and fancied all she needed was a little sleep; her extremities were warm, and every feature bore the aspect of comfort and health. This being my first case, I fancied my patient secure, and from my great need of a little repose, left her in charge of the hospital surgeon; but I had not been long gone, ere the vomiting and purging recurring soon reduced her to her former state of debility. I was not apprised of the event, and she sunk in five and a half hours after I left her . . . . I have no doubt the case would have issued in complete reaction, had the remedy, which already had produced such effect, been repeated."

Writing to express his pleasure at hearing Latta's results, O'Shaughnessy could not resist making some further therapeutic suggestions, including minute doses of astringents and stimulants (ammonia carbonate intravenously based on its toleration by horses, quinine sulfate, dilute spirits and weak herbal decoctions ([30], p. 281).

Refining Latta's therapeutic recommendations, Lewins ([31], pp. 243–244) noted that "a large quantity must be injected, from five to ten pounds in an adult and repeated at longer or shorter intervals as the state of the pulse and other symptoms may indicate; whenever the pulse fails, more fluid ought to be thrown in to produce an effect . . . without regard to quantity." However, no treatment omitting the quantities of the fluid losses or replacing all the losses as they occurred could lower CFRs.

Influenced by the prevailing concept of cholera as a disease with the three phases of premonitory, collapse and reaction, treatment began too late and was focused on correcting the collapse stage, which initial intravenous boluses appeared to do, after which Latta recommended astringent enemas, hoping to stop the diarrhea and prevent recurrent shock ([15], p. 276).

The concept of continuous maintenance therapy after correction of shock to prevent its recurrence, obvious in retrospect, had not occurred to anyone at this point. As Latta reported, the initial startling improvement following such I.V. infusions was usually followed by recurrences of collapse with frequent fatal termination. The actual average volumes of I.V. saline given, though sufficient to transiently restore blood pressure and pulse, were far below the amounts needed to replace the total volume of ongoing cholera fluid losses.

Two translation-blocking factors prevented Latta from achieving reliable recoveries and wider acceptance of his innovation. Though he recognized that the patients who died after initial I.V. saline infusions resuscitated them did so because of lack of timely repetition of the infusions, the lack of a therapeutic method ensuring effective and timely maintenance therapy after initial rehydration ensured continued high CFRs. Though serum sp.gr. was measurable, its use as a monitoring tool to guide therapy escaped notice and/or actual practice. Additionally, Latta's sharp clinical eye, proven by his vivid descriptions, did not lead to a standard method of monitoring clinical signs (changes in degree of sunkenness of eyes, tenting of skin, etc.) to guide maintenance therapy. Without a means to monitor ongoing losses and replace them in a timely manner, severely ill cholera patients invariably faced multiple episodes of recurrent dehydration and shock, most ending fatally.

Though Latta described using "warm" I.V. saline infusions, the problem of the late often fatal "febrile stage" indicates that the solutions and implements used were not accidentally sterilized as might have happened had he first boiled the water, then allowing it to cool to the desired "warm" temperature.

Regardless of the lethality of repeated rehydration rather than maintenance therapy after rehydration, medical microbiology remained undiscovered, leading to a "typhoidal" stage of fatal sepsis after I.V. injections of unsterile solutions. Lethal air emboli were another impediment to wide acceptance [10].

Secondary factors which contributed to the stagnation of Latta's I.V. saline therapy for cholera were his death in 1833, the waning of the 1831–1833 cholera epidemic in the U.K. and Europe and, when it returned, the continued popularity among physicians of bleeding and myriad ineffective, often harmful traditional remedies and procedures. Practitioners trying I.V. saline infusions reported mixed, usually transient results ([31], pp. 292–293) followed by deaths. CFRs were acutely typically 70% or more; no method of measuring input and output was developed. Controversy over Latta's treatment preceded his death from tuberculosis in 1833 [32].

Another less recognized factor was the "tinkering effect", or the misguided modifications of formula or methods by various medical authorities introducing inadequately evaluated innovations, whether useless, harmful or beneficial. For example, the use of I.V. albumin by Parkes ([10], p. 391) and others or of I.V. milk infusions by Bovell ([10], p. 394) had disastrous effects, helping to discredit the method.

I.V. saline was tried in Madras Presidency in 1832 but abandoned, although transient improvement was reported [32]. O'Shaughnessy went to India in 1833, where he helped introduce the telegraph and practiced an early form of photography ([33]). Though a medical officer, no evidence exists that he continued cholera studies or altered the beliefs or practices of colonial administrators or physicians during the annual cholera epidemics, though Macgregor in 1838 in South India indicated he would use Mackintosh's version of I.V. therapy (vide infra) in "bad" cases [32]. An interesting example of post-Latta practice was the work of William Marsden, who published a summary of his cholera treatments from 1832 to 1834, with follow-up editions from 1848 to 1865 after cholera recurrences [34].

He notes O'Shaughnessy's publications and, while ignoring Latta's, espouses I.V. saline infusions for advanced-stage cholera. He noted patients' extreme thirst, but proscribed oral fluids, fearing vomiting, while continuing to recommend Stevens' "saline" treatment, water (to clean the bowels) and also the purgatives and 2 h hot baths containing 7–14 pounds of salt for relief of cramps. He shared the opinion of those suggesting a (mesenteric) neuronal mechanism of cholera. Marsden recommended Stevens' oral salt powders dissolved in a small quantity of water q 15 min (p. 46) to suppress the disease in the first stage (before collapse) and larger saline solutions (followed by water) to clean the intestines. If the patient remained pulseless, he followed O'Shaughnessy's recommendation of "fluid corresponding in character as nearly as possible to the serum of the blood, injected in sufficient quantity to fully restore the pulse". Afterwards, opium (otherwise condemned) and quinine, and then for survivors, rice, other farinaceous puddings and malt liquor. A subsequent septic "typhoid" stage was again noted. His CFRs ranged from 31 to 90% in patients receiving various treatments ([34], p. 61). One series with remarkably high survival rates clearly included only patients with non-cholera diarrheas.

Like Latta, Marsden gave I.V. saline chiefly to terminal cholera patients after pulse disappeared, noting that attending physicians must not be away for over two hours to avoid losing patients due to unattended relapses; but his CFRs indicate that such absences were the rule rather than the exception.

Marsden's use of rectal cannulas for I.V. infusions is notable in the days before autoclaving. Sepsis due to unsterile infusions and a faulty method of replacing the large unmeasured ongoing losses, by waiting for shock to recur, remained key translational blocks to widespread adoption of I.V. saline as the treatment of choice. The same faulty therapeutic methodology would ensure high CFRs until after 1959 [29].

In the decades after Marsden, numerous practitioners tried various I.V. and oral treatments, among them MacIntosh, Magendie, Broussais, Lizard, and Wall. MacIntosh, in 1836, used an I.V. solution close to normal saline and, like Latta, added bicarbonate. An experimental addition of I.V. egg albumen was quickly abandoned. CFR was 84% ([10], p. 391) but this was attributed to tardy treatment, the ill-fated but often repeated practice recognized by Latta. Magendie's cure-all "punch" contained a pint of chamomile infusion, 2 oz. of alcohol, 1 oz. of sugar and lemon juice, along with frictions and heat. No method of administration was indicated; 27% survival was claimed [35]. Broussais [36], like many others, advocated what he called his "physiologic method", including vapor baths, leeches, plasters and sweet drinks, the latter given to induce vomiting rather than rehydrate. He reported 97.5% survival using these treatments, but the Gazette Medical reported only 17%. Lizard [37], following Delpech, reported success in 30 cases with intravenous saline and oral alkali. In 1893, Wall used an I.V. solution similar to MacIntosh's but with more bicarbonate (24 mEq/L.) [38], and added gelatin. CFR was 70% [39]. Lewis [40] used oral alkali.

Borne by trade and the burgeoning shipping industry linking endemic to non-endemic areas, cholera revisited England and the continent repeatedly during the 19th c., with Latta and Lewins' urging of persistent fluid replacement being ignored, little or no effective treatment and a resurgence of maniacal or quack "cures": extract of lamb testicle can be added to Jones' tally [41], along with a costly venerable concoction attributed to Galen, called Theraica, consisting of wine, spices, purgatives and viper's broth [42]. Stevens' blood color-changing "salines" continued to be debunked ([43], p. 64–65). Amid this morass, Pacini, who discovered cholera vibrio, also advocated I.V. saline replacement therapy [44] using a formula close to normal saline. Sterilization by boiling of water to prepare solutions for I.V. use gained usage by 1892 ([45], p. 151) though pyrogens, while not usually fatal, were not removed until 1938 ([46], p. 784).

The medical establishment continued to ignore or reject sound therapeutic paradigms; and medical textbooks such as Osler's ([47] p. 232–233) in 1907 advocated apocryphal treatments such as morphine, reduced or enhanced oral intake (ice, brandy or coffee and other drinks), cocaine, hot water lavage, heat, hot baths, hypodermic injections of ether and enteroclysis with warm water and soap or tannic acid (3–4 L), as in the 1902 edition [10]. The sign that the enteroclysis had been thoroughly accomplished was when the patient vomited the tannic acid bowel irrigant. S.C. saline infusions (4 g/L) and I.V. milk were recommended "until the pulse returned". Relying on return of a failing pulse to guide repeat infusions [48] failed to save patients, as in Lewins' day.

9. 20th Century: Rogers

Sellards' advocacy of bicarbonate or base precursors [38,49], used eighty years earlier by Latta [15], led Rogers to add alkali to his hypertonic saline regimen, though Sellards' advocacy was based chiefly on the mistaken idea that the alkali would prevent uremia. When Osler's text was updated by McCrae [50], revised recommendations included alkaline stomach washes, hot baths, abdominal heat, castor oil or calomel purgatives, opium, kaolin, potassium permanganate and pituitary extract and caffeine in case of collapse, and Rogers' hypertonic saline injections (I.V., rectal, intraperitoneal (I.P.) or subcutaneous (S.C.)) [51,52], repeated as needed to keep the blood pressure above (a mere) 70 and the sp.gr. below 1.063. If uremic, the saline plus bicarbonate solution was recommended.

Rogers saw the gut as a passive osmotic membrane, assuming that I.V. hypertonic saline would draw the diarrheal fluid back into the blood, preventing death [51]. This in fact did not occur, nor did it account for potassium or bicarbonate losses or for adverse effects of large infusions of hypertonic saline. Serum sp.gr. was used to estimate initial degree of dehydration and rehydration fluid needs but was not consistently used to monitor hydration status continuously to match I.V. fluid volumes to losses to reduce CFRs; sp.gr. was eventually omitted from Rogers' cholera treatment recommendations [53]. Fixed amounts (4 pints) of I.V. hypertonic saline were given during the collapse or "algid" stage, then stopped [53]. CFRs rarely fell below 30% [52], far above those ultimately achievable with further advances in replacement solutions and therapeutic methodology.

Rogers' methods were becoming more critically viewed, and modern methods of analysis were reapplied to studies of cholera pathophysiology. Recommendations from the British War Office as late as 1946 [53] noted that drugs were chiefly of little use, but the traditional castor oil purgative (with brandy) and morphine for vomiting were retained. Oral glucose was permitted, with Coramine, kaolin and pituitary extract for persistent hypotension. Rogers' I.V. saline with bicarbonate (and rectal saline) were noted, guided by blood sp.gr. and blood pressure, but blood pressure monitoring replaced sp.gr. for faster mass treatment, and the need for hypertonic saline and alkali solutions was questioned; normal saline being simpler to formulate and more rapidly administered. I.V. glucose (10–25%) or 4.5% S.C. without rationale was strongly advocated, However, archaica such as essential oils, mixtures (opium, bismuth salicylate, chloroform, etc.) and rectal tannin enemas, poultices and dry cupping over the kidneys, persisted, and waiting for blood pressure to fall risked fatalities if used as the sole monitoring method without intake and output measurements.

10. Robert A. Phillips

Phillips and co-workers in the U.S. Navy clarified the composition of cholera's "rice water" diarrhea and provided guidelines for appropriate I.V. replacement solutions. Applying the balance study technique, they developed optimal methods for rehydration and maintenance of patients with severe dehydration due to cholera and other severe NDDs.

Phillips had devoted his professional life to research on cholera and its effects on intestinal absorption of water and electrolytes. In 1948 [54], he and coworkers used modern analytic methods to precisely compare the electrolyte content of cholera patients' blood and "rice water" diarrhea. They used I.V. normal saline with added bicarbonate and potassium to replace the water and electrolyte losses [55]. However, their method of therapy was based on bladder catheters to monitor urine output; and after initial rehydration, they gave maintenance fluids only when urine output fell after severe dehydration recurred, too late to totally eliminate fatalities. Though Phillips had developed the copper sulfate method of measuring blood sp.gr. (other solutions had been used earlier), it was not used in Egypt to closely monitor hydration status, nor were diarrhea fluid volumes measured. Patients were at risk of recurrent severe dehydration, and 3 of 40 patients died [55].

Contemporaneously, several authors, perhaps inspired by parallel pediatric recommendations, suggested calf or human [56] plasma infusions for cholera. Total I.V. requirements were estimated from initial serum or plasma sp.gr. or monitored by venous pressure.

Both oral and I.V. glucose with half-strength saline were recommended by Chaudhuri [57], equally with oral plain saline, water or other beverages.

Continuing his pursuit of better treatments at NAMRU II in Taipei with Watten and colleagues, the method of measuring the actual volumes of diarrhea and vomitus of cholera patients (along with plasma sp.gr. monitoring) and replacing them with matching volumes of I.V. fluids containing appropriate electrolyte content was developed further. As in the earlier Egyptian studies, they used chiefly normal saline, later adding sodium bicarbonate and potassium chloride as needed to correct acidosis and hypokalemia [29]. This method could eliminate fatalities if delivered in a timely manner, with I.V. rehydration followed by I.V. maintenance therapy given continuously to match diarrhea and vomitus losses and avoid recurrent dehydration, shock and renal failure. Monitoring clinical signs could obviate plasma sp.gr. measurements for routine clinical use [58–60].

A wood-frame ("Watten") cot with a covering plastic sheet with a sleeve entering a calibrated translucent bucket or one with a dip stick below [59] facilitated both balance studies and management of cholera epidemics, and could be mass manufactured on short notice. Physicians or nurses could monitor the level of diarrheal fluid lost q4–6 h by glancing at the bucket and checking that the volume of I.V. fluids matched volume of losses.

Later, at the Pakistan-SEATO Cholera Research Hospital (PSCRL) in Dacca (now the International Center for Diarrheal Diseases Research, Bangladesh, or ICDDRB, Dhaka, Bangladesh), Robert Gordon and colleagues introduced a single I.V. solution matching the electrolyte composition of adult cholera patients [60], and usable in pediatric cholera patients, whose rice water diarrhea contained moderately less sodium chloride and more potassium. This original "Dacca Solution" contained bicarbonate, but later versions replaced non-sterile B.P. grade sodium bicarbonate (requiring special equipment to sterilize) with a base precursor such as acetate [61] or citrate [62], both ingredients simpler to autoclave. Lactate also had adherents [58] but etched glass I.V. bottles. Oral citrate had been used earlier in an incomplete formula [63].

11. Parenteral to Oral Therapy: From Glucose for Calories to Glucose–Sodium Coupled Transport

The translational mishaps that marked the historical path toward an I.V. treatment and method reducing cholera CFRs virtually to zero were paralleled by a similarly complicated series of events and non-events characterizing the development of a safe and effective oral therapy for cholera and NDDs [6,7].

The Lancet statement that "The discovery that . . . glucose accelerates absorption of solute and water . . . was potentially the most important medical advance this century" [3] focuses on the scientific advances in understanding of intestinal absorption mechanisms, particularly the co-transport of glucose and sodium ions, enhancing salt and water absorption. The statement reinforces the conventional translational paradigm of bench to bedside, based on the assumption that the in vitro or animal model studies starting from 1959 [64] linking sugar and salt absorption led directly to the demonstration of an oral therapeutic paradigm and method capable of reducing [2,65] or eliminating [66,67] the requirement for I.V. therapy and were the sine qua non of oral therapy's translational success.

In fact, the historical sequence illustrates that empirical clinical observations rather than basic science discoveries led to new pathophysiologic and therapeutic paradigms. Key insights into therapeutic methodology then rescued advances from failures. The prevailing wisdom that oral intake would aggravate diarrhea during the acute phase of illness had to be overcome by the marriage of empirical clinical research and post facto confirmatory basic science to establish that while the accurate therapeutic paradigm remained essential, the key to translational success was not the route of delivery per se, but the absorbability of the delivered fluid and an effective therapeutic methodology ensuring net positive gut balance, i.e., that intake exceeded output.

As early as 1824 in India, where British health workers almost universally advocated bleeding cholera patients and withholding all oral fluids, William Scot [68], considering the latter highly questionable, stated that "are we to pay no attention to the dreadful feeling of thirst, which forms so general and so distressing a symptom of the disease, and are we to disregard the state of the body, robbed, as it evidently is, in most instances, of all its serous and aqueous parts?..." The free use of diluents is indicated by the raging thirst, which prevails, and by the extent of the discharges, which evidently drain the system of a large portion of its serous or watery parts. He recommended tepid diluent fluids such as acidulated water, barley, rice, sago or arrow root decoction, chicken water or beef tea given freely from onset (wine or spirits to be diluted in arrowroot or sago). Rice water or pepper water could obviate caste restrictions on other liquids. Unfortunately, no methods or quantitative advice were included, and he proceeded with recommending the litany of opium, calomel, bleeding, and ipecac.

As noted above, Latta, in 1831–1832, had correctly reported [15] the failure of plain oral (and rectal) saline to benefit cholera patients; and while Stevens had reported its "miraculous" benefits, his work had been discredited, though some continued to believe it.

The first study linking salt with enhanced glucose absorption was published by Reid in 1901 [69] but led to no oral therapy breakthrough, because Reid focused on the increase in glucose absorption in the presence of salt, overlooking the obverse effect of glucose on salt and water absorption. Considering salt entering the lumen to be a sign of deterioration of his dog loop model, he curtailed his studies. There was apparently no awareness that this was the normal role of sodium and chloride in intestinal osmoregulation.

Neither Reid nor anyone in the medical world was studying cholera pathophysiology or new treatments; Rogers' hypertonic saline was soon to become the accepted therapeutic modality. The prevailing colonial order had little or no concern about cholera in the native populations not served by any adequate medical facilities. Mortality from NDDs was very high in the U.S. and Europe at the time, but pediatric therapy was based on avoiding oral intake in the belief that oral intake would aggravate diarrhea during the acute phase of disease. Reid's discovery is an example of how a potentially ground-breaking basic science observation published in a contextual vacuum can lead nowhere.

12. Hospital-Based Use of Oral Electrolyte Solutions with Glucose Added to Boost Caloric Intake

Up to the mid-20th C., pediatric diarrhea therapy included an initial period with no food given for 24 h and often longer. The treatment of cholera recommended by Osler in 1902 has been recorded by Howard-Jones [10]. By 1907, his treatment of pediatric NDDs included alkaline stomach washes with castor oil or calomel purgatives with opioids and chloroform, including laudanum enemas at six hourly intervals [47]—for alkaline stools (then regarded as a sign of protein decomposition), carbohydrates (barley water); and for acid stools, "beef juice". Water and bicarbonate was delivered by mouth or bowel (for acidosis) and normal saline by the slowly absorbed S.C. route, which had highly undesirable effects including pain, infection and tissue damage.

As noted earlier, dietary recommendations per se, though perennially popular, are not equivalent to effective treatments, i.e., use of a given food or solution is not by itself, without a linked effective methodology and proof of maximal reduction in case fatality rates, a harbinger of later medical breakthroughs.

Brown and Boyd [70] in 1922 advocated 12–48 h starvation, allowing oral water, S.C., I.P. and I.V. saline and glucose, and exsanguinating transfusions to remove supposed toxins; CFRs were 39–80%. The ill-defined and inappropriate concept of "infantile intestinal intoxication" long persisted as a clinical misnomer.

Powers in 1926 [71] recommended blood transfusions and starvation up to 12 days. The rationale for blood or plasma transfusions was never clear, but was regarded as a way to correct "shock", actually caused by severe water and electrolyte loss leading to severe dehydration, not by blood loss. Regarding oral fluids, he stated "By mouth ... we give water; we have tried Ringer's solution and 2 to 5% glucose both in water and in Ringer's solution. We have been unable to observe, as yet, any advantage in any solution over water." CFR was 33%.

The fundamentals of pediatric diarrhea therapy for decades remained the withholding of oral intake for a variable period [70–92]. Gamble in 1943 suggested up to 20 days without oral intake and some considered adequate oral intake sometimes impossible even without vomiting [72]. Administration of electrolyte solutions *or* glucose by I.V., slow S.C. or hazardous I.P. routes, along with plasma or whole blood transfusion, was considered standard therapy. Resumption of oral intake could begin after correction of dehydration using parenteral routes, but the lack of knowledge about the role of glucose in intestinal salt absorption led variously to recommendations for oral glucose, plain water, plain saline, half-strength Hartmann's solution, glucose with saline or sucrose with saline [73,76]. Some of these recommendations were potentially harmful by augmenting diarrhea or sodium losses and by aggravating negative nutritional balance. While the non-absorbability during cholera of oral plain saline without glucose was shown in balance studies, such studies were rarely performed in non-cholera pediatric NDDs. Multiple antibiotics were used [84] in the era before rotavirus and other viral enteric pathogens were discovered, despite no benefit for most patients.

Use of oral glucose as part of cholera or NDD treatment continued as a recommendation without provision of objective evidence of caloric or absorptive efficacy or net gut balance studies. Such dietary recommendations, along with many other oral foods or liquids (including oral plain saline without glucose) were unaccompanied by any reproducible method or objective results in terms of reducing or eliminating I.V. fluid requirements or eliminating high CFRs. If vomiting occurred, parenteral infusions were given, often for many days.

There were no descriptions of any therapeutic method of administration linking input to output or reference to any objective evidence of effect on outcomes. Formulaic rules for parenteral therapy in hospitals or rehydration centers were often bewilderingly complex [89].

Powers' recommendations dominated pediatric NDD therapy over five decades, including the inappropriate use of blood transfusions or plasma, which must have spread untold infections with hepatitis C and B and other blood-borne diseases. Liberal use of plain water by mouth or nasogastric tube during the first 48 h risked hyponatremia, and slowly absorbed, painful I.P. and S.C. infusions were easily infected and disfiguring (especially S.C. 5–10% glucose). Treatment often included prolonged starvation and restriction of oral solutions to the mildest cases or in late maintenance largely as a bridge to resumption of diet. Sugars were often omitted from oral electrolyte solutions without determining absorbability without them. Vomiting was widely regarded as an absolute contraindication to oral intake without determining quantity and clinical importance. Antibiotic use was indiscriminate, though few cases involved susceptible microorganisms (rotavirus and other enteric viral pathogens had not yet been discovered.)

The overwhelming concern about vomiting, effect of oral intake on stool volume and the belief in the ameliatory effect of starvation provided a strong negative bias against expansion of oral rehydration and maintenance therapy during diarrhea. Globally, the devastating effect on nutritional status of repeated episodes of starvation therapy on infants experiencing ten or more diarrhea episodes per year was long ignored.

Darrow's influential publications [74,75,79,82,88] employed an initial 2–5 day starvation period, but his I.V. and oral potassium balance studies demonstrated the importance of replacing potassium adequately (still an issue today) but did not include studies of complete oral rehydration or maintenance solutions. Inadequacy of potassium replacement persisted, particularly in areas of widespread potassium deficiency, due partly to reaction to deaths from overaggressive potassium infusion [75]. Through the 1950s and 1960s, parenteral fluids were usually continued for 2 days or occasionally for 3–5 days [90]. Harrison recommended 12 days of parenteral therapy [84], including blood, plasma and I.V. glucose-electrolyte infusions in severely dehydrated cases. CRFs remained relatively high despite reductions with improved parenteral therapy [88]. Withholding of food and oral fluids for variable periods remained part of routine therapy and continued feeding in early diarrhea was considered irrational [86,90] even after the nutritional benefits of early feeding were demonstrated [80,87]. It was stated that "in most cases diarrhea ceases after suspension of oral intake and start of parenteral therapy" [89].

In patients with mild or absent dehydration, most of short duration, almost any oral fluid intake that does not aggravate diarrhea or electrolyte inbalance is safe to recommend, and continued feeding avoids the harmful effects of starvation therapy. The repeated stress on "resting the stomach", "N.P.O", and the like as an essential part of the therapeutic approach to dehydrated pediatric diarrhea patients, and the concern that oral intake would aggravate vomiting and diarrhea placed barriers blocking use of oral rehydration or oral maintenance therapy as initial treatment for patients with profuse dehydrating diarrhea prior to convalescence.

For years after the sugar/sodium transport literature grew, the pediatric literature reflected little or no awareness of the effect of those sugars on intestinal absorption or net gut balance. Sugar concentrations in oral solutions used for caloric purposes were excessively high, leading to complications when absorptive capacity was exceeded [86].

While oral solutions with sugars added for caloric content in convalescent or mild, non-dehydrated patients reportedly began in the U.S. in 1946 [91], oral intake continued to be restricted during early hours of therapy and transfusions of blood, plasma or albumen persisted [90] when dehydration was detected.

In contrast, "oral" (actually almost always nasogastrically administered) solutions were used in South America at least as early as 1943 [93] initially using electrolyte solutions with or *without* sugars, with no balance studies to demonstrate efficacy. As noted above, oral plain electrolyte solutions aggravate cholera, and while not properly studied in pediatric diarrheas before 1968, the same was true in one published case [89]. The rationale in 1943 was partly to avoid the harm resulting from infusions by S.C. and I.P. routes [93].

In the 1950s and 1960s, the use of electrolyte solutions, often but not always with glucose or sucrose added as a source of calories, had wide application in South and Central America [93–101] and So. Africa (102–104), administered chiefly by nasogastric tube to infants with relative mild dehydration. Fixed volumes were given without reference to actual volume of losses. Failures were promptly hospitalized; but even with close supervision, CFRs were as high as 6.3%, compared to under 1% using modern rehydration and maintenance therapy, though a significant improvement over prior local interventions. With 24 h coverage at one hydration center, 20.4% were hospitalized and follow-up revealed a 14% CFR after hospital discharge [99]; 77% were successfully treated by monitoring clinical signs, but 7.4% required re-admission.

Various nasogastric or oral solution formulations were used in addition to I.V. therapy [94,95], the oral fluids ranging from water, to tea, Ringer's or other saline solutions with or without sugar, sugar solutions with low sodium, etc. One formula closely matched one shown effective in modern studies [96,97], albeit using sucrose instead of glucose, sucrose being less effective [98] though usable if glucose is unavailable.

The reliance on gastroclysis necessitated administration in hospitals or special rehydration centers with insufficient staff to cover night and holiday shifts adequately [99]. Patients were intermittently unattended and mothers were on their own for prolonged periods if they were permitted to participate at all. The nasogastric tubes obviated direct maternal control of therapy and required restraining infants by wrapping them in sheets to prevent pulling out nasogastric tubes or turn to a position impeding flow ([99], see Figure 1). Occasional deaths occurred when restrained infants aspirated regurgitated fluids. Complex formulas used to calculate fluid requirements ensured dependence on the medical supervision which was intermittently absent. Actual volumes of diarrheal and vomitus losses usually went unmeasured, nor were intake and output routinely monitored. There was also no published rigorous system of monitoring clinical signs of hydration status on a continuous basis during therapy.

ORAL THERAPY SHEET

TIME	I·V·	ORAL GIVEN	VOMIT	INTAKE MINUS VOMIT	STOOL	GUT NET	CUMULATIVE GUT NET	URINE
11 AM	3	← ADMISSION REHYDRATION (Wt· = 30 Kg·)						
12 NOON	0	START ORAL SOLUTION						
6 PM	0	3	0·5	2·5	2	+0·5	+0·5	0·2
12 MN	0	2	0	2	1·8	+0·2	+0·7	0·25
6 AM	0	2	0	2	1·5	+0·5	+1·2	0·24

Figure 1. ORT I & O SHEET: figures in liters.

Chlorophenothiazine was often used in attempting to control vomiting as a cause of failure, despite a 23% incidence of significant side effects [100]. Antibiotics were given frequently, and it took years to recognize their lack of benefit in most cases [100]. Gastroclysis was never intended for use in severely dehydrated patients for either rehydration or maintenance fluid and electrolyte therapy and was eclipsed by the rapid development of centers relying on I.V. infusions. The use of oral glucose for calories, along with electrolytes beginning after the acute phase, remained essentially a dietary therapeutic recommendation. Lower CFRs were achieved chiefly at centers employing improved use of I.V. electrolyte therapy. The efficacy of gastroclysis relative to patients' degree of dehydration and balance data was never objectively established, though high rates of treatments avoiding parenteral fluids were reported from some centers [99,100]. Attempts to transfer therapy to homes were problematic for infants with profuse diarrhea in the absence of clear guidelines for mothers and depended on elaborate personnel and referral facilities needed to ensure success [95].

In the U.S., distribution of high-sugar commercial formulas and maternal errors in preparing safe solutions led to epidemics of hypernatremia [86,91], and later of hyponatremia due to use of low-sodium (30 mEq/L) oral solutions [92]. Hospitalization for even relatively mild dehydration was far more profitable even when outpatient treatment would have sufficed, and the decreased incidence of severe dehydrating diarrhea diminished staff expertise in its management and triage.

In the U.K. [78], Lawson used oral half-strength Hartmann's solution (no sugar) in the mildest cases, but gave serum I.V. Vomiting was considered an absolute contraindication to oral feeding. CFR was 7%. In South Africa, oral Darrow's solution was given after S.C. infusions [102]. CFR was 14%. Another center [103] used oral or nasogastric half-Darrow's solution with glucose for up to 48 h. CFRs were omitted. Bowie [104] reported a regime of half-strength Darrow's solution in 1.5% dextrose by mouth for 24 h unless vomiting persisted. CFR was, nevertheless, 9.5%.

13. Chatterjee

A widely quoted misinterpretation regarding the origins of modern oral rehydration and maintenance therapy arose from H.N. Chatterjee's 1953 Lancet article [105] titled "Control of vomiting in cholera and oral replacement of fluid." No balance data were presented to establish that net absorption was occurring in the small number of selected convalescent or mildly ill patients treated orally. He described the use of promethazine and chlorotheophylline ("Avomine") to treat vomiting in cholera patients. The patients selected for treatment were those whose condition was "relatively satisfactory". Vomiting stopped after one Avomine tablet in mild cases, and up to six tablets were given to patients whose vomiting persisted 24 h. In modern studies, vomiting stops quickly after rapid rehydration and correction of acidosis in most cases, rarely persisting up to 24 h after admission. So the value of "Avomine" was not in fact established by its uncontrolled use. Chatterjee claimed, however, that Avomine use permitted oral therapy with a hypotonic solution (NaCl 4 g, 25 g glucose and later 2 g KCl per L) by stopping vomiting. Cholera diarrhea, however, continued, for which he gave the juice of crushed leaves of *Coleus aromaticus*, an antidiarrheal folk remedy which is rich in forskolin, a cyclic AMP enhancer [106]. This in theory should aggravate diarrhea as do cholera toxin or VIP, but Chatterjee claimed it controlled the diarrhea, permitting oral therapy. (No controlled clinical trial confirming his claims was performed.) He stated that 33 mild cases among 1093 cholera patients (3%) were successfully treated using this tripartite regimen and an additional 153 moderately severe cases received oral and *rectally* administered glucose-saline solution. Only 17% of the 1093 cholera patients received no I.V. therapy, the majority of his patients receiving only I.V. therapy. As there is no evidence that rectal glucose-saline solutions have any beneficial effect in cholera, his reported success, with no balance data, probably was due to his choice of mildly ill patients rather than his treatment regimen. His solution contained 68 mEq/L Na$^+$ vs. 133 in adult cholera stool.

Without balance data, the amount of net absorption of Chatterjee's oral solution is unknown. His report is anecdotal rather than evidentiary, even for his selected non-severe patients. His choice of glucose was not based on any effect on intestinal absorption, as such data did not appear until 1959 [64].

Separately [107], he reported that antibiotics, including tetracyclines, did not check the diarrhea or reduce mortality in cholera (proof that antibiotics did in fact shorten cholera diarrhea duration and volume appeared later). Therefore, he gave crude juice from *Coleus aromaticus* to 200 cholera patients whose diarrhea stopped within 24 h in 40%, 48 h in 74% and 72 h in 92.5%. Controls (every 6th case) received kaolin and bismuth suspension, and their diarrhea stopped within 24 h in 55%, 48 h in 12.5% and 73 h in 30%. Both groups received routine treatment of shock, presumably with I.V. therapy. Patients also received antihistamines (then believed protective against uremia) and vitamin C. Whether the *Coleus* extract had an antidiarrheal or antibacterial effect remains unknown; Chatterjee noted that it caused an early appearance of rough colonies of *V. cholerae*, whereas smooth colonies persisted in the control group.

14. The Translational Steps Leading to Modern Oral Rehydration and Maintenance Therapy

The advance to a successful practical oral rehydration and maintenance therapy has been meticulously recorded by Joshua Ruxin based on tape recordings of all the principle workers involved in its evolution [108]. This documents the essential links between empirical and laboratory basic science and the crucial role of clinical insight and methodology. A brief summary with some additional details will illustrate some parallels between the evolution of I.V. and oral treatments for cholera and NDDs.

In the early 1960s, Phillips and coworkers measured changes in net diarrheal losses during intestinal perfusion of plain saline in cholera patients and found it unabsorbable [109]. This was consistent with the paralyzed sodium pump theory of cholera pathophysiology. Potassium and bicarbonate were found to be absorbable during cholera. He reported that plain water was also absorbable, but this observation was possibly incorrect, based on mistaken interpretation of the finding that the patients given plain water to drink developed a slight increase in urinary output of low sp.gr.

Given the derangement of intestinal osmoregulation by cholera toxin demonstrated in the dog cholera model [110], hypotonic intestinal saline solutions are not absorbable, but their luminal tonicity is adjusted by increased plasma to lumen sodium chloride secretion. In cholera patients, this leads rapidly to marked negative sodium and chloride balance. Resulting hyponatremia triggers ADH suppression and consequent increased hypoosmolar urine output [111] that Phillips took as proof of water absorption. His studies had shown major net sodium losses and rising plasma sp.gr. during intestinal plain water perfusions [109]. Thus, the extent, if any, of plain water absorption during cholera remains an open question. His statement that a patient drinking water was maintained in water balance is contradicted by the rise in plasma sp.gr. during the oral period.

Phillips then added glucose to the perfused saline solution and observed for the first time that the glucose was absorbed and induced a reduction in the net rate of sodium ion losses, indicating that the coupled glucose-saline transport mechanism was not inactivated in cholera [16]. According to several sources [108] and as Phillips stated [16], his choice of glucose to add to plain saline solutions for intestinal perfusion of cholera patients was to determine the intestinal response to raising the saline solution tonicity with a nonelectrolyte. The effect of glucose on water absorption was not mentioned, since he believed that plain water was absorbable by itself in cholera [109].

Phillips' observations in the early 1960s were made at the very beginning of what afterwards became a vast literature on coupled substrate/sodium absorption, but little had been published at the time, and the early studies were in vitro and in animal models, published in journals unlikely to have been available to NAMRU-2 in Taipei, since in those days journals arrived many months late. His early work omitted those references, suggesting, as he indicated, that his glucose observation was empirical, exploratory, investigational and open ended. After observing the decreased net salt losses accompanying the addition of glucose to the saline perfusions, he proposed a new therapeutic paradigm: to use glucose to *stop* the cholera diarrhea by promoting reabsorption of intestinal luminal fluid. The question of the ongoing effects of cholera toxin on the intestinal mucosa was not addressed:

"We also demonstrated that dextrose when given by mouth is absorbed and in its absorption sodium and chloride ions are absorbed along with water, with an amelioration of the diarrhea. This is a dose-dependent response but unfortunately, if sufficient dextrose is given to *stop the diarrhea* (italics mine), most patients develop nausea and vomiting. Thus the hope for a simple method of treating cholera by this procedure did not materialize." [112]. Translational progress was derailed by a faulty therapeutic paradigm: he believed that glucose could promote absorption to such an extent as to *stop* the cholera diarrhea abruptly; patients would reabsorb their own diarrhea fluid. Intake and output measurements would be obviated, along with the need for medical staff, hospitals and I.V. fluids. To achieve this, he devised a highly concentrated glucose and electrolyte solution to be given to acute phase cholera patients by oral or nasogastric routes.

Though he was later characterized by some as uninterested in practical applications and in pursuit of only basic science goals [108], he was in fact eager to test the glucose finding a potential treatment breakthrough, and sent a team to test the concentrated glucose and saline solution during a cholera outbreak in the Philippines.

The Philippine trial was a failure, and 5 of some 30 patients died. Deaths were attributed by a visiting observer to cardiopulmonary decompensation from overhydration due to combined absorption of the oral or nasogastric solution plus continued excessive I.V. infusions [108]. A likely precipitating factor was massive net water loss into the intestinal lumen precipitated by the hyperosmolar concentrated solution used. The defect in osmoregulation of luminal contents in cholera, in which hypertonic solutions are adjusted chiefly by rapid luminal influx of water [110], was not yet identified.

Ironically, Phillips, whose work led to the modern I.V. therapy of cholera based on balance studies and intake and output measurements, had not conceived of the alternative paradigm of using an isotonic oral glucose-electrolyte solution for replacing ongoing losses of water and electrolyte balance after correcting shock with I.V. rehydration fluids (or rehydrating and maintaining patients not in shock with the oral solution alone).

The most likely reason for this failure was Phillips' assumption that the solution would stop the diarrhea by causing patients to reabsorb their own rice water fluid [112]. The alternative of having patients drink up to 100 L of an absorbable solution to replace their fluid losses must have been viewed, if at all, as impossible to implement in most cholera-affected areas, which had no medical personnel, supplies and equipment to implement the matching principle. The possible solution of tying the amount of oral solution to be imbibed to the patient's clinical signs of hydration status was not then considered. Another factor may have been his adherence to the theory of the paralyzed sodium pump theory of cholera pathophysiology [113]: if glucose freed up the paralyzed pump, it might stop the diarrhea. However, glucose was not an antidote in the traditional sense; it could enhance salt and water absorption to replace diarrheal losses, not stop them.

Importantly, the adjuvant value of antibiotics in shortening the duration of cholera had not yet been discovered. Many antibiotic trials had "failed" due to flawed designs in which mortality was the endpoint in studies in which fluid and electrolyte therapy was inadequate. In that setting, the value of adequate antibiotics could not be revealed. Only after the use of tetracycline (and later other appropriate antibiotics) along with rehydration and maintenance I.V. therapy was tested in 1964 could the shortening of diarrhea from a mean of 1.8 down to 0.8 days be revealed [114,115]. Before this beneficial effect of antibiotic therapy on cholera duration was demonstrated, the prospect of up to 9 days of large volume oral therapy probably seemed unachievable.

Phillips' research strategy was notable for n of 1 studies, which he used effectively when studying basic physiological functions which varied little between subjects. If the result came up positive, a larger confirmatory study could be performed; if negative, further studies would await additional supportive data. Many of his cholera studies were performed on one or two subjects.

In 1965, Love at NAMRU II, using the n of 1 approach, referenced the active transport literature and reported that in the rabbit ileal loop cholera model, net water and salt absorption followed use of a glucose-containing electrolyte solution, noting the apparent contradiction of the sodium pump paralysis concept [116]. He also used the solution orally in a single (relatively mildly ill) cholera patient to demonstrate brief achievement of net positive gut balance. Love mentioned the therapeutic potential, but his report did not lead to renewed interest in a clinical trial based on the new principle, suggesting that the negative aftermath of the failed Philippine clinical trial persisted.

The shock of the failed trial was traumatic enough to bias Phillips against allowing any further attempt to develop an oral therapy for cholera, and there the matter might well have ended had David Sachar not arrived on the scene to serendipitously revive interest in the glucose issue that Phillips had serendipitously discovered.

As Ruxin noted [108], Sachar and Hirschhorn were among the series of young investigators sent abroad to conduct research on diseases which were of military importance. At the time, such assignments at NIH in the Public Health Service satisfied the requirement for military service during the Vietnam war. Sachar's study in cholera patients would extend Love's findings in the rabbit model and one cholera patient and would again test Phillips' theory that cholera resulted from paralysis of "the sodium pump". He trained to measure intestinal transmural electrical potentials at Ussing's lab in Denmark, and arrived with an apparatus to do so in cholera patients. When glucose or galactose was added to the luminal saline solution, an increased potential appeared, indicating sodium absorption [117]. Hirschhorn, observing Sachar's results, recognized the potential importance of this finding beyond the conflict it created with the paralyzed sodium pump theory, and asked Phillips' permission to study it further. Phillips had, after publishing the brief mention of the glucose effect in 1964 [16], suppressed information about the failed Philippine oral therapy trial and withheld approval, sharing with Hirschhorn the failed Philippine ORT trial as an indication that the oral route would never be safe or effective.

However, Hirschhorn convinced a reluctant Phillips to permit a further study not for any therapeutic goal, but to explore further the absorption of glucose and other sugars in cholera patients. Communications exchanged between the investigators at the PSCRL, Dacca (now Dhaka) and the Johns Hopkins Center for Medical Research and Training (JHCMRT), Calcutta (now Kolkata) led to a study confirming achievement of positive net gut balance during glucose-electrolyte perfusion periods, as Love had shown in a single patient. The link to the transport literature was now firm Hirschhorn was about to return home, as were the lead ICMRT investigators, and the final translational step remained uncertain and unrealized.

At the 1967 U.S.–Japan cholera conference in Los Altos, brief abstracts of the two groups' findings were presented, stating that: "Glucose and galactose (two sugars associated with the enhanced active transport of sodium) markedly reduce the stool output in actively purging cholera patients when given by mouth along with isotonic electrolyte solution in large quantities" [118].

Actually, it was net diarrhea fluid losses, not stool output per se that was reduced, and the sugar-electrolyte solutions were given not by mouth but solely by nasogastric or intestinal tubing. Net positive gut balance was not actually mentioned.

The ICMRT abstract stated that "Significant absorption of water, glucose and electrolytes was observed which varied with glucose concentration" [119]. It is notable that nothing but these two brief abstracts were published or made available in draft form before the successful spring 1968 oral maintenance trial in Dhaka was complete.

In final published form in July, 1968, the findings were summarized somewhat differently: "The rate of intestinal fluid loss was decreased significantly . . . .when electrolyte solutions containing glucose were administered intragastrically or into the intestine for periods of 12 to 32 h [120]" and "A study of patients with severe cholera has demonstrated absorption of glucose and a definite improvement in net water and electrolyte balance during intragastric infusion of glucose-electrolyte solution. In most patients studied, water, electrolyte and acid-base balance were maintained satisfactorily for 12 h (out of a total 48 h study period) solely by the intragastric infusion of glucose-electrolyte solution." [121]. The two reports concluded that "further investigation of the role [of oral solutions] was warranted but cautioned that intravenous solutions remain the mainstay of the successful treatment of cholera" [120], and "The results suggest that oral glucose therapy could be of value in the treatment of cholera and that the requirement for expensive and scarce I.V. fluids may be reduced thereby" [121]. The possibility that the findings might have significance for NDDs beyond cholera was not mentioned.

In sum, the studies of Hirschhorn, Pierce and co-workers confirmed and expanded Phillips' earlier report of the glucose effect in cholera patients, but did not constitute or demonstrate the efficacy of oral or nasogastric fluids for eliminating the need for intravenous maintenance or rehydration therapy. This time the added linkage to the factor of the "intact" (vide infra) active transport mechanism of sodium, and with it chloride and water, during cholera when glucose was present shifted the therapeutic paradigm from stopping the diarrhea to diminishing the net fluid and electrolyte losses by infusing glucose plus electrolyte solutions via intragastric or intraintestinal tubes. The losses were still huge and prolonged, and it was not clear how this would become a useful practical treatment.

Oral therapy per se did not yet exist, since both Hirschhorn and Pierce and colleagues had kept patients on I.V. fluid drips during the study, and the study periods with gastric or intestinal perfusion via plastic tubes were alternated with lengthy periods of I.V. maintenance therapy. Neither report included the volumes of I.V. fluids the patients received. Patients' fluid losses were huge and long-lasting, and the problem of vomiting and the methodological context remained unresolved issues. Importantly, Hirschhorn, Pierce and colleagues had shifted away from the therapeutic paradigm of stopping the diarrhea, while illuminating a broader range of responses to sugars in cholera patients. Demonstration of the (clinical bedside) success of oral rehydration or maintenance therapy per se and proofs of efficacy and of effectiveness in the field were still awaited, but without Hirschhorn's and Fierce's finding that intragastric glucose-electrolytes infusions improved sodium absorption and net water and salt balance during cholera, Phillips' finding that glucose did not stop the diarrhea might have kept the oral therapy concept buried as a few lines in the literature, as quoted above.

In recent years, it has been found that substrate-enhanced active sodium transport in cholera is not merely intact as previously thought, but is in fact *increased* [122]. This fascinating paradox of increased absorption of sugars (and some amino acids) enhancing active transport of salt and, with it, water during the most profound diarrhea, arising from chloride secretion linked by the cystic fibrosis transmembrane regulator (CFTR), awaits further research in the quest for a therapeutic intervention capable of quickly stopping cholera diarrhea, as sought from O'Shaughnessy's to Phillips' time and today.

The fall of 1967 arrived with a unique absence of cholera in Dacca (now Dhaka). PSCRL staff, equipment and supplies were moved to Malumghat, between Chittagong and Cox's Bazaar to help manage a cholera outbreak near the Christian Memorial Hospital located there. On arrival, we found the wards empty; local mullahs had warned the affected Muslim village populations against entering the Christian hospital, claiming the "sign of the pig" would be put on their foreheads. As cholera was seen as always fatal, they were persuaded to let their beloved family members die in the huts. Dr. Zahidul Haque, a Chittagonian dialect speaker, joined a visit to the affected villages to convince the elders to permit treatment of their affected family members. Ultimately, convincing them necessitated starting I.V.s in the huts, demonstrating, as Latta had described, the apparent miracle of the almost dead rising back to life within minutes. The hospital wards soon filled up [123].

The former Director General of Health of East Pakistan, Dr. Fahimuddin, led a visit to the local thana (police station) to check the scope of the epidemic. The officer in charge was relaxing with his feet crossed up on his desk. As Fahimuddin had a quiet, unassuming manner, the officer did not budge until we informed him who Fahimuddin was, upon which he hastily jumped to his feet and nervously asked how he could assist us. His response to Fahimuddin's question as to the extent of cholera in the area was to insist that there was none, though we had been treating patients there. This gave immediate insight into the total lack of reporting of cases and the absence of any governmental will, compassion, organizational ability and resources to prevent cholera deaths. The thought of the patients dying unattended in their village huts reinforced the urgency of developing a treatment that would overcome the factors preventing life-saving medical care from reaching them: cost, non-availability of supplies, lack of trained personnel and governmental inaction. It could be available in every village Additionally, if it worked in cholera, it would work in all the less profuse, albeit lethal NDDs affecting both children and adults.

No publication on the glucose effect in cholera was yet available except Phillips' original observation and the brief abstracts presented at Palo Alto. However, Rafiqul Islam, a PSCRL staff clinician, had authored a protocol to be implemented at the Malumghat hospital, of the feasibility of a nasogastrically administered glucose solution whose electrolyte composition, though low in potassium, approximated that of cholera diarrhea. The version implemented differed in minor details from the version included in the PSCRL 1967 Technical Committee Report [124]. The method, apparently adopted from that used in Hirschhorn's study, was flawed in that patients were given fixed quantities of the solution with no matching between volumes of losses and of oral fluid intake. After intravenous fluids corrected shock, patients who lost a liter per hour but were given the fixed volume of 500 or 750 mL of oral solution per hour (depending on weight) became rapidly dehydrated and slipped back towards shock, necessitating termination of the study. Patients who lost 250 mL per hour but received 500–750 mL per hour of oral solution soon became edematous due to overhydration. This was the second oral therapy study to fail, due partly to the idea that only a highly simplified method, requiring only a fixed oral dose with the fewest measurements or clinical skills, could possibly be useful. Even though the annual increases in patient admissions to the cholera hospital's wards in Dhaka had reached levels challenging the ability of the hospital to meet I.V. fluid production needs, the use of oral maintenance therapy as a means of drastically reducing those needs remained unrealized.

When the trial was terminated, careful review of the data made the pattern of failure evident: underhydration, overhydration, underhydration, overhydration . . . yielding the insight that oral therapy *had* to work if only a method of matching the losses with equal volumes of an oral glucose plus electrolytes solution closely matching the electrolyte composition of cholera diarrhea was used. Being new to cholera and having just mastered basic intake and output monitoring of cholera patients, using Watten cots and I.V. therapy with 5-4-1 solution for both rehydration and maintenance, the crucial oral therapeutic methodology fell into place. A new revised oral maintenance therapy protocol was drafted using a matching volumes method.

Patients either drank the solution or received it or by nasogastric tube: the results were the same, showing that nasogastric tubes were unnecessary. Intravenous needs of the most severely dehydrated patients in shock were reduced by 80%. Subsequent studies showed that most patients with non-cholera diarrheas could be rehydrated and maintained with oral fluids alone, using the new methodology. Vomiting, which had posed a psychological barrier to oral intake, proved to constitute in the majority of patients an insignificant fluid volume, not a barrier to positive fluid balance, at this stage of disease. Future training in ORT technique would focus on this point.

The translational development of an absorbable oral solution and an effective methodology of administering it addressed the persistent unavailability of the intravenous fluids and therapeutic methodology (persisting even today as reflected by the CFRs in some recent cholera and AWD outbreaks). Eight years passed from Phillips' first observation that cholera patients' intestine could absorb oral saline if glucose was present to the first translation into an effective therapeutic method was published in the Lancet 17 August 1968 [3]. Further studies proved that most cholera and NDD patients not in shock, and even those with severe dehydration and moderate hypotension [9,66,67,125–127] could be rehydrated and maintained using oral glucose-electrolytes solutions alone. Today, over 90% of patients can be rehydrated and maintained with ORT alone. An exception is patients early in the course of severe cholera with early massive vomiting [128].

The development of modern oral glucose-electrolyte rehydration and maintenance therapy as initial treatment, and the completion of treatment within a relatively short period, radically altered therapy and made it possible to extend it beyond hospitals and treatment centers into homes.

The final translational breakthrough was the realization that volume of oral intake had to match volume of losses. Since, with tetracycline, diarrhea volume decreased in each successive 4–6 h monitoring period, matching previous periods' losses ensured positive gut net water and electrolyte balance and maintenance of hydration (Figure 1).

Treatment monitoring forms were used in the pivotal first successful oral therapy study using an ORS averaging the adult and pediatric cholera stool electrolyte compositions [2]. After correction of shock with initial I.V. rehydration, patient received the oral glucose-saline solution to drink. Diarrhea and vomitus volumes were measured using Watten cots, calibrated stool buckets and bedside basins. Volume of oral solution to drink was matched to volume of losses in the previous 4 or 6 h intake and output (I & O) period. Tetracycline given orally after rehydration ensured duration would average 32 h [114,115], during which gut net balance (oral solution volume imbibed minus diarrheal losses in the bucket) was monitored. (Other antibiotics can be used based on vibrio antimicrobial sensitivities, particularly for children.)

Note that the I & O record shows that matching the volume oF ORS to drink to the volume of losses in the previous I & O period results in sustained positive net gut balance, since cholera diarrhea volume decreases with successive I & O periods when adjuvant antibacterials are given. In most cases, vomitus losses proved negligible compared to diarrhea losses.

In retrospect, this seems an obvious conclusion, already employed for intravenous therapy, but it had escaped a series of investigators skilled in the field, due in part to the magnitude of losses, the exaggerated fear of vomiting compared to actual vomitus losses of patients at this stage of their disease, the hesitation to accept the feasibility of using such a method outside of the hospital orbit, and the bias towards attempts to stop rather than replace the outflow of water and salts. The traditional framework of hospital-based rather than home-based treatment also played a role.

The matching principle employed an ORS formulation containing electrolyte concentrations close to those in cholera stool. Use of lower concentrations requires cholera patients to drink volumes exceeding losses, to avoid electrolyte imbalances, a method that may exceed patients' drinking capacity and possibly raise risk of overhydration. For use in pediatric NDDs, the 2:1 ratio of oral solution intake to water was successful in many studies, while avoiding (and even treating) clinically significant hypernatremia or hyponatremia [98,125–127].

The puzzle of how to successfully extend such a therapy to patients at home and before dehydration became clinically significant depended on a method of using the therapeutic paradigm and effectively adapting it to clinical signs and symptoms of hydration status recognizable by mothers, enabling them to use the ORS successfully at home. It could reach every village. Additionally, if it worked in cholera, it would work in all the less profuse, albeit lethal non-cholera AWDs affecting both children and adults.

A successful large field trial conducted at the rudimentary Matlab Bazaar field treatment center using paramedical workers and nurses [65] set the stage for the use of oral rehydration and maintenance therapy in a epidemic of cholera (79% in one sample of 100 patients) and cholera-like ADWDs under disaster conditions. Indira Gandhi's office was notified of the potential for the new ORT method to ameliorate the cholera epidemic then in the refugee camps near Kolkata during the 1971 refugee crisis in India precipitated by the Bangladesh independence war, and forwarded the information to the Indian Ministry of Health on or before 21 June 1971 [129]. Shortly afterwards, Dilip Mahalanabis and colleagues arrived and utilized the WHO formulation of ORS (90 mEq Na^+) to save many cholera patients' lives in the camps with limited amounts of I.V. fluid available, extending the use of oral maintenance to using family members and paramedicals to keep patients drinking, and oral rehydration alone in milder cases. CFR was 3.6% among 3700 patients treated, compared to an estimated 30% in the camps in general [130].

The success in treating the 3700 refugees (79% confirmed cholera in 100 sampled) helped secure the strong support of the WHO, UNICEF, the USAID to mount a global ORT program with enormous impact. Adaptation of the ORT method was extended to less profuse but still often fatal NDDs in hospitals, field treatment centers and in homes with a strong emphasis on effective maternal instruction and substituting monitoring of clinical signs of hydration status for intake and output measurements [131].

Annual mortality from diarrheal diseases among under-5-year-olds fell from five million to under 500,000 by 2018 [6,7].

15. Conclusions

What does the review of the history of development of I.V. and oral rehydration and maintenance therapy tell us about translational medicine? Among the factors blocking translational success were the entrenched erroneous concepts and opinions regarding pathophysiologic and therapeutic paradigms and their undue establishment in the medical literature, which, even in the modern era, has been noted to contain a significant proportion of erroneous information [132].

Lapses in clinical methodology also negated correct paradigms, some of them, in retrospect, seemingly simple and obvious. Just as the need to replace water and electrolyte losses orally with volumes of glucose-electrolyte solutions matching those of the preceding I & O period was missed, so was the necessity for maintenance I.V. fluids to prevent recurrent dehydration and shock in the 19th C. development of I.V. therapy, due probably to the prevalent misconception of cholera as a "three-stage" disease terminating in "collapse".

Clinical science was ahead of the as yet unborn sciences of microbiology and biomedical engineering, referred to by Howard-Jones as the "interdependence" of the different branches of science. This posed the anti-translational barriers of sepsis and air emboli.

The effect of serendipitous empirical observations such as Phillips' glucose findings revealed a mechanism allowing intestinal absorption in cholera patients, bringing science to the bedside. However, a faulty therapeutic paradigm interrupted translational progress.

The science of active transport, though not in the historical chain of events leading to Phillips' initial observation of the glucose effect was nonetheless influential in sustaining support for the rationale of oral rehydration and maintenance therapy, even though the heightening of this effect above normal levels in cholera was not recognized until oral therapy was already widely used.

Active transport research also led directly to testing amino acids [17] and other substrates and optimizing electrolyte and substrate concentrations in the ongoing quest for an ORS capable of reducing duration and volume of diarrhea.

Realization of the social and societal consequences of centuries of neglect of the population at risk played a role in the prioritization of the effort to develop an inexpensive and readily available oral therapy, and helped overcome the relatively low priority given applied medicine relative to basic science in the research establishment.

Lastly, the completion of the revolution in diarrhea therapy was the result of translational "side effects", including abandonment of traditionally recommended but unnecessary blood and blood product transfusions, reduced harm associated with I.V. therapy (multiple venepunctures, need for restraints, overhydration with edema, infection and thromboemboli) and the transfer from hospital/treatment center to home therapy. Additionally the traditional use of oral electrolytes without substrates and of high calorie-oriented glucose or sucrose concentrations prolonging diarrhea and electrolyte imbalance was phased out.

16. Afterword

The decimation of annual under 5 AWD deaths from 5 million to approximately half a million by 2020 [6,7] was achieved with the original WHO Oralyte formulation containing 90 mEq/L of sodium. The Oralyte formulation was adaptable for treatment of both cholera and NDD patients, both adults and children, the former when patients drank one and one half times their fluid losses and the latter matching losses using the 2:1 method [9].

Regretfully, the excellent global track record of highly satisfactory effectiveness and safety has undergone retro-translational alterations, and the historical tendency toward "innovations" as "improvements" has resulted in altering the original WHO ORS formulation to a "low" sodium formulation inadequate to maintain sodium balance in cholera patients, in whom the "low-sodium ORS" confers no benefit but has potential for harm from sodium depletion [9]. Its safety in cholera and NDDs has been inadequately studied [9]. Where antibiotic-resistant *V. cholerae* are prevalent, diarrhea persists for 9–10 days and patients receiving oral or nasogastric replacement with the low-sodium ORS will develop severe and life-threatening sodium losses. The low-sodium ORS for cholera and severe NDDs puts at risk the global translational benefits achieved for both cholera and pediatric severe NDDs with the original single Oralyte ORS formulation. A more rational modification, if one were deemed necessary, would be to promote two different ORS formulations, one for cholera and one for NDDs.

Funding: This research received no external funding.

Institutional Review Board Statement: Not applicable.

Informed Consent Statement: N.A. Ethical review and approval were waived for this study since it is purely a historical review.

Acknowledgments: The work of the WHO, UNICEF, the USAID, the BRAC and dedicated national government health ministries resulting in the use of ORT to bring annual under 5 diarrheal deaths from five million to some 500,000 between 1978 and 2021 is a monumental success of public health in the 21st century.

Conflicts of Interest: The author declares no conflict of interest.

References

1. Rosenfeld, L. Cholera, acidosis and fluid-electrolyte therapy in 1832 Chapter VIII. In *Four Centuries of Clinical Chemistry*; Gordon and Breach Science: Singapore, 1999; pp. 151–155.
2. Nalin, D.; Cash, R.; Islam, R.; Molla, M.; Phillips, R. Oral Maintenance Therapy for Cholera in Adults. *Lancet* **1968**, *292*, 370–372. [CrossRef]
3. Series, E. Water with sugar and salt. *Lancet* **1978**, *2*, 300–301.
4. Howard-Jones, N. Cholera nomenclature and nosology: A historical note. *Bull. World Heal. Organ.* **1974**, *51*, 317–324.
5. Marie, A.; Roos, E. Biomedicine and Health: Galen and Humoral Theory. In *Scientific Thought*; Lerner, K.L., Lerrer, B.W., Eds.; Gale: Farmington Hills, MI, USA, 2009.
6. Nalin, D.R.; Cash, R.A. 50 years of oral rehydration therapy: The solution is still simple. *Lancet* **2018**, *392*, 536–538. [CrossRef]
7. Glass, R. Oral rehydration therapy for diarrheal disease: A 50 year perspective. *JAMA* **2018**, *320*, 865–866. [CrossRef]
8. Woodward, J.J. Treatment of diarrhea and dysentery. In *Medical and Surgical History of the War of the Rebellion*; Gov't. Printing Office: Washington, DC, USA, 1879; Volume 1, pp. 666–667, Second issue; Chapt. 1, Section iv.
9. Nalin, D. Issues and Controversies in the Evolution of Oral Rehydration Therapy (ORT). *Trop. Med. Infect. Dis.* **2021**, *6*, 34. [CrossRef] [PubMed]
10. Howard-Jones, S.N. Cholera therapy in the 19TH century. *J. Hist. Med.* **1972**, 373–395. Available online: https://archive.org/details/b22334671/page/34/mode/2up (accessed on 12 March 2022).
11. Editorial. *Lancet* **1831**, *2*, 285.
12. Stevens, W. *Observations on the Healthy and Diseased Properties of the Blood*; J. Murray: London, UK, 1832; p. 504.
13. Stevens, W. *Observations on the Nature and the Treatment of the Asiatic Cholera*; Hippolyte Bailliere: London, UK, 1853; p. 475.
14. Hermann, R. Considerations sur la nature et sur le traitement du cholera Analyses Chimiques (pp. 1–40) and Quelques considerations sur la nature et sur le traitement du cholera, pp. 41–149. In *Rapport Sur le Cholera-Morbus de Moscou*; Markus, F.C.M., Ed.; Auguste Semen: Moscow, Russia, 1832; p. 153, Nabu public domain reprints, USA.
15. Latta, T. Saline venous injection in cases of malignant cholera performed while in the vapour-bath. *Lancet* **1832**, *2*, 208–209. [CrossRef]
16. Phillips, R.A. Water and Electrolyte Losses in Cholera. *Fed. Proc.* **1964**, *23*, 705–712.
17. Nalin, D.R.; Cash, R.A.; Rahaman, M.; Yunus, M. Effect of glycine and glucose on sodium and water absorption in patients with cholera. *Gut* **1970**, *11*, 768–772. [CrossRef] [PubMed]
18. Speelman, P.; Butler, T.; Kabir, I.; Ali, A.; Banwell, J. Colonic dysfunction during cholera infection. *Gastroenterology* **1986**, *91*, 1154–1170. [CrossRef]
19. Torres-pinedo, R.; Conde, E.; Robillard, G.; Maldonado, M. Studies on infant diarrhea. III. Changes in composition of saline and glucose-saline solutions instilled into the colon. *Pediatrics* **1968**, *42*, 303–311. [CrossRef] [PubMed]
20. Daly, W.J.; DuPont, H.L. The controversial and short-lived early use of rehydration therapy for cholera. *Clin. Infect. Dis.* **2008**, *47*, 1315–1319. [CrossRef]
21. Finberg, L. The early history of the treatment for dehydration. *Arch. Pediatr. Adolesc. Med.* **1998**, *152*, 71–73. [CrossRef]
22. Lamontagne, F.; Fowler, R.A.; Adhikari, N.K.; Murthy, S.; Brett-Major, D.M.; Jacobs, M.; Uyeki, T.M.; Vallenas, C.; Norris, S.L.; Fletcher, T.E.; et al. Evidence-based guidelines for supportive care of patients with Ebola virus disease. *Lancet* **2018**, *391*, 700–708. [CrossRef]
23. Johnson, S. Stevens's experiments on the blood. *Lancet* **1831**, *17*, 376–378. [CrossRef]
24. Jaehnichen, F. Quelques considerations sur la nature et sur le traitement du cholera. In *Rapport Sur le Cholera Morbus de Moscou*; Markus, F.C.M., Ed.; Auguste Semen: Moscou, Russia, 1832; p. 153, Nabu public domain reprints.
25. Afroze, F.; Bloom, S.; Bech, P.; Ahmed, T.; Alam Sarker, S.; Clemens, J.D.; Islam, F.; Nalin, D. Cholera and pancreatic cholera: Is VIP the common pathophysiologic factor? *Trop. Med. Infect. Dis.* **2020**, *5*, 111. [CrossRef] [PubMed]
26. Weissbach, H.; King, W.; Sjoerdsma, A.; Udenfriend, S. Formation of Indole-3-acetic acid and tryptamine in animals: A method for estimation of indole-3-acetic acid in tissues. *J. Biol. Chem.* **1959**, *234*, 81–88. [CrossRef]
27. O'Shaughnessy, W.B. Proposal of a new method of treating the blue epidemic cholera by the injection of highly-oxygenated salts into the venous system. *Lancet* **1831**, *17*, 366–371. [CrossRef]
28. O'Shaughnessy, W.B. Experiments on the blood in cholera. *Lancet* **1831**, *17*, 490. [CrossRef]
29. Watten, R.H.; Morgan, F.M.; Songkhla, Y.; Vanikiati, B.; Phillips, R.A. Water and electrolyte studies in cholera. *J. Clin. Investig.* **1959**, *38*, 1879–1889. [CrossRef] [PubMed]
30. O'Shaughnessy, W.B. Note from Dr. O'Shaughnessy. *Lancet* **1831**, *2*, 281.

31. Lewins, R. Injection of saline solutions in extraordinary quantities into the veins in cases of malignant cholera. *Lancet* **1832**, *18*, 243–244. [CrossRef]
32. Greig, E.D.W. The treatment of cholera by intravenous saline injections; with particular reference to the contributions of Dr. Thomas Aitchison Latta of Leith (1832). *Edinb. Med. J.* **1946**, *53*, 256–263. [PubMed]
33. Moon, J.B. Doctors afield. Sir William Brooke O'Shaughnessy—The foundations of fluid therapy and the indian telegraph service. *NEJM* **1967**, *276*, 283–284. [CrossRef] [PubMed]
34. Marsden, W. *Symptoms and Treatment of Malignant Diarrhea: Better Known by the Name of Asiatic or Malignant Cholera, as Treated in the Royal Free Hospital during the Years 1832, 1833, 1834, 1848 and 1854*; Henry Renshaw: London, UK, 1865; Nabu Public Domain Reprints 2021.
35. Olmstead, J.D. François Magendie: Pioneer in Experimental Physiology and Scientific Medicine in XIX Century France. *J. Nerv. Ment. Dis.* **1947**, *105*, 97.
36. Broussais, F.J.V. *Le Cholera-Morbus Epidemique, Observe et Traite Selon la Methode Physiologique*; Delaunay: Paris, France, 1832.
37. Dodin, A.; Brossollet, J. Therapeutiques au cours de l'epidemie de cholera de 1832. *Bull. Societe Pathologie Exotique* **1971**, *64*, 613–623.
38. Sellards, A.W. Tolerance for alkalies in Asiatic cholera. *Phil. J. Sci.* **1910**, *5*, 363–390.
39. Wall, A.J. *Asiatic Cholera: Its History, Pathology and Modern Treatment*; Forgotten Books: London, UK, 1893.
40. Lewis, D. Alkaline remedies in malignant cholera. *Lancet* **1832**, *19*, 22. [CrossRef]
41. Guspenski, D.M. Le Traitement du cholera asiatique par des injections sous-cutanees de l'emulsion testiculaire. *C. R. Soc. Biol.* **1892**, *4*, 321–326.
42. Jameson, J. *Report on the Epidemic Cholera Morbus as it Visited the Territories Subject to the Presidency of Bengal in the Years 1817, 1818 and 1819*; Government Gazette Press Calcutta: Calcutta, India, 1820; p. 245.
43. Parkin, J. *The Antidotal Treatment of the Epidemic Cholera*, 4th ed.; David Bogue: London, UK, 1883; pp. 165–173, Kessinger Legacy Reprints.
44. Friedrichs, R. Who Discovered Vibrio Cholera? Available online: https://www.ph.ucla.edu/epi/snow/firstdiscoveredcholera.html (accessed on 3 March 2022).
45. Stockwell, G.A. *Cholera: Its Protean Aspects and Its Management*; Davis: Detroit, MI, USA, 1893; Volume 2, p. 151. Classic Reprint Series; Forgotten Books, FB and C LTD, London 2015.
46. Pollitzer, R. *Cholera*; WHO Monograph Series No. 43; WHO: Geneva, Switzerland, 1959; p. 782.
47. Osler, W. *Principles and Practice of Medicine*, 6th ed.; Appletons: New York, NY, USA, 1907.
48. Nichols, H.J.; Andrews, V.L. The Treatment of Asiatic Cholera during the Recent Epidemic. *Philipp. J. Sci. Sec. B* **1909**, *4*, 81–97.
49. Sellards, A.W. The relationship of the renal lesions of Asiatic cholera to the ordinary nephritides with especial reference to acidosis. *J. Trop. Dis.* **1914**, *2*, 104–117.
50. McCrae, T. *Osler's Principles and Practice of Medicine*, 11th ed.; Appleton: New York, NY, USA; London, UK, 1930.
51. Rogers, L. *Cholera and Its Treatment. Oxford Medical Publications*; Frowde, H., Ed.; Hodder & Stoughton: London, UK, 1911.
52. Rogers, L. The treatment of cholera by injections of hypertonic saline solutions with a simple and rapid method of intrabdominal administration. *Phil. J. Sci.* **1909**, *4*, 99–104.
53. *Memoranda on Medical Diseases in Tropical and Subtropical Areas*, 8th ed.; HM Stationery Office: London, UK; War Office: London, UK; War Office: London, UK, 1946; pp. 84–86.
54. Weaver, R.H.; Johnson, M.K.; Phillips, R.A. Biochemical studies of cholera. *J. Egypt. Public Health Assoc.* **1948**, *23*, 511.
55. Johnson, M.E.; Weaver. R.H.; Phillips. The treatment of cholera. *J. Egypt. Public Health Assoc.* **1948**, *23*, 15–37.
56. Ghanem, M.H.; Mikhail, M.N. Clinical and biochemical studies in cholera and the rationale of treatment. *Trans. R. Soc. Trop. Med. Hyg.* **1949**, *43*, 81. [CrossRef]
57. Chaudhuri, H.N. Notes on some remedies. 34. Dehydration and its treatment. Part 5. Treatment of cholera. *Indian Med. Gaz.* **1950**, *85*, 257–260.
58. Carpenter, C.C.J.; Mitra, P.P.; Dano, P.E.; Weeks, S.N.; Chaudhuri, R.N. Clinical evaluation of fluid requirements in Asiatic cholera. *Lancet* **1965**, *1*, 726–728. [CrossRef]
59. Phillips, R.A. Asiatic cholera with emphasis on pathophysiological effects of the disease. *Ann. Rev. Med.* **1968**, *19*, 69–79. [CrossRef]
60. Gordon, R.S., Jr.; Greenough, W.G.; Lindenbaum, J. The management of epidemic cholera. *Mil. Med.* **1965**, 475–479. [CrossRef]
61. Cash, R.A.; Nalin, D.R.; Toaha, K.M.M.; Huq, Z. Acetate in the correction of acidosis secondary to diarrhea. *Lancet* **1969**, *294*, 302–303. [CrossRef]
62. Islam, M.R. Citrate can effectively replace bicarbonate in oral rehydration salts for cholera and infantile diarrhea. *Bull. WHO* **1986**, *64*, 145–150.
63. Gupte, P.B. Cholera and summer diarrhea. *Antiseptic* **1948**, *45*, 328–330. [PubMed]
64. Riklis, E.; Quastel, J.H. Effects of cations on sugar absorption by isolated surviving guine pig intestine. *Can. J. Biochem. Physiol.* **1958**, *36*, 347–362. [CrossRef] [PubMed]
65. Cash, R.A.; Nalin, D.R.; Rochat, R.; Reller, B.; Haque, E.; Rahman, M. A clinical trial of oral therapy in a rural treatment center. *Am. J. Trop. Med. Hyg.* **1970**, *19*, 653–656. [CrossRef] [PubMed]

66. Cash, R.A.; Nalin, D.R.; Forrest, J.; Abrutyn, E. Rapid correction of the acidosis and dehydration of cholera with an oral solution. *Lancet* **1970**, *2*, 549–550. [CrossRef]
67. Nalin, D.R.; Cash, R.A. Oral or nasogastric maintenance therapy for diarrheas of unknown etiology resembling cholera. *Trans. R. Soc. Trop. Med. Hyg.* **1970**, *64*, 769–771. [CrossRef]
68. Scot, W. *Report on the Epidemic Cholera as It Has Appeared in the Territories Subject to the Presidency of Fort St. George*. Asylum Press: Madras, India, 1824; p. 118, pp. lxv–lxxli and 178–8.
69. Reid, E.W. Intestinal absorption of solutions. *J. Physiol.* **1902**, *28*, 241–256. [CrossRef] [PubMed]
70. Brown, A.; Boyd, G. Acute intestinal intoxication in infants:Analysis of 75 cases treated in the hospital for sick children, Toronto during the summer of 1922. *Can. Med. Assoc. J.* **1923**, *13*, 800–806.
71. Powers, G.F. A comprehensive plan of treatment for the so-called intestinal intoxication of infants. *Am. J Dis. Child.* **1926**, *32*, 232–257. [CrossRef]
72. Gamble, J.L. Deficits in diarrhea. *J. Pediatri.* **1943**, *30*, 488–494. [CrossRef]
73. Segar, L. Alimentary intoxication. In *Therapeutics of Infancy and Childhood*; Litchfield, H.R., Dembo, L.H., Eds.; FA Davis Company: Philadelphia, PA, USA, 1942; p. 3658, Chapt 23 Nutritional disorders.
74. Darrow, D.C. The retention of electrolyte during recovery from severe dehydration due to diarrhea. *J. Pediatri.* **1946**, *28*, 515–540. [CrossRef]
75. Govan, C.D.; Darrow, D.C. The use of KCl in the therapy of the dehydration of diarrhea in infants. *J. Pediatri.* **1946**, *28*, 541–549. [CrossRef]
76. Frant, S.; Abramson, H. Diseases of the newborn:Epidemic diarrhea of the newborn. Chapter xviii. In *Therapeutics of Infancy and Childhood*; Litchfield, H.R., Dembo, L.H., Eds.; FA Davis Company Philadelphia, PA, USA, 1947; pp. 384–394
77. Ibid. Chapt. 22. In *Nutritional Disorders. Alimentary Intoxication*; pp. 490–491.
78. Lawson, D. Management of gastroenteritis at the Hospital for Sick Children, Great Ormond Street 1948–49. *Great Ormond Street J.* **1951**, *2*, 110–114.
79. Darrow, D.C.; Pratt, E.L.; Flett, J.; Gamble, A.H.; Wiese, H.F. Disturbances of water and electrolytes in infantile diarrhea. *Pediatrics* **1949**, *3*, 129–156. [CrossRef] [PubMed]
80. Chung, A.W.; Viscorova, B. The effect of early oral feeding versis early oral starvation on the course of infantile diarrhea. *J. Pediatri.* **1948**, *33*, 14–22. [CrossRef]
81. Finberg, L. Measures promoting recovery from the physiologic disturbances of infantile diarrhea. *Pediatrics* **1952**, *9*, 519–533.
82. Darrow, D.C. Therapeutic measures promoting recovery from the physiologic disturbances of infanitale diar-rhea. *Pediatrics* **1953**, *1*, 519–533.
83. Franz, M.H.; Segar, W.E. The association of various factors and hypernatremic diarrheal dehydration. *AMA J. Dis. Child.* **1959**, *97*, 298–302. [CrossRef]
84. Harrison, H.E. The treatment of diarrhea in infancy. *Pediatri. Clin. N. Am.* **1954**, *1*, 335–348. [CrossRef]
85. Hirschhorn, N. The treatment of acute diarrhea in children: An historical and physiological perspective. *Am. J Clin. Nutr.* **1980**, *33*, 337–363. [CrossRef] [PubMed]
86. Finberg, L. The possible role of the physician in causing hypernatremia in infants dehydrated from diarrhea. *Pediatrics* **1958**, *22*, 2–4. [CrossRef] [PubMed]
87. Holt, E. Oral feeding in diarrhea and hypertonic dehydration. *Pediatrics* **1958**, *22*, 1024–1025. [CrossRef]
88. Darrow, D.C.; Welsh, J.S. Recent experience in the therapy of diarrnea in infants. *J. Pediatr.* **1960**, *56*, 204–210. [CrossRef]
89. Kooh, S.W.; Metcoff, J. Physiologic considerations in fluid and electrolyte therapy with particular reference to diarrheal dehydration in children. *J. Pediatri.* **1963**, *62*, 107–113. [CrossRef]
90. Finberg, L. The management of the critically ill child with dehydration secondary to diarrhea. *Pediatrics* **1970**, *45*, 1029–1036. [CrossRef] [PubMed]
91. Finberg, L. Editorial: The role of oral electrolyte- glucose solutions in hydration for children-international and domestic aspects. *J. Pediatri.* **1980**, *96*, 51–54. [CrossRef]
92. Finberg, L. Editorial: Too little water has become too much. *AJDC* **1986**, *140*, 524. [CrossRef] [PubMed]
93. Arriagada, P. Hydratacion en gota a gota continua por sonda rinoesofagica. *Rev. Chil. Pediatría* **1943**, *14*, 436–442.
94. Yankauer, A.; Ordway, N.K. Diarrheal disease and health services in Latin America. *Public Health Rep.* **1964**, *79*, 917–924. [CrossRef] [PubMed]
95. Meneghello, J.; Rosselot, J.; Aguilo, C.; Monckeberg, F.; Undurage, O.; Ferreiro, M. Infantile diarrhea and dehydraticn: Ambulatory treatment in a hydration center. *Adv. Pediatr.* **1960**, *11*, 183–206.
96. Mariotte, O.C.; Ceballos, C.V. Rehidratacion oral casera. Ensayo piloto en una zona rural de mexico. *Bol. Epidemiol.* **1961**, *25*, 104–108.
97. Toro, R.O.; Cervantes, V.C. La disminucion de la mortalidad infantile por diarrhea mediante la rehid-ratacion oral temprana. Observaciones de un ano de trabajo. *Bol. Epidemiol.* **1962**, *26*, 17–27.
98. Nalin, D.R.; Mata, L.; Vargas, W.; Loria, A.R.; Levine, M.M.; de Cespedes, C.; Lizano, C.; Simhon, A.; Mohs, E. Comparison of sucrose with glucose in oral therapy of infant diarrhea. *Lancet* **1978**, *312*, 277–279. [CrossRef]
99. Meneghello, J.; Rosselot, J.; Undurraga, O.; Aguilo, C.; Ferreiro, M. Experiencia tecnica en administrative en el funcionamiento de un centro de hidratacion. *Boletín. Oficina Sanit. Panam.* **1958**, *45*, 402–411.

100. De la Torre, J.A.; Larracilla-Alegre, J. La via oral para la hidratacion y correccion del desiquilibriohidroeletro-litico en enfermos ambulatorios, menores de dos anos con "diarrhea". *Bol. Med. Hosp. Infant.* **1961**, *18*, 151–163.
101. Larracilla-Alegre, J. A 50 anos de iniciada la hidratacion oral voluntaria en ninos con diarrheas. *Rev. Mex. Pediatr.* **2011**, *78*, 85–90.
102. Truswell, A.S. Results of out-patient treatment of infantile gastro-enteritis. *S. Afr. Med. J.* **1957**, *31*, 446–451. [PubMed]
103. Hansen, J.D.L. Outpatient or home treatment of severe gastro-enteritis with dehydration in infants. *S. Afr. Med. J.* **1957**, *31*, 452–454.
104. Bowie, M.D. The management of gastro-enteritis with dehydration in out-patients. *S. Afr. Med. J.* **1960**, *34*, 344–348.
105. Chatterjee, H.N. Control of vomiting in cholera and oral replacement of fluid. *Lancet* **1953**, *ii*, 1063. [CrossRef]
106. Alasbahi, R.H.; Melzig, M.F. Forskolin and derivatives as tools for studying the role of cAMP. *Pharmazie* **2012**, *67*, 5–13. [PubMed]
107. Chatterjee, H.N. Therapy of diarrhea in cholera. *Lancet* **1953**, *ii*, 1045–1046. [CrossRef]
108. Ruxin, J.N. Magic Bullet: The history of oral rehydration therapy. *Med. Hist.* **1994**, *38*, 363–397. [CrossRef]
109. Phillips, R.A.; Wallace, C.K.; Blackwell, R.Q. Water and electrolyte absorption by the intestine in cholera. In Proceedings of the Cholera Research Symposium, Honolulu, HI, USA, 24–29 January 1965; Dept, of Health, Education and Welfare, PHS: Washington, DC, USA; pp. 299–308.
110. Nalin, D.R.; Ally, K.; Hare, K.; Hare, R. Effects of cholera enterotoxin on jejunal osmoregulation of mannitol solutions in digs. *J. Infect.Dis.* **1972**, *125*, 528–532. [PubMed]
111. Sahay, M.; Sahay, R. Hyponatremia: A practical approach. *Indian J. Endocrinol. Metab.* **2014**, *18*, 760–771. [CrossRef] [PubMed]
112. Phillips, R.A. Twenty years of cholera research. *JAMA* **1967**, *202*, 610–614. [CrossRef] [PubMed]
113. Huber, G.S.; Phillips, R.A. Cholera and the sodium pump. In Proceedings of the SEATO Conference on Cholera, Dacca, Pakistan, 5–8 December 1960; NIH: Bethesda, MD, USA, 1962; pp. 37–40.
114. Greenough, W.B., III.; Rosenberg, I.S.; Gordon, R.S.; Davies, B.I. Tetracycline in the treatment of cholera. *Lancet* **1964**, 355–357. [CrossRef]
115. Carpenter, C.C.J.; Sack, R.B.; Mitra, P.P.; Mondal, A. Tetracycline for treatment of cholera. *Bull. Calcutta Sch. Trop. Med.* **1964**, *12*, 30.
116. Love, A.H.G. The effect of glucose on cation transport. In Proceedings of the Cholera Research Symposium, Honolulu, HI, USA, 24–29 January 1965; No. 1328. Dept. of Health, Education and Welfare, PHS: Washington, DC, USA; pp. 144–147.
117. Sachar, D.; Taylor, J.O.; Saha, J.R.; Phillips, R.A. Intestinal transmural electric potential and its response to glucose in acute and convalescent cholera. *Gastroenterology* **1969**, *56*, 512–521. [CrossRef]
118. Hirschhorn, N.; Kinzie, J.L.; Sachar, D.B.; Taylor, J.O.; Northrup, R.S.; Phillips, R.A. Reduction of Stool Output in Cholera by Glucose and Electrolyte Lavage. In Proceedings of the Symposium on Cholera, Palo Alto, CA, USA, 26–28 July 1967; U.S.-Japan Cooperative Medical Science Program, Office of International Reesearch, NIH: PBethesda, MD, USA; p. 37.
119. Pierce, N.F.; Banwell, J.G.; Mitra, R.C.; Caranasos, G.J.; Keimowitz, R.I.; Mondal, A.; Manji, P.M. Oral maintenance of waterelectrolyte and acid-base balance in cholera: A preliminary report. *Indian J. Med. Res.* **1968**, *56*, 640–645. [PubMed]
120. Hirschhorn, N.; Kinzie, J.L.; Sachar, D.B.; Northrup, R.S.; Taylor, J.O.; Ahmad, Z.; Phillips, R.A. Decrease in net stool output in cholera during intestinal perfusion with glucose-containing solutions. *NEJM* **1968**, *279*, 176–181. [CrossRef] [PubMed]
121. Pierce, N.F.; Banwell, J.G.; Mitra, R.C.; Caranasos, G.J.; Keimowitz, R.I.; Mondal, A.; Manji, P.M. Effect of intragastric glucose-electrolyte infusion upon water and electrolyte balance in Asiatic cholera. *Gastroenterology* **1968**, *55*, 333–343. [CrossRef]
122. Nalin, D. Cholera pathophysiology: Have we missed the boat? *Acad. Lett.* **2021**, *9766*, 1–4. [CrossRef]
123. Woodward, B.; Shurkin, J.; Gordon, D. *Scientists Greater than Einstein: The Biggest Lifesavers of the 20th Century*; Quilldriver Books: Fresno, CA, USA, 2006; pp. 107–142.
124. Islam, R. Research Protocol. Oral Lavage of a Solution Containing Glucose, Electrolytes and Tetracycline as a Method of Treatment of Acute Cholera. Pakistan-SEATO Cholera Research Laboratory. In Proceedings of the Technical Committee Meeting Proceedings, Dacca East Pakistan, 27–29 November 1967. C1/P4.
125. Pizarro, D.; Posada, G.; Mata, L.; Nalin, D.; Mohs, E. Oral rehydration of neonates with dehydrating di-arrheas. *Lancet* **1979**, *314*, 1209–1210. [CrossRef]
126. Pizarro, D.; Posada, G.; Nalin, D.R.; Mohs, E.; Levine, M. Evaluation of oral therapy for infant diarrhea in an emergency room setting: Utilization of acute episode for instructing mothers in oral therapy method. *Bull. WHO* **1979**, *57*, 983–986. [PubMed]
127. Nalin, D.R.; Levine, M.M.; Mata, L.; de Cespedes, C.; Vargas, W.; Lizano, C.; Loria, A.R.; Simhon, A.; Mohs, E. Oral rehydration and maintenance of children with rotavirus and bacterial diarrheas. *Bull. WHO* **1979**, *57*, 453–459. [PubMed]
128. Nalin, D.R.; Levine, M.M.; Hornick, R.; Bergquist, E.; Hoover, D.; Holley, H.P.; Waterman, D.; Van Blerk, J.; Matheny, S.; Sotman, S.; et al. The problem of emesis during oral glucose-electrolyte therapy given from the start of severe cholera. *Trans. R. Soc. Trop. Med. Hyg.* **1979**, *73*, 10–14. [CrossRef]
129. Malhotra, M. *Letter from Prime Minister Indira Gandhi's Secretariat*; Indian Ministry of Health: New Delhi, India, 1971.
130. Mahalanabis, D.; Choudhuri, A.B.; Bagchi, N.G.; Bhattacharya, A.K.; Simpson, T.W. Oral fluid therapy of cholera among Bangladesh refugees. *Johns Hopkins Med. J.* **1973**, *132*, 197–205.
131. Chowdhury, A.M.R.; Cash, R.A. *A Simple Solution: Teaching Millions to Treat Diarrhoea at Home*; University Press Ltd.: Dhaka, Bangladesh, 1996.
132. Ioannidis, J.P.A. Why most published research findings are false. *PLoS Med.* **2005**, *2*, e124. [CrossRef] [PubMed]

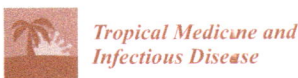 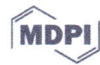

Article

Using Oral Rehydration Therapy (ORT) in the Community

Richard A. Cash

Department of Global Health and Population, Harvard T.H. Chan School of Public Health, Boston, MA 02115, USA; racash@hsph.harvard.edu

Abstract: For ORT to have a maximum impact on public health it should be used in the community, in the home. A number of programs have been developed over the years to extend ORT to home use. One of the most successful approaches was the Oral Therapy Education Program (OTEP) developed by BRAC, the world's largest NGO. Mothers were taught in the home by an OTEP worker using seven simple messages and a demonstration. The program, which led to high levels of use and knowledge retention, is described. What the OTEP and other successful home-based programs have demonstrated is that home care of diarrhea using ORS can be effectively implemented and can have a positive impact on the reduction of diarrhea morbidity and mortality.

Keywords: oral rehydration solution (ORS); oral rehydration therapy (ORT); community-based care; OTEP; BRAC

1. Introduction

The development and proof-of-concept of oral rehydration solution (ORS) and the treatment package of oral rehydration therapy (ORT) were many years in the making, from physiologic studies to the first clinical applications in 1968 [1]. The reasoning behind this effort was to expand therapy to those areas where intravenous (IV) fluid, needles, and IV tubing were not available and where health personnel were in very short supply—that is, in most countries where cholera was a significant health problem. ORS was to be an intervention for use not only in health facilities but also in the home. Though ORS was originally developed for cholera, there is increasing evidence that it is effective in all types of infectious diarrheas, ranging from rotavirus to the recent demonstrations of its effectiveness in Ebola-related diarrhea. It seems to be a universal treatment.

For ORS to be most effective in reducing diarrhea morbidity it has to be used where cases occur. This article examines efforts to extend the use of ORS to the community—to local practitioners and mothers and other home-based care givers.

2. Early Efforts

Soon after the clinical studies demonstrated the effectiveness of ORS in treating adult and childhood cholera and non-cholera diarrhea, efforts began to extend care to rural treatment centers and the home. Early interventions focused on producing packets of electrolytes and glucose for wide distribution. Packets were originally designed to be added to one liter of potable water, with instructions written on the packet. The World Health Organization (WHO) heavily endorsed this concept, and training courses were set up worldwide to teach doctors how to use ORS. The United Nations Children's Fund (UNICEF), under the leadership of Jim Grant, established a number of facilities for the production of ORS packets. The United States Agency for International Development (USAID) was a major contributor to conferences and workshops to help disseminate knowledge about ORS and to support programs to expand distribution. Packets were an attractive idea as they standardized the composition of ORS, were easy to distribute, and could be sold by shops and pharmacies. There were flaws in this strategy, however, especially in the poorest countries. A mother or other child caregiver had to be literate to

Citation: Cash, R.A. Using Oral Rehydration Therapy (ORT) in the Community. *TMID* **2021**, *6*, 92. https://doi.org/10.3390/tropicalmed6020092

Academic Editors: David Nalin and John Frean

Received: 12 April 2021
Accepted: 24 May 2021
Published: 29 May 2021

Publisher's Note: MDPI stays neutral with regard to jurisdictional claims in published maps and institutional affiliations.

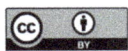

Copyright: © 2021 by the author. Licensee MDPI, Basel, Switzerland. This article is an open access article distributed under the terms and conditions of the Creative Commons Attribution (CC BY) license (https://creativecommons.org/licenses/by/4.0/).

read the instructions; the person making up the solution had to have a liter container to mix the water and salts; and there had to be an effective distribution system to send the packets to the village and home. Despite these issues, WHO was initially opposed to any other methods of delivery and any change in the formula. One size was designed to fit all, including the size of the packet.

Use of ORS in the community was less extensive than might have been expected both because of these limitations and the resistance of some health providers, especially doctors. To many it seemed counterintuitive to give oral fluids when the child had diarrhea, and there was little money to be made in selling such an inexpensive product. This led a number of governments and community-based organizations to try other methods of delivering ORS and increasing use. Rather than attempting to review these many efforts to increase community and home-based use, this article will focus on one program that used innovative strategies to greatly increase use in a very large population—the Oral Therapy Education Program (OTEP) of BRAC, a large Bangladeshi non-governmental organization (NGO) [2].

3. The BRAC OTEP Program

Founded in 1972, BRAC is a Bangladeshi NGO that is presently the largest in the world and has been ranked the number-one NGO globally over the past 5 years. BRAC is especially known for scaling up programs to reach millions, whether it be through microcredit, mobile banking, primary education, water and sanitation, health interventions, or multiple other development programs. In 1980 OTEP began a 10-year effort to educate every Bangladeshi mother about ORS and to teach them how to prepare and use the solution.

As in so many low-income countries, diarrhea was the cause of up to 30% of infant and child deaths. There was a significant shortage of MBBS physicians (the degree of a trained allopathic doctor), estimated at less than 1 per 10,000 in rural areas, and fewer nurses, with most care delivered by unlicensed village doctors (or village "quacks") or through local drug sellers in village shops. Based on the WHO approach, the government established the National Oral Rehydration Program (NORP) which was designed to distribute the oral therapy packets to pharmacies and treatment facilities, and to teach doctors throughout the country. The number of treatment facilities was limited and most did not have a full complement of health personnel. Female literacy was less than 5% and there were no standard 1-liter containers in the countryside. It was no wonder that knowledge and use with respect to ORS were limited. BRAC concluded that the only means of spreading the use of ORS to reduce diarrhea morbidity and mortality was to teach women, all women, how to prepare and use ORS in the village, in the home.

Treatment was literally put in the hands of the mother. A local experiment indicated that a 3-finger pinch of salt (labon) and a hand scoop of raw sugar (gur, which is half glucose and half fructose but also contains potassium) dissolved in a half a liter of water (500 cc) produced an oral solution with a sodium content of approximately 50 mEq/liter. This labon-gur solution (LGS) was tested in adult patients with non-cholera diarrhea treated at the Cholera Research Laboratory in Dhaka (now the icddr,b). The outcome was similar to that of a group with mild to moderate diarrhea given the standard WHO-recommended solution. Though WHO had serious reservations about promoting incomplete home-based solutions, BRAC began field tests, convinced that successful treatment of child diarrhea lay in convincing the mother to hydrate with an available and appropriate solution, and that the packet-based program would not work in rural Bangladesh.

Though a national program was not yet being considered by BRAC there were four questions that remained to be answered in designing their program: What should be the message content? Who should be the recipients of the message? What should be the method of teaching? Who should be the teachers? The response to each of these questions would shape the creation of the program and how it was to be evaluated.

Mothers were the obvious recipients of the message, and given that less than 5% were literate, the message had to be crafted so that literacy was not required. To reach mothers in the village, teaching had to be provided in the home by women. Lastly, the message had to be simple and practical, with a primary focus on teaching how to prepare the solution. Originally, in the program it was decided that the message would involve 17 points. The message was reduced to 10, and finally 7 essential points (see Box 1) [2]. What is not often appreciated is that it takes much more skill to simplify than to complicate. This is often true of public health messaging, which often suffers from providing unnecessary information in a long format.

Box 1. The 7 points to remember in the BRAC OTEP program were as follows.

| 1. Defining different terms for diarrhea—i.e., "dud haga", "ajirno", "amasha", "daeria", or "cholera" and their effects |
| 2. Symptoms of diarrhea |
| 3. Simple management of loose motions (replacing salt and water in the body) |
| 4. Preparing ORS (3-finger pinch of salt, 1 fistful of gur/sugar, dissolved in 1 half-seer of water or 500 cc |
| 5. Administration of ORS |
| 6. Advice on nutrition (continued breastfeeding, rice, curry, other household foods) |
| 7. Prevention (drinking water from a safe source, keeping food clean, breastfeeding) |

Teachers were called oral replacement workers (ORW). The ORWs were all women recruited from the districts in which the program was conducted. They were 20–35 years of age, had about 10 years of schooling, and did not have children younger than 3 years of age. The original training was for 5 days and focused on teaching techniques and recordkeeping. There were daily feedback meetings and a 1-day refresher course every 3 months.

Each ORW visited up to 10 women a day with each encounter lasting about 20 min. All the ORWs were recruited from the villages. The ORW would go house to house, teaching the method of a 3-finger pinch of salt (labon) and a fistful of raw sugar (gur) or refined sugar to each half-liter of water. This will be referred to as the "labon-gur" solution. To ensure the mother had a half-liter container, the ORW carried the proper-sized cup. She requested the mother to bring any container from the kitchen into which a half a litter of water was poured and a scratch mark made on the pot to designate how much water should be used. The water used was the best available drinking water normally used in the home. Boiling the water was not encouraged as it added another step, increased fuel consumption, and there were no studies indicating that childhood diarrhea would worsen if contaminated water was used.

The ORWs were not given a fixed salary but were paid on the basis of their performance as educators. That is, the more the mothers learned, the more they were paid. To do this it was necessary to develop an effective monitoring system. Each ORW kept a list of the mothers she taught. A supervisor would randomly select a 10% sample that would be given to the monitor to visit and interview. All monitors were young men who could travel from village to village, something that a single woman could not do. The monitors had no direct contact with the ORWs.

The mother was asked about the 7 points and to prepare the labon-gur solution. Her responses were graded according to the following criteria: A—answered 6–7 questions and prepared the solution; B—answered 4–5 questions and prepared the solutions; C—answered 2–3 points and prepared the solution; D—could not prepare the solution. From these results the ORW salary was calculated. For all mothers graded as A, the worker received Taka (Tk) 4 (USD 0.025 using the 1980 exchange rate) multiplied by the number of mothers she had seen in a given period of time; for B she received Tk 2; for C she received Tk 1; and for those graded D she received no compensation. Major emphasis was placed on ensuring that the mother knew how to correctly prepare the labon-gur solution.

If the program maximized worker payments it was because mothers were learning. The incentive system resulted in more attention being given to improving the teaching technique, and suggestions came from the bottom up. As the ORW demonstrated and then asked the mothers to prepare the solution, communication with the mother increased, as did interest in the teaching session.

4. Scaling Up the OTEP

The mantra of the BRAC founder, F.H. Abed, was "Small is beautiful but big is necessary".

When the pilot program of OTEP demonstrated that ORS could be prepared by village women who remembered the 7 points, the next step was to plan to teach every mother in the country in order to scale up the program. Small groups of 6–10 ORWs fanned out across the country, spending 4 weeks at a community facility at the union level (a union is the smallest administrative unit in Bangladesh and is composed of 9 villages). They were accompanied by a cook and a chowkidar (watchman). From the community center they reached all the villages in a union. As the program expanded it continued to evolve based on feedback from the OTEP staff, the Technical Advisory Committee, and the Research and Evaluation Division of BRAC. Some important changes included: establishing field labs to monitor the quality of the ORS; revising the 7 points; involving men at village markets; teaching about ORS in schools; increasing the length of stay in a union from 4 to 6 weeks; teaching small groups rather than individuals; improved monitoring; and experimenting with cereal-based ORS. As men were often the decision makers deciding what treatment should be given to the child, they also had to be informed of the method and its value.

Factors affecting the successful scaling-up of OTEP can be summarized as follows: management; performance-linked salary; planning; recruitment; training and staff development; communication; logistics; feedback and coordination; staff commitment; government support; international support; use of outside expertise; and funding.

Was the OTEP a success? As the objective of the OTEP was to teach each and every mother in Bangladesh to prepare and use ORS to treat diarrhea, success could be measured by different criteria: coverage; knowledge; management; use, impact; replication; and sustainability. In the evaluation of any intervention, time is a critical factor. How long should it take to change ideas and practice? The OTEP program lasted 10 years, so it should be evaluated over that period of time. OTEP field workers visited all the villages (except a few in tribal districts where there was civil unrest), which translated into 12 million households, though the number of women taught was higher as some households had more than 1 woman. Over 90% of mothers knew of and could prepare ORS, and the vast majority of them were capable of preparing a clinically safe and effective solution. Even 15 years after the initial encounter with an OTEP worker, ~70%, reported knowledge and use.

An important indicator of success is how frequently and the degree to which ORT is used in treating an episode of diarrhea. If all types of diarrheas—mild, moderate, or severe, watery or non-watery—were included in the denominator, about half of the episodes were treated with ORT (LGS, packet ORS, or other rehydrating fluids). If the denominator was more rigidly defined as only more severe cases, use increased to 82%. Today, Bangladesh has the highest use rate of ORT to treat diarrhea of any country.

Measuring mortality from a constellation of conditions like diarrhea is problematic as there are many causes and contributing factors to overall mortality, especially in environments where mortality is high. Studies examining "process" measures (retention of knowledge, use rates, perception, etc.) have been far more useful and much less costly. If mothers retain the knowledge, they are more likely to use ORT with increased frequency and volume if diarrhea appears to be more severe. Evidence suggests that in higher-risk groups (infants, children, and the elderly), diarrhea-related mortality was reduced and there's no doubt that ORT use has contributed to lowering overall diarrhea mortality [3,4].

There are many lessons from the BRAC experience with ORT in developing the message, spreading the message, increasing use, and scaling up health education projects. One observation is that mothers, regardless of their degree of literacy, have the capacity to learn given the right kind of teaching. The message was based on previous experiences (childcare and cooking), addressed the well-recognized problem of child diarrhea, and was culturally acceptable. By preparing the solution at home using ingredients usually available, no money had to be spent by the mother unless she had to purchase gur or sugar. Simplifying the message was essential; a guiding principle of health education should be to keep the necessary ideas and discard the others. Simplifying is not "dumbing down".

In spreading the message in the community, different strategies were used. Firstly, the quality of teaching was linked to the salary of the ORW. This led to suggestions coming from the "bottom up" as there was a strong incentive for workers to improve their performance. The more the mothers learned, the higher the salary. The OTEP messages were reinforced through education of the men, school programs, and the use of newspapers, radio, and TV, though the latter was not widely available in rural areas. Programs were designed to reach local health care providers, with most being in the informal sector, and drug sellers. Even though there was limited monetary gain associated with increased home use of ORT, the outreach to health providers reinforced the messages, limited negative pushback, and increased their skill set. Packets of ORS salts in Bangladesh are now designed to be dissolved in a half-liter of water rather than the standard liter packet, demonstrating the degree to which the message has been adopted.

Knowledge led to increased use, which was measured in various ways but most importantly by first asking women. The use of ORT can also be deduced by the numbers of children coming to hospital with diarrhea and the state of hydration of these children. The number of visits should be reduced and the level of dehydration should improve. Measuring mortality is often at the request of a donor, but process measurements proved to be far more important.

What are the lessons regarding the scaling up of programs such as OTEP? Observations from BRAC have been framed as follows [5]:

Innovation is a process of iteration, learning, evaluation, and implementation, requiring patience;

We should start by learning and recognize that social innovation is a constant adjustment;

We should focus on what needs to be reduced, not added—simple solutions scale easier;

Get decision makers to pay attention;

The goal is improvement, not total change.

BRAC has a clear institutional vision—the alleviation of poverty—and a commitment to scaling up. Pilot programs were developed with robust monitoring, evaluation, and research as critical components. Scaling up was achieved through a simple message and information was delivered directly. Staff were trained prior to scaling up. As a learning institution, BRAC embraced feedback and failure. Like any implementation program there were tensions within the strategy, but the program was flexible. BRAC also worked with the government, not in competition, so programs complimented each other.

A number of global initiatives were taking place when the OTEP program began, which lent credibility to their effort and others to increase community use (see Box 2). That a simple solution could have such an impact on infant and child health and that this technology could be put in the hands of mothers changed the meaning of primary health care.

Box 2. Policies and programs that contributed to increasing community use of ORT.

1. Alma Ata and "Health for All";
2. WHO's commitment to expanding the use of ORS;
3. UNICEF and its Growth monitoring, Oral therapy, Breast feeding and immunization (GOBI) program;
4. The role of NGOs (such as BRAC), other NGOs, and GNGOs;
5. Global meetings (e.g., ICORT I, II, III);
6. Inter-sectoral collaboration and increased support for applied research; and
7. Private sector marketing and distribution of ORS.

There were many other country programs developing their own strategy to spread the use and message of ORT. As the distribution of packets and the availability of standard containers became more widespread there was probably less need for the "pinch and scoop" method of the labon-gur approach. Packets do provide a more complete solution, with both bicarbonate and potassium in the mix. In addition to packets, some programs have focused on using cereals as a substitute for glucose (gur or sugar). Rice has been a favorite. BRAC recognized that the price of even gur was often beyond the means of the very poor and when rice/rice powder was found to be effective [6] (more so in cholera and non-vibrio cholera) and more universally available than sugar or gur, BRAC began to recommend rice for ORT [7]. As fuel must be used to cook the rice, this proved to be a disincentive for some mothers, and many preferred to use sugar. The basic message of using water and electrolytes with an absorbable substrate (e.g., glucose, sucrose, rice) to prevent dehydration, overcome deficit, and replace losses from diarrhea remained the same for all methods and has persisted. Hydrate, hydrate, hydrate. That is the important message that programs must deliver to the community.

A final thought by Albert Einstein might summarize the BRAC experience; "Everything should be as simple as possible but not one bit simpler."

Funding: OTEP was funded primarily from the Swiss Development Cooperation (SDC) with additional funding being provided by the ODA (UK), the Swedish Free Church Aid, and the Swedish International Development Agency (SIDA).

Institutional Review Board Statement: Not applicable.

Informed Consent Statement: Not applicable.

Conflicts of Interest: The author declares no conflict of interest.

Abbreviations

ORS	Oral rehydration solution
ORT	Oral rehydration therapy, which is based on the proper use of ORS and includes nutrition advice during diarrhea
OTEP	Oral Therapy Education Programme (of BRAC)
BRAC	A Bangladeshi Non-Government Organization (NGO)
UNICEF	United Nations Children's Fund
icddr,b	International Centre for Diarrhea Disease Research, Bangladesh

References

1. Nalin, D. Issues and controversies in the evolution of oral rehydration therapy (ORT). *Trop. Med. Infect. Dis.* **2021**, *6*, 34. [CrossRef] [PubMed]
2. Chowdhury, A.M.R.; Cash, R.A. *A Simple Solution: Teaching Millions to Treat Diarrhoea at Home*; The University Press Limited: Dhaka, Bangladesh, 1996.
3. Munos, M.K.; Walker, C.L.F.; E Black, R. The effect of oral rehydration solution and recommended home fluids on diarrhoea mortality. *Int. J. Epidemiol.* **2010**, *39* (Suppl. 1), i75–i87. [CrossRef] [PubMed]
4. Billah, S.M.; Raihana, S.; Ali, N.B.; Iqbal, A.; Rahman, M.M.; Khan, A.N.S.; Karim, F.; Karim, M.A.; Hassan, A.; Jackson, B.; et al. Bangladesh: A success case in combating childhood diarrhoea. *J. Glob. Health* **2019**, *9*, 020803. [CrossRef] [PubMed]
5. Aslam, A.; BRAC-Bangladesh; (Google Foundation, San Francisco, CA, USA). Personal communication, 2017.
6. Molla, A.M.; Ahmed, S.M.; Greenough, W.B., 3rd. Rice-based oral rehydration solution decreases stool volume in acute diarrhoea. *Bull. World Health Organ.* **1985**, *63*, 751–756. [PubMed]
7. Chowdhury, A.M.; Karim, F.; Rohde, J.E.; Ahmed, J.; Abed, F.H. Oral rehydration therapy: a community trial comparing the acceptability of homemade sucrose and cereal-based solutions. *Bull. World Health Organ.* **1991**, *69*, 229–234. [PubMed]

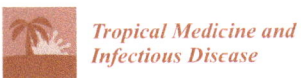

Review

Issues and Controversies in the Evolution of Oral Rehydration Therapy (ORT)

David Nalin

Albany Medical College, Albany, NY 12208-3478, USA; nalindavid@gmail.com

Abstract: The original studies demonstrating the efficacy of oral glucose-electrolytes solutions in reducing or eliminating the need for intravenous therapy to correct dehydration caused by acute watery diarrheas (AWD) were focused chiefly on cholera patients. Later research adapted the oral therapy (ORT) methodology for treatment of non-cholera AWDs including for pediatric patients. These adaptations included the 2:1 regimen using 2 parts of the original WHO oral rehydration solution (ORS) formulation followed by 1 part additional plain water, and a "low sodium" packet formulation with similar average electrolyte and glucose concentrations when dissolved in the recommended volume of water. The programmatic desire for a single ORS packet formulation has led to controversy over use of the "low sodium" formulations to treat cholera patients. This is the subject of the current review, with the conclusion that use of the low-sodium ORS to treat cholera patients leads to negative sodium balance, leading to hyponatremia and, in severe cases, particularly in pediatric cholera, to seizures and other complications of sodium depletion. Therefore it is recommended that two separate ORS packet formulations be used, one for cholera therapy and the other for non-cholera pediatric AWD.

Keywords: cholera; non-cholera acute watery diarrheas (AWDs); oral rehydration solutions (ORS); ORS formulations; sodium balance; hyponatremia; hyponatremic seizures; hyponatremic sequelae

1. Introduction

Since 1990, controversies in the field of oral rehydration therapy (ORT) have arisen concerning efforts to preserve a single formulation for cholera and non-cholera acute watery diarrheas (AWD) in patients of all ages, while modifying the original WHO (Oralyte) oral rehydration solution (ORS) formulation containing 90 mEq/L Na$^+$, to address three goals: (1) to safely provide effective rehydration and maintenance therapy for both cholera and non-cholera AWDs; (2) to reduce duration and volume of diarrhea and (3) to reduce the need for restarting intravenous fluids after completing rehydration, during the oral maintenance period [1,2]. The treatment of dysentery and inflammatory diarrheal diseases in which dehydration is not the main focus of therapy is beyond the scope of this report.

This paper will offer a critical review of the major studies done to support the above goals, focusing on those studies chosen for the 2011 Cochrane review [3–10]. The Cochrane-reviewed studies, and others referenced in this review, dealt mainly with patients seen in hospital settings in a research context who had severe dehydration due to profuse adult or pediatric cholera and/or non-cholera AWD. It is chiefly in such patients that otherwise academic discussions of different ORS formulations and ORT methods translate into significantly different clinical outcomes. Optimal treatment of hospitalized patients with severe dehydration due to diarrhea requires measurement of intake and output using essential equipment such as Watten cholera cots [11] and ample supplies of appropriate I.V. and oral replacement fluids. Home or outpatient therapy of less severely dehydrated patients requires use chiefly of clinical signs of hydration status to monitor therapeutic status, and is best addressed in detail in a separate review.

The Cochrane review covered structural aspects of the studies, but did not comment in detail on the quality of the design, clinical research methods or analytic approach to

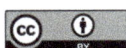

the data, aspects of which will be the subject of this report. This review will also provide context by considering the fundamentals of ORT and ORS composition and the history of ORS evolution, special characteristics of cholera pathophysiology, limitations of prior studies and implications for future safety studies.

2. Basic Principles of Oral Therapy Methodology

Oral rehydration and maintenance therapy for significantly dehydrating AWD is not a magic bullet which works simply by giving patients ORS to drink; achieving optimal results requires administering the oral solutions according to the following well established ORT methodologic principles. Effective and safe ORT rests on the basic principle of AWD treatment: *timely replacement of the water and electrolyte losses of AWD with matching volumes of an absorbable ORS with electrolyte content sufficient to replace the electrolyte losses of AWD*. Deviation from this principle has resulted either in higher ORT failure rates with reversion to I.V. therapy and/or electrolyte abnormalities with potentially serious and avoidable sequelae of severe hyponatrema or hypernatremia.

Gross diarrhea rate (GDR), or the volume of diarrheal stool passed over a given unit of time, is far less important for successful ORT and optimal success rates than net gut balance, or the difference between diarrheal volume and volume of ORS intake in a given observation period. An excess of ORS intake volume over diarrheal volume during a given observation period, usually 4 or 6 h, is called *positive net gut balance (PNGB)*, and early achievement of PNGB is key to successful ORT [12]. Moderate increases in *GDR* are of negligible consequence if exceeded by ORS intake.

Initial diarrhea rates after hospital admission for AWD determine subsequent total stool volume [13]. Two methods of prestratification of patients entered in research studies ensure validity of comparison groups: entry only of patients in shock due to dehydration, or, more elegantly, allocating patients after confirming comparable GDR rates during the several hours required for initial intravenous rehydration. Allocation based on any other criteria often leads to an imbalance in disease severity between comparison groups which can bias the outcomes and accounts for a significant amount of variability seen between different results from the different centers conducting these studies.

When severely dehydrated patients arrive at treatment centers for rehydration, they are generally at or past their peak diarrhea rate. At this point vomiting, sometimes massive at disease onset (e.g., cholera [14]), is waning, and may wane more rapidly with correction of acidosis using ORS or, if patients are in shock due to dehydration, using I.V. fluids containing bicarbonate or a base precursor [15]. Vomiting quickly subsides soon after initiating treatment of most patients arriving at treatment centers, and measured vomitus volumes are generally small in relation to diarrhea volumes in most patients. Failure to correct acidosis in severely dehydrated patients leads to increased risk of pulmonary edema during I.V. rehydration [16].

Maintaining PNGB using proper ORT methodology will allow sufficient net fluid absorption to replace insensible losses and, in addition, promote sufficient net absorption to permit use of ORS with sodium content modestly lower than that of diarrhea fluid (e.g., 120 mEq/L. in cholera patients), while maintaining positive electrolyte balance [17].

If inadequate oral intake results in delayed or failed achievement of PNGB, additional I.V. fluid will be needed. This can arise rarely from excess vomiting or more commonly from inadequate monitoring or supervision, leading to failure of pediatric patients to be given or to drink sufficient ORS. Also, pediatric diarrhea patients in endemic areas not uncommonly have malabsorption of glucose and dietary sugars [18,19] and will be at higher risk of ORT failure and hypernatremia due to excess water loss in diarrheal stools. Caregivers should be alert to such patients, who may require I.V. therapy, though they can respond to ORS formulations with glycine replacing glucose. Researchers must be careful to avoid disproportionately allocating such patients among comparison groups, to avoid confounding interpretation of outcome results.

Claims have been made, without presentation of objective quantitative evidence, that mothers are aware of gross stool volume. In the writer's opinion, based on extensive experience, mothers are aware of time since onset and of subsequent duration of diarrhea, and of course would prefer to see it stop if asked; but this is different from perception of the small difference in stool volume measured in most studies of modified ORS formulations [20].

Even trained clinicians are unable to accurately guess diarrheal volumes without stool volume measurements, as shown when they were asked to guess the volume of synthetic diarrhea fluid tossed onto a bedsheet. Estimates were wildly inaccurate (Dr. Norbert Hirschhorn, personal communication). Mothers (and clinicians) would doubtless like to have available a drug which could stop the diarrhea in minutes, but no currently available ORS formulation does that.

Experience from many studies have confirmed that the taste and appearance of plain ORS do not influence ORS acceptability among moderately and severely dehydrated patients, consistent with a recent report regarding milder cases [21]. Sweetening the ORS has had a negative effect [22]. The enormous benefits of ORS result from preventing and quickly correcting signs of dehydration, which parents fully appreciate.

3. Home Therapy with the WHO 90 ORS Using the 2:1 Regimen

When no I.V. is available, patients need the early positive balance and superior retention this regimen affords, to *replace* pretreatment deficits and *maintain* positive water and electrolyte balance (Figures 1–7).

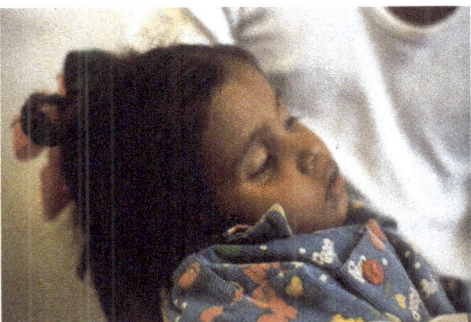

Figure 1. Severely dehydrated child in Greentown, Lahore, Pakistan. Note deeply sunken eyes and obtunded appearance. Etiology unknown.

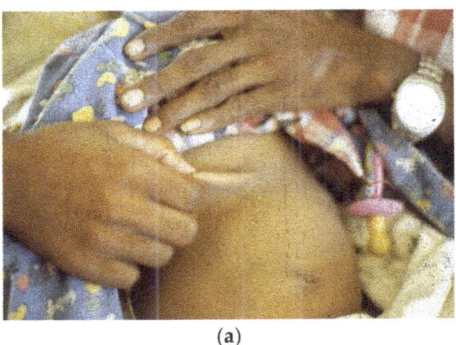 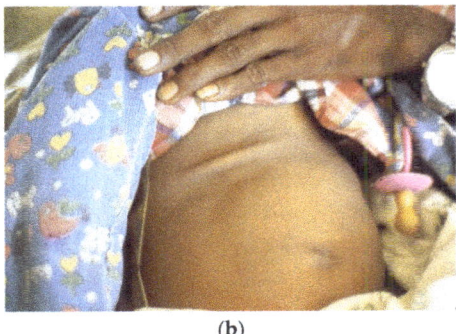

(a) (b)

Figure 2. (a) Father pinches abdominal skin as instructed, (b) showing tenting indicating decreased elasticity after withdrawing hand.

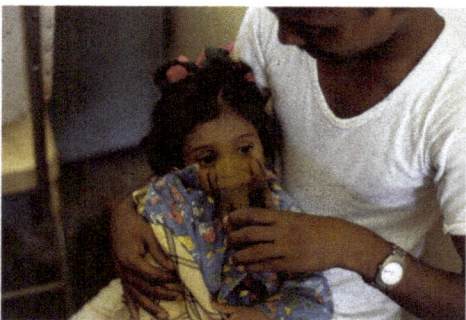

Figure 3. Father begins to offer patient oral rehydration solution (ORS) (WHO 90 formulation) to drink.

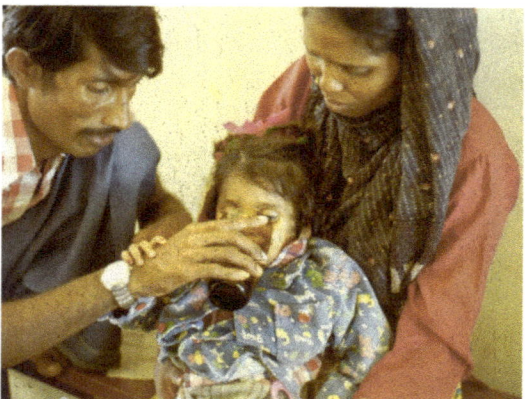

Figure 4. Patient continues to drink, using hand to keep ORS coming.

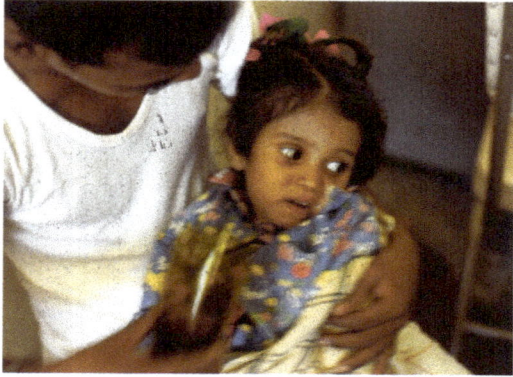

Figure 5. Patient now more alert, eyes less sunken at 1 h after starting ORS.

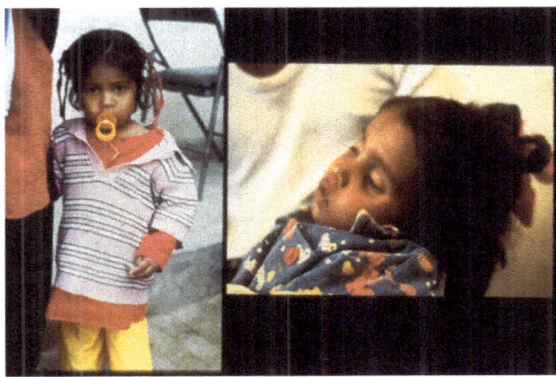

Figure 6. Patient after recovery, with pretreatment appearance on right.

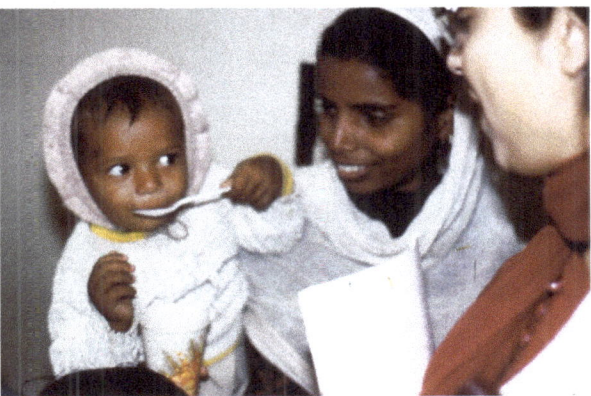

Figure 7. The ultimate goal: another child with acute watery diarrheas (AWD) starting ORS to prevent becoming dehydrated.

4. The Evolution of ORT and ORS

The first successful clinical trial of ORT [17] was successful based on the combination of an appropriate ORS and, importantly, an effective *method* of administering the solution. The ORS formulation used had an electrolyte content approximating that of cholera diarrheal fluid losses, with sodium halfway between that of pediatric and adult cholera diarrhea fluid, and 110 mMol/L. glucose, without which the patients could not absorb the sodium, chloride and water essential to effective therapy.

ORS formulations using a range of sodium levels, chiefly 90 mEq/L with glucose as the substrate and additional water intake (or breast milk feedings) permitted, have proven effective in treating dehydration in patients with cholera, nonvibrio cholera (caused by enterotoxigenic *Escherichia coli* and other organisms producing cholera toxin analogs) and non-cholera AWD including rotavirus diarrhea [23] and have decimated global under-five AWD mortality [24,25]. However, ORS formulations with Na^+ content significantly below patients' stool Na^+ losses lead to negative sodium balance, Na^+ depletion with hyponatremia and heightened risk of hyponatremic complications, whether combined with glucose, rice or other substrates [6,9].

The therapeutic method which proved essential [12,17] to overcoming the failures of earlier ORT trials [26] consisted of rapid initial correction of shock when present on admission, using I.V. rehydration. Oral therapy began *as soon as* shock was corrected, generally after administering I.V. fluid equivalent to 10% of admission body weight (in populations with BMIs (body mass index) below Western levels.) Initially, oral therapy was administered at a rate of 0.5 to 0.75 L/h in adults, based on body weight [17]. If the GNB (gut net balance: see PNGB above) monitored during the first 4 h indicated a fluid requirement greater than that estimated on admission, oral therapy was increased to match the volume of losses. Hydration status was monitored by checking plasma sp. gr. during the transition to oral maintenance. A rise over 1.030 was an indication for additional I.V. fluids to avoid progression to severe dehydration, estimation of hydration status based on clinical signs alone being less sensitive and more dependent on variable subjective criteria.

The ORS formulation used contained 120 mEq/L of Na^+ (ORS 120), suitable for treating cholera and nonvibrio cholera patients. Using this method, total I.V. fluid requirements of cholera patients admitted in shock averaged 80% less than in controls and plasma Na^+ remained normal. Patients not in severe shock were rehydrated and maintained in water and electrolyte balance using ORT alone without I.V. fluids [27,28]. Since cholera patients given effective adjunct antibiotic therapy [29], and most hospitalized non-cholera AWD patients, have steadily declining stool volume after treatment begins [13], closely matching ORS volume and composition imbibed in each sequential 4 or 6 h period to volume and composition of losses in the prior period by using fluids of appropriate composition ensures maintenance of PNGB of both water and electrolytes [12]. In the first large-scale field trial using this method [30], total I.V. requirements averaged 3.0 L in cholera patients arriving in shock whose average admission weight was 40 kg. Nonvibrio cholera patients not in shock on admission were successfully treated using glucose or glucose+glycine ORT alone with no I.V. fluids. Plasma sodium remained normal [28].

The ORS 90 formulation with 90 mEq/L of sodium (abbreviated "WHO 90" here because the Oralyte name has been copied by other ORS brands) was devised as a "compromise" between a formulation approximating the mean composition of cholera diarrhea fluid and that of noncholera pediatric AWDs. Since diarrheal stool content of sodium (directly) and potassium (inversely) correlate closely with diarrhea rate [31] (Figure 8) and cholera diarrhea rates are greatly in excess of average non-cholera AWD rates, the "compromise" provided excess sodium and insufficient potassium for pediatric non-cholera AWD patients and insufficient sodium for pediatric and adult cholera patients, if the method of matching fluid losses with equal volumes of ORS was used. After the initial clinical trial of the WHO ORS 90 formulation [32], it was noted [33] that, to maintain positive sodium balance using this formulation in cholera patients, the patients would have to drink an amount of the ORS equivalent to one and one-half times their diarrhea volume of the previous intake and output period, rather than simply matching that volume, in order to avoid negative Na^+ balance and hyponatremia. Some patients would be unable to imbibe such large volumes over 24–32 h, leading to increased failure rates. However, the 1.5 X losses requirement was not promoted for general use, though it obviated the need for a separate ORS formulation for cholera. In research studies, however, it has been often matched or exceeded, somewhat confounding the conclusions regarding formulation impact *per se* [7–9,34].

The WHO 90 formulation was nonetheless highly successful in reducing global diarrheal mortality, since it was within the range of effective formulations suitable for most mild and moderate AWDs, in which ORS intake is limited by low diarrhea volume and short duration; any "extra" sodium in that formulation is needed to replace pretreatment losses when ORS 90 is used for both rehydration *and* maintenance without I.V. rehydration. In addition, allowance of extra free water (or breast milk [35]) given to pediatric AWD patients, either permissively ("ad libitum") or in the fixed 2:1 ratio [36] prevented hypernatremia, the 2:1 method having the added safety factor of offering protection against instances of wrongly mixed hyperconcentrated ORS preparations. Also, the 90 mEq/L ORS proved safe and effective for treatment of noncholera AWDs in neonates and of children with hypo- or hypernatremia on admission when the 2:1 regimen was used [37]. The 2:1 regimen permitted use of the WHO 90 ORS packet in noncholera pediatric diarrhea patients and had the advantage of promoting early PNGB while avoiding transient hypernatremia [38].

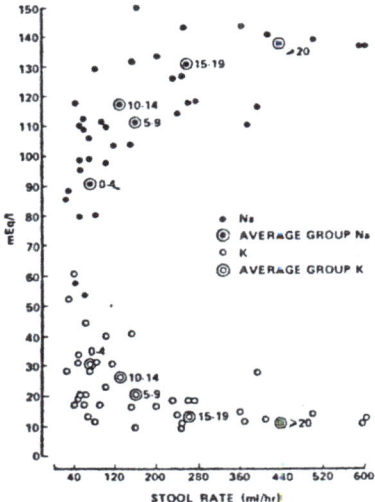

Figure 8. Relationship of diarrheal sodium and potassium losses (mEq/L) to stooling rate in 37 cholera patients during a period of maximum diarrhea 12–24 h after admission. At all ages, stool sodium tends to rise and potassium to fall at higher diarrhea rates. The numbers of patients were: 12 (0–4 yrs old), 10 (5–9 yrs), 6 (10–14 yrs), 2 (15–19 yrs), 7 (20 yrs and over). From Lancet, 30 October 1976, p. 957.

In cholera patients, the inevitable high incidence of negative sodium balance, hyponatremia and, in some patients, seizures and other complications of hyponatremia, was overlooked until 2006 (10) due to lack of sodium balance studies plus inadequate safety surveillance for several decades in those areas where cholera was highly prevalent. The fundamental differences between cholera (including nonvibrio cholera) and other AWDs in magnitude of losses and pathophysiology underline the inferior efficacy for maintenance of Na^+ balance and for avoidance of hyponatremia when ORS formulations with glucose or rice with ORS 90 or less are used to treat cholera patients.

5. Major Differences in Pathophysiology of Cholera and Non-Cholera AWDs

Recent studies have found that absorption of sugars and amino acids promoting active transport of sodium is not merely intact but is *increased* in response to cholera toxin [39–45]. This provides an explanation for the fact that oral therapy using ORS formulations with combined glucose and glycine [46,47], alanine [48] or glutamine [49] and other similar substrate combinations, and rice-based ORS (34) (furnishing glucose and amino acids on hydrolysis [50] are all capable of enhancing absorption and reducing diarrhea duration and volume in cholera and nonvibrio cholera but appear to *have no such effect* in noncholera AWD, particularly in children [51–55] and notably in rotavirus diarrhea [56], in which glucose ORS is effective [23], although glucose is often detectable in the stools. Rotavirus diarrhea may represent a distinct pathophysiology in which added glycine or other actively transported amino acid, or added rice, does not yield any significant advantage. The pathophysiology of this and of other noncholera AWDs may also limit absorption of amino acids by effects on villus function [57], as do some antibiotics used in ORS clinical trials [58]. In acute porcine viral enteritis, sodium-dependent alanine transport in the brush border membrane is reduced [59], suggesting one mechanism possibly explaining the lack of alanine, glycine or glutamine efficacy in human noncholera, notably viral, AWD.

In both the normal and the diarrhea-affected small bowel, sodium secretion into the lumen proceeds according to its *chemical* gradient, *not* the osmolar gradient per se. In the normal small bowel, osmoregulation of luminal contents is achieved by a combination of sodium excretion into the lumen according to the chemical gradient of sodium, and water absorption or secretion into the lumen according to the osmolar gradient. Animal studies have shown that cholera deranges normal small bowel osmoregulation due largely to interference with the absorptive component, with the effect that, in cholera, osmoregulation is accomplished solely by altering the rate of net *secretion* of water and salt. While rate of net water secretion into hypotonic lumenal solutions is reduced, rate of salt excretion is increased [60].

Repeated concern in the literature about the osmolality of ORS has persistently ignored the fact that the most successful ORS for cholera, containing glucose and glycine, has the *highest* osmolality of any successful ORS to date, proving that *absorbability trumps osmolality* as regards success rates of different ORS formulations. [46,47]. The same probably holds true for rice ORS, since the only available evidence indicates that rice, like sucrose, must be hydrolyzed in the intestinal lumen before the products of digestion are absorbed [61]. Rice is also reported to contain an antidiarrheal agent possibly interfering with adenyl cyclase [62,63], but such an agent would not be effective in diarrhoeal disorders related to other biochemical mechanisms, consistent with the clinical benefits of rice ORS being confined to cholera.

While reports are conflicting as to whether a rice (or rice product) diet has any additional effect on patients receiving ORS with glucose or other non-rice substrates [64,65], the effects of a rice diet on outcomes in patients receiving other ORS formulations have not been reported. However, it is counterintuitive, if rice has a positive beneficial effect, that giving a rice diet to patients receiving ORS without rice would have no effect.

In an effort to promote a single global ORS formulation, international bodies have recommended [1] a single ORS formulation with lower glucose, lower sodium (75 mEq/L.) and lower osmolality ("75 ORS"), based primarily on a modest and often clinically insignificant diminution in GDR, diarrhea duration and (variably in some studies) so-called "unscheduled" I.V. fluids, or I.V. fluids resumed post-rehydration, these modest advantages occurring *only* in noncholera pediatric populations, *not* in cholera patients [1].

An alternative mechanism explaining the apparent "benefits" of reduced diarrhea rates when hypoosmolar ORS is used is that the induction of hyponatremia by such formulations itself lowers diarrhea rate [66].

The "low glucose, low sodium, low osmolarity" ORS formulation is suboptimal for adults and children with cholera, because it contains sodium and chloride content far below that lost in cholera diarrhea. Use of the 75 ORS formulation in the majority of adult and pediatric cholera patients is, like WHO90, suboptimal in replacing sodium losses and causes even greater negative sodium balance with very large net sodium losses, which will lead to hyponatremia and, in a subset of cholera patients so treated, to seizures and other symptoms of severe hyponatremia.

Unlike the case with the WHO 90 ORS using the 2:1 regimen [34], the safety of ORS 75 in terms of net sodium balance when treating AWD in neonates or treating children with pre-existing hyponatremic or hypernatremic dehydration (a very high percentage of AWD patients at some centers) [67] has not been determined.

The assumption that cholera patients made hyponatremic rarely suffer adverse outcomes rests on no evidence, since, despite the magnitude of sodium losses using 75 ORS (Table 1), these have not been systematically looked for using established standardized tests of the well-known serious sequelae of hyponatremia [68–70] in any follow-up studies of hyponatremic pediatric or adult cholera patients.

Table 1. Comparison of calculated net sodium losses in cholera patients treated with ORS containing 75 vs. 90 mEq/L. sodium. The 8 L total stool volume is an example based on figures in J. Pediatrics 78: 355–358, 1971. * Na⁺ in mEq. Stool sodium levels from Table 11-2, P.225, in Cholera, Eds. Barua and Burrows 1974. W.B. Saunders Co.. Philadelphia.

	Na⁺ Losses in Cholera Patient Given (ORS75 vs. ORS90)	
	ADULTS	CHILDREN
Stool Na⁺ (mEq/L)	140	101
ORS Na⁺	75 vs. 90	75 vs. 90
Na⁺ Loss	−65 vs. −50	−26 vs. −10
Stool Vol. (L)	25	8
Total Na⁺ loss (mEq) *	−1625 vs. −1250	−208 vs. −80

Furthermore, the seizures seen in cholera patients made hyponatremic by use of this formulation have been arbitrarily attributed to other causes. For example, shigellosis is listed as a possible cause, whereas seizures are not a feature of shigellosis in the absence of hyponatremia [71]. Additionally, the "withdrawal" from analysis of patients with complicating other disorders transferred to the ICU [6,10] has the effect of obscuring the degree of harm caused by hyponatremia in the most vulnerable patients [72,73] who have a case fatality rate of 10% [74].

6. Limitations of Existing Studies

The Cochrane reviewed reports subdivided the international definition of hyponatremia (<135 mEq/L.) arbitrarily into cutoffs of 130, 127 or 125 mEq/L. of sodium [5–7,9,10], but. as previously noted: "neurocognitive deficits are evident, even in apparently asymptomatic patients, when such changes are specifically probed for." Such deficits occur after hyponatremia of diverse causes in adults and children [68,69]. Detection of such deficits, which have been associated not only with seizures and stupor, but with less obvious signs and symptoms (e.g., headache, muscle cramps, weakness, restlessness, disorientation, depressed reflexes, gait disturbances, developmental retardation) require detailed examination and use of sensitive clinical tests, including the Mini-Mental State Examination, the Clock Completion test, the Audio Recording Cognitive Screening tool and a battery of attention tests (Visual Vigilance, Working Memory or Digit Span, Go/No Go, Intermodal Comparison, Divided Attention and Phasic Alert). No such screening was conducted in any of the Cochrane reviewed studies, whether in hyponatremic patients with or without seizures in hospital or in follow-up after discharge. The assumption stated in some reports indicating that dietary sodium should correct sodium deficits is by no means guaranteed and does not obviate the need to thoroughly check for hyponatremia-induced neurologic and developmental deficits. Furthermore, the assumption of dietary correction is particularly doubtful in severely malnourished diarrhea patients [67] and those with multiple AWD episodes per annum, which can number nine or more in some areas [75].

Unlike the case with the WHO 90 ORS using the 2:1 ratio [36], safety of ORS 75 in terms of net sodium balance when treating neonates or treating children with pre-existing hyponatremic or hypernatremic dehydration has not been tested. Safety studies over time in children with chronic hyponatremia or multiple AWD episodes annually are also needed.

Part of the confusion over this issue arises from the incomplete design of studies aiming to demonstrate "low" seizure rates in such patients, without follow-up for more long-term harmful effects. The only published large-scale survey compared seizure rates in cholera patients-treated chiefly (92%) with the low-sodium *rice* ORS to those treated in a prior year with the original glucose WHO 90 ORS. However as noted above, the WHO 90 formulation was significantly deficient in sodium compared to the sodium content of cholera diarrhea and was bound to cause negative sodium balance leading to hyponatremia in cholera patients unless, rather than simply matching their losses, they drank an amount equivalent to at least one and one-half times the volume of their diarrhea fluid, as originally noted soon after the formulation adopted by WHO was tested [31]. This would exceed drinking capacity in profusely purging patients, and the need to drink more of that formulation than with the earlier cholera ORS formulations in order to avoid hyponatremia was largely ignored. However in one Cochrane-reviewed study, remarkably, patients were given *twice* or *thrice* the amount of ORS to drink compared to the volume of their losses [7], a methodology placing a huge burden on patients and one sure to lead to increased failure rates in the field.

Other differences in methodology between study centers, confounding interpretation of ORS formulation effects, include the different quantities and duration of I.V. fluids given in the "rehydration" phase [5–9], percentage of severely dehydrated patients (4 vs. 23% [3]) or inclusion [4] vs. exclusion [3] of severely malnourished patients and identification [4–9] or lack thereof [3] of concurrent antibiotic therapy (erythromycin may inhibit jejunal D-galactase and sucrase [58]), omission of patient weights [3,4,7,10], inclusion or omission [7–10] of foods given during studies, of stool volume [4,10] or plasma sp. gr. measurements [3,5,6], use of different therapeutic methods (matching intake with output vs. giving a fixed number of ORS packets regardless of diarrhea duration [3,5]; allowing patients to become severely dehydrated after initial dehydration before resuming I.V. fluids [3,5,6], inclusion vs. exclusion of complete data on long-duration and high volume diarrhea patients [7], and reporting only 24 h serum Na^+ levels in studies lasting 43–44 h [6].

Discrepant results include more unscheduled I.V. fluid needed in the low Na^+ group [4,6] and highly variable disease severity (total stool volumes) between different centers' outbreaks [3–10]. In one rice ORS study [8], stool volume fell 17% but inexplicably ORS volume fell 27%, suggesting lax management. These and other methodologic variations between centers in patient selection and management undoubtedly account for the considerable variability in results obtained. Many studies comparing different ORS formulations suffer from similar deficiencies and it is not surprising that conflicting results are not uncommon, chiefly from failure to prestratify by initial stool rates in most studies and use of different rehydration and maintenance methods and percent of breast-fed or food-fed infants.

In the Cochrane-reviewed studies, clinically estimated state of hydration (actually of severe dehydration) was used as the criterion for resuming I.V. fluids, called "unscheduled I.V.s", but the data on specific clinical signs triggering I.V. resumption were omitted. The fact that in some studies severe dehydration could be permitted to recur [3,5,6] suggests a failure to respond to lesser degrees of recurrent dehydration or lapses in monitoring of the clinical signs of dehydration, which could have been more accurately and objectively accomplished by monitoring plasma sp. gr. levels.

Interpretation of results is also clouded by several other issues. Studies ostensibly comparing 75 with 90 mEq/L. formulations actually compared 75 or 90 mEq/L. Na^+ given together with dietary rice preparations or noodles and salt [3–10]. Additionally, total quantities of I.V. fluids given after rehydration, representing additional salt loading offsetting sodium deficits, were not presented [3–10]. One study substituted stool frequency for stool volumes [4], but stool frequency can be high in low-volume inflammatory AWD, so the validity of this substitution is questionable, and frequency has not been correlated directly with total stool volume. The range of etiologic agents also differed between centers and seasons [3,4]. A claim that use of the lower Na^+ ORS would reduce blood-borne diseases [6] is without any basis.

7. Discussion

Despite these limitations, most studies in pediatric or adult cholera patients concluded that the efficacy of 75 and 90 mEq/L. Na^+ ORS formulations was similar, with neither ORS superior. Most studies showed no clinically or statistically significant differences in key parameters like total stool volume and duration, vomiting incidence and unscheduled I.V.

rate. However, the obvious fact that the efficacy in terms of maintaining sodium balance was inadequate in both groups went unstated.

Since both the 75 and the 90 mEq/L. sodium ORS glucose formulations lead to hyponatremia when given to cholera patients losing 100–145 mEq/L of sodium, it was to be expected that the *rates* of hyponatremia would be the same using either of the two formulations. In that light, the comparisons of hyponatremia rates using 75 ORS vs. 90 ORS to show no significant differences was a straw-man hypothesis. The unmeasured net *negative sodium balance* will certainly be greater using the 75 than using the 90 mEq/L. ORS formulation (see Table 1 above).

Surprisingly, from both the efficacy and safety perspectives, not a single sodium balance study was conducted prior to promoting the low-sodium glucose (or rice)-based ORS formulations for use in cholera patients, and none has appeared since. No sufficiently sized and powered properly controlled sodium balance efficacy and safety study comparing results with ORS containing 75 vs. 90 mEq/L. Na+ has been done with either rice or glucose as substrates. Two such studies formerly said to be planned (2, see pp. 34–35 for studies #NCDT00490932 and NCT 00672308) apparently have not been published, if indeed completed as reported [2].

The danger of profound iatrogenic sodium losses and hyponatremia complications resulting from treatment of pediatric and adult cholera patients treated with the 75 mEq/L. ORS sodium formulation will be even more pronounced when treating patients harboring antibiotic resistant *V. cholerae*, who may need up to 100 L of ORS to replace their stool losses after initial I.V. rehydration [76].

Serum sodium in adults does not decline until there is more than 200 mEq net sodium loss. Monitoring only serum sodium does not give a correct estimate of total body sodium loss. Cholera patients of all ages have massive sodium losses using the low-sodium ORS, leading to serum sodium declining to hyponatremic levels in >50% of adult cholera patients treated with ORS 90 with glucose (Nalin D, unpublished data). This results in a cutoff of antidiuretic hormone (ADH) with resulting polyuria even during dehydration, and this has been misinterpreted in clinical studies of low-sodium ORS as a sign of good hydration [5,7] which it is not. This exemplifies the clinical misinterpretation resulting from the polyuria, which use of the low-sodium solution can lead to.

In the settings of rural cholera treatment centers or home treatment, management of hypernatremic seizures and related complications is likely to have serious consequences which are attributable only to the use of this formulation instead of one matching more closely that of cholera diarrhea. Such a formulation should contain 120 mEq/L. of sodium, providing that ORS substrates, which in cholera alone enhance salt absorption more than glucose alone, are used in the ORS, including formulations with glucose plus glycine or rice powder (which yields glucose, amino acids and antidiarrheal components on hydrolysis [50,62,63]). The price of glycine has been mistakenly mentioned as a reason not to use it for cholera patients, but in fact glycine and glucose are available in bulk as food additives on the global wholesale market at about the same price, such as $1/kg [77,78]. Other amino acids which also promote active transport are far costlier. Rice or glucose plus glycine ORS packets would also offer savings in reduced hospitalization time; whether rice or glucose plus glycine ORS has any advantage in terms of commercial packet shelf life, and whether all of the many varieties of rice are equally effective, have not been determined. Results obtained using rice ORS or glycine–glucose ORS have been generally similar in that the advantages with either ORS are reproducible only in studies with a majority of cholera and/or nonvibrio cholera patients, not in patients with AWDs of other etiologies. This again underlines the pathophysiologic peculiarities of diarrhea-caused *V. cholerae* or by strains of enterotoxigenic *E. coli* and related pathogens producing cholera toxin analogs, versus other diarrheal pathogens.

Rice is also ineffective in patients with rice carbohydrate malabsorption [79], in which boiled rice fed to children with cholera leads to increased volume and duration of diarrhea [80]. Lastly, a Cochrane review concluded that the advantages of rice ORS, like those of glycine–glucose ORS, are seen in cholera or nonvibrio cholera but not in other types of AWD [81].

8. Conclusions

In sum, fear of what has turned out to be chiefly transient mild or moderate hypernatremia has led to ORS formulations inducing high prevalence hyponatremia, notably at a time when pediatric recommendations for intravenous fluid therapy have shifted to higher sodium I.V. solutions [82–85]. Ironically, hypernatremic seizures, feared when glucose ORS with 90 mEq/L. Na^+ is used in noncholera AWD patients, appeared in only 1 of 48,511 WHO 90-treated patients surveyed in the largest series, compared with 47 hyponatremic seizures [10]. The incidence rates reported in that study were minimized by using a denominator including a majority of nondehydrated or mildly dehydrated patients not in the risk pool for hyponatremia. When the denominator was restricted to severely dehydrated patients, the hyponatremic seizure rate was 0.15% in the study group, but the comparable rate in the comparison group was omitted. In another study [3], one out of every 13 children with serum $Na^+ < 125$ had seizures. Projected on a global basis, this represents a very significant morbidity burden linked with this formulation.

The dichotomy in efficacy of the low Na^+ ORS formulation between cholera and non-cholera AWDs presents a paradox: in cholera, the goal of an ORS with 120 mEq/L. Na+ and either rice or glycine–glucose, which significantly reduce both duration and volume of diarrhea safely and without profound net sodium losses, is an attractive option. In noncholera pediatric AWDs, the ORS with 3 lowered parameters appears to offer similar benefits but has inferior efficacy for maintaining sodium balance and leads to an iatrogenic increased incidence of hyponatremic toxicity when used for cholera. Perhaps studies in which less than three variables are changed would be useful. In cholera, 75 ORS with rice also causes hyponatremia [9].

Outcomes of ORS formulation studies are etiology-dependent, cholera and related diseases benefiting very significantly from glucose ORS with added actively transport-promoting amino acids, benefits not seen in rotavirus and related noncholera AWDs in which absorption of glucose is sufficient for successful ORT [23], but absorption of added amino acids is evidently blocked by pathogenetic factors.

Cholera outbreaks have occurred in recent years in Haiti, Yemen and many African countries and are quickly recognized. A choice is at hand between two different oral treatment modalities for cholera, an ORS with 120 mEq/L. Na^+ plus rice or glucose-glycine, vs. one using 75 ORS with glucose or rice. The 75 ORS option is significantly less effective in maintaining sodium balance and has a less favorable though inadequately monitored safety profile. No clinical trials to date have employed standard sensitive neurologic tests [68,69] to monitor for adverse effects of hyponatremia other than seizures, including long-term effects on developmental parameters and delayed mortality. If 75 ORS is to be promoted for cholera, its safety profile should be firmly established as indicated in Table 2.

Table 2. Comprehensive safety studies recommended to fully assess safety of hyponatremia induced or aggravated in cholera patients receiving ORS 75. For standard tests, see [68,69].

Recommended Safety Studies of 75 ORS in Cholera Patients	
STUDIES	PURPOSE
Na^+ Balance	Determine size of Na^+ deficite
Clinical Sequelae	R/O acute sequelae using standard tests
Follow-up Studies	R/O developmental deficits and excess post-convalescent mortality

It is in the long-term public health interest to choose the safer and more effective ORS formulation for cholera. Even a "low" percentage of hyponatremic seizures and other neurologic and developmental sequelae translates globally into thousands of cases annually, a major avoidable morbidity. The time has come to recognize that two different ORS formulations are needed, one with rice or with glucose plus glycine for use in cholera epidemics, and one for noncholera AWDs. Both rice and glycine–glucose ORS have advantages in cholera, but for use in packets glycine, which does not require boiling, may be advantageous, and may have superior shelf life before and after mixing [86], while preserving the savings in reduced hospitalization time for patients at cholera treatment centers when either ORS is used.

However, if glucose-ORS alone is to be globally recommended and if the programmatic goal of promoting only a single ORS packet is the overweening concern, another possible alternative meriting clinical trials would be to alter the volume of water used to dilute the ORS packets when confronting cholera. For example, an ORS suitable for use in cholera can be made by reconstituting four WHO 90 packets in 3 L of potable water (Table 3). The dilutional water volume can easily be measured, as now, using household containers, or standardized by use of calibrated plastic bags [87]. A similar solution has been found suitable for use in hospitalized cholera patients of all ages when the matching method is used to balance intake with output [88]. The resulting glucose content is close to that found optimal in early balance studies [32].

Table 3. How 4 ORS 90 packets could be dissolved in 3 L of water to make a solution more suitable for replacing cholera patients' electrolyte losses. Using ORS 75 packets with 2.6 g NaCl each, a similar solution could be prepared by dissolving four packets in 2.5 L of water.

ORS Suitable for Cholera Patients	
Dissolve 4 Packets of 90 ORS in 3 L Water	Resulting ORS Concentrations
	Na$^+$ 120 *
	K$^+$ 27 *
	Cl$^-$ 107 *
	Citrate 13@
	Glucose 147@

* mEq/L, @mMol/L.

Funding: This research received no external funding.

Institutional Review Board Statement: Not applicable.

Informed Consent Statement: Figures 1–7: At the time, the parents provided verbal consent for both the child and themselves to be photographed, likewise for the other photographed subjects. It is necessary to show the patient's face to demonstrate the clinical features of the condition under discussion. The photographs were taken a long time ago and it is not possible to trace the subjects and obtain retroactive specific written permission for publication.

Conflicts of Interest: The authors declare no conflict of interest.

Abbreviations

AWD	Acute Watery Diarhhea
ORS	Oral Rehydratation Solution
ORT	Oral Rehydratation Therapy
ORS75	ORS with 75 mEq/L Sodium (Na$^+$)
ORS90	ORS With 90 mEq/L Sodium (Na$^+$)
ORS120	ORS With 120 mEq/L Sodium (Na$^+$)
GDR	Gross Diarrhea Rate, ml/hr
NGB	Net Gut Balance (oral intake) − (stool+vomitus) in Liters
PNGB	Positive Net Gut Balance
CHOLERA	AWD Caused by *Vibrio cholerae*
ETEC	Enterotoxigenic *Escherichia coli*
NONVIBRIO CHOLERA	Severe AWD Due to ETEC or Bacteria with Cholera Toxin Analogs

References

1. WHO. Reduced Osmolarity Oral Rehydration Salts (ORS) Formulation; Department of Child and Adolescent Health and Development. Available online: https://apps.who.int/iris/handle/10665/67322 (accessed on 20 October 2020).
2. Musekiwa, A.; Volmink, J.; Cochrane Infectious Diseases Group. Oral Rehydration Salt Solution for Treating Cholera: ≤270 mOs/L solutions vs. ≤310 mOsm/L Solutions. *Cochrane Database Syst. Rev.* **2011**, *2011*, CD003754. [CrossRef]
3. CHOICE Study Group. Multicenter, randomized, double-blind clinical trial to evaluate the efficacy and safety of a reduced osmolarity oral rehydration salts solution in children with acute watery diarrhea. *Pediatrics* **2001**, *107*, 613–618. [CrossRef]
4. Alam, S.; Afzal, K.; Maheshwari, M.; Shukla, I. Controlled trial of hypo-osmolar versus world Health Organization Oral rehydration solution. *Indian Pediatrics* **2000**, *37*, 952–960.
5. Pulungsih, S.P.; Punjabi, N.H.; Rafli, K.; Rifajati, A.; Kumala, S.; Simanjuntak, C.H.; Yuwono Lesmana, M.; Subekti, D.; Sutoto; Fontaine, O. Standard WHO_ORS versus reduced-osmolarity ORS in the management of cholera patients. *J. Health Popul. Nutr.* **2006**, *24*, 107–112.
6. Alam, N.H.; Majumder, R.N.; Fuchs, G.J.; The CHOICE study group. Efficacy and safety of oral rehydration solution with reduced osmolarity in adults with cholera: A randomized double-blind clinical trial. *Lancet* **1999**, *354*, 296–299. [CrossRef]
7. Faruque, A.S.G.; Mahalanabis, D.; Hamadani, J.D.; Zetterstrom, R. Reduced osmolarity oral rehydration salt in cholera. *Scan. J. Infect Dis.* **1996**, *28*, 87–90. [CrossRef] [PubMed]
8. Bhattacharya, M.K.; Bhattacharya, S.K.; Dutta, D.; Deb, A.K.; Deb, M.; Dutta, A.; Saha, C.A.; Nair, G.B.; Mahalanabis, D. Efficacy of oral hyposmolar glucose-based and rice-based oral rehydration salt solutions in the treatment of cholera in adults. *Scan. J. Gastroent.* **1998**, *33*, 159–163. [CrossRef]
9. Dutta, M.K.; Bhattacharya, M.K.; Deb, A.K.; Sarkar, A.; Chatterjee, A.; Biswas, A.B.; Chatterjee, K.; Nair, G.B.; Bhattacharya, S.K. Evaluation of oral hypo-osmolar glucose-based and rice-based oral rehydration solutions in the treatment of cholera in children. *Acta Paediatr.* **2000**, *89*, 787–790. [CrossRef]
10. Alam, N.H.; Yunus, M.; Faruque, A.S.G.; Gyr, N.; Sattar, S.; Parvin, S.; Ahmed, J.U.; Salam, M.A.; Sack, D.A. Symptomatic hyponatremia during treatment of dehydrating diarrheal disease with reduced osmolarity oral rehydration solution. *JAMA* **2006**, *296*, 567–573. [CrossRef]
11. Phillips, R.A. Asiatic cholera. *Ann. Rev. Med.* **1968**, *19*, 69–79. [CrossRef]
12. Nalin, D.R. Oral therapy for diarrheal diseases. *J. Diarrheal Dis. Res.* **1987**, *5*, 283–292.
13. Hirschhorn, N.; Kinzie, J.I.; Sachar, D.B.; Northrup, R.S.; Taylor, J.O.; Ahmad, S.Z.; Philllips, R.A. Decrease in net stool output in cholera during intestinal perfusion with glucose-containing solutions. *NEJM* **1968**, *279*, 176–181. [CrossRef]
14. Nalin, D.R.; Levine, M.M.; Hornick, R.; Bergquist, E.; Hoover, D.; Holley, H.P.; Waterman, D.; Van Blerk, J.; Matheny, S.; Sotman, S.; et al. The problem of emesis during oral glucose-electrolytes therapy given from the onset of severe cholera. *Trans. Roy. Soc. Trop. Med. Hyg.* **1979**, *73*, 10–14. [CrossRef]
15. Cash, R.A.; Nalin, D.R.; Toaha, K.M.M.; Huq, Z. Acetate in the correction of acidosis secondary to diarrhea. *Lancet* **1969**, *294*, 302–303. [CrossRef]
16. Harvey, R.M.; Enson, Y.; Lewis, M.L.; Greenough, W.B.; Ally, K.; Panno, R.A. Hemodynamic studies on cholera, Effects of hypovolemia and acidosis. *Circulation* **1968**, *37*, 709–728. [CrossRef]
17. Nalin, D.R.; Cash, R.A.; Islam, R.; Molla, M.; Phillips, R.A. Oral maintenance therapy for cholera in adults. *Lancet* **1968**, *292*, 370–373. [CrossRef]
18. El-Mougi, M.; Hendaw, A.; Koura, H.; Hegazi, E.; Fontain, O.; Pierce, N.F. Efficacy of standard glucose-based and reduced-osmolarity maltodextrin-based oral rehyration solutions: Effect of sugar malabsorption. *Bull. WHO* **1996**, *74*, 471–477.
19. Lifschitz, F.; Coello-Ramirez, P.; Gutierrez, L.L.C. Monosaccharide intolerance and hypoglycemia in infants with diarrh74, 471-477.ea: Metabolic studies in 23 infants. *J. Peds* **1970**, *77*, 604–612. [CrossRef]
20. Hirschhorn, N.; Nalin, D.R.; Cash, R.A. CHOICE Study Group Trial. *Pediatrics* **2002**, *109*, 713–715. [CrossRef]
21. Saniel, M.C.; Zimicki, S.; Carlos, C.C.; Maria, A.C.S.; Balis, A.C.; Malacad, C. *J. Diarrhoeal Dis. Res.* **1997**, *15*, 47–52.
22. Isolauri, E. Evaluation of an oral rehydration solution with Na+ 60 mmol/L. in infants hospitalized for acute diarrhea or treated as outpatients. *Acta Paediatr. Scand* **1985**, *74*, 643–649. [CrossRef]
23. Nalin, D.R.; Levine, M.M.; Mata, L.; de Cespedes, C.; Vargas, W.; Lizano, C.; Loria, A.R.; Simhon, A.; Mohs, E. Oral rehydration and maintenance of children with rotavirus and bacterial diarrheas. *Bull. WHO* **1979**, *57*, 453–459.
24. Snyder, J.D.; Merson, M.H. The magnitude of the problem of acute diarrheal disease: A review of active surveillance data. *Bull. WHO* **1982**, *60*, 506–513.
25. GBD 2016 Diarrhoeal Disease Collaborators. Estimates of the global, regional and national morbidity, mortality and aetiologies of diarrhea in 195 countries: A systematic analysis for the Global Burden of Disease Study 2016. *Lancet* **2018**, *18*, 1211–1228. [CrossRef]
26. Ruxin, J. Magic Bullet: The history of oral rehydration therapy. *Med. Hist.* **1994**, *38*, 363–397. [CrossRef] [PubMed]
27. Cash, R.A.; Nalin, D.R.; Forrest, J.; Abrutyn, E. Rapid correction of the acidosis and dehydration of cholera with an oral solution. *Lancet* **1970**, *296*, 549–550. [CrossRef]
28. Nalin, D.R.; Cash, R.A. Oral or nasogastric maintenance therapy for diarrheas of unknown etiology resembling cholera. *Trans. Roy. Soc. Trop. Med. Hyg.* **1970**, *64*, 769–771. [CrossRef]

29. Greenough, W.B.; Gordon, R.S., Jr.; Rosenberg, I.S.; David, B.I.; Benenson, A.H. Tetracycline in the treatment of cholera. *Lancet* **1964**, *1*, 335–337. [CrossRef]
30. Cash, R.A.; Nalin, D.R.; Rochat, R.; Reller, B.; Haque, E.; Rahman, M. A clinical trial of oral therapy in a rural cholera treatment center. *Am. J. Trop. Med. Hyg.* **1970**, *19*, 653–656. [CrossRef]
31. Nalin, D.R.; Cash, R.A. Sodium content in oral therapy for diarrhea. *Lancet* **1976**, *2*, 957. [CrossRef]
32. Pierce, N.F.; Banwell, J.G.; Mitra, R.C.; Caranasos, G.J.; Keimowitz, R.I.; Mondal, A.; Manji, P.M. Effect of intragastric glucose-electrolyte infusion upon water and electrolyte balance in Asiatic cholera. *Gastroenterology* **1968**, *55*, 333–344. [CrossRef]
33. Nalin, D.R. Oral Cholera Therapy. *Ann. Intern. Med.* **1970**, *72*, 288–289. [CrossRef]
34. Molla, A.M.; Ahmed, S.M.; Greenough, W.B., III. Rice-based oral rehydration solution decreases the stool volume in acute diarrhea. *Bull. WHO* **1985**, *63*, 751–756.
35. Roy, S.K.; Rabbani, G.H.; Black, R.E. Oral rehydration solution safely used in breast-fed children without additional water. *J. Trop. Med. Hyg.* **1984**, *87*, 11–13. [PubMed]
36. Nalin, D.R.; Levine, M.M.; Mata, L.; de Cespedes, C.; Vargas, W.; Lizano, C.; Loria, A.R.; Simhon, A.; Mohs, E. Comparison of sucrose with glucose in oral therapy of infant diarrheas. *Lancet* **1978**, *312*, 277–279. [CrossRef]
37. Pizarro, D.; Possada, G.; Villavicencio, N.; Mohs, E.; Levine, M.M. Hypernatremic and hyponatremic diarrheal dehydration. Treatment with oral glucose-electrolyte solution. *Am. J. Dis. Child.* **1983**, *137*, 730–734. [CrossRef] [PubMed]
38. Nalin, D.R.; Harland, E.; Ramlal, A.; Swaby, D.; McDonald, J.; Gangarosa, R.; Levine, M.; Akierman, A.; Antonine, M.; Mackenzie, K.; et al. Comparison of low and high sodium and potassium content in oral rehydration solutions. *J. Pediatr.* **1980**, *97*, 848–853. [CrossRef]
39. Clancy, B.M.; Czech, M.P. Hexose transport stimulation and membrane redistribution of glucose transporter isoforms in response to cholera toxin, dibutyryl cyclic AMP and insulin in 3T3-L1 adipocytes. *J. Biol. Chem.* **1990**, *265*, 12434–12443. [CrossRef]
40. Nath, S.K.; Rautureau, M.; Heyman, H. Emergence of Na+-glucose cotransport in an epithelial secretory cell line sensitive to cholera toxin. *Am. J. Physiol.* **1989**, *1069*, G335–G341. [CrossRef]
41. Moule, S.K.; Bradford, N.M.; McGivan, J.D. Short-term stimulation of Na+-dependent amino acid transport by dibutryl cyclic AMP in hepatocytes. Characteristics and partial mechanism. *Biochem. J.* **1987**, *241*, 737–743. [CrossRef]
42. Tai, Y.H.; Perez, E.; Desjeux, J.F. Cholera toxin and cyclic AMP stimulate D-glucose absorption in rat ileum. In *Ion Gradient-Coupled Transport*; Alverado, F., Van Os, C.H., Eds.; Elsevier: Amsterdam, The Netherlands, 1986; pp. 403–406.
43. Wright Em Hirsh, J.R.; Loo, D.D.; Zampighi, G.A. Regulation of Na+/glucose cotransporters. *J. Exp. Biol.* **1997**, *200*, 287–293.
44. Flach, C.F.; Lange, S.; Jennische, E.; Lonnroth, I. Cholera toxin induces expression of ion channels and carriers in small intestinal mucosea. *FEBS Lett.* **2004**, *561*, 122–126. [CrossRef]
45. Schiller, L.E.; Santa Ana, C.; Porter, J.; Fortran, J.S. Glucose-stimulated sodium transport by the human intestine during experimental cholera. *Gastroenterology* **1997**, *112*, 1529–1535. [CrossRef]
46. Nalin, D.R.; Cash, R.A.; Rahaman, M.; Yunus, M. Effect of glycine and glucose on sodium and water absorption in patients with cholera. *Gut* **1970**, *11*, 768–772. [CrossRef] [PubMed]
47. Patra, F.C.; Mahalanabis, D.; Jalan, K.N.; Sen, A.; Banerjee, P. In search of a super solution: controlled trial of glycine-glucose oral rehydration solution in infantile diarrhea? *Acta Pediatr. Scand* **1984**, *73*, 18. [CrossRef] [PubMed]
48. Patra, F.C.; Sack, D.A.; Islam, A.; Alam, A.N.; Mazumder, R.N. Oral rehydration formula containing alanine and glucose for treatment of diarrhea: A controlled trial. *BMJ* **1989**, *298*, 1353–1356. [CrossRef] [PubMed]
49. Punjabi, N.H.; Kumala, S.; Rasidi, C.; Witham, N.D.; Pulungsih, S.P.; Rivai, A.R.; Sukri, N.; Burr, D.H.; Lesmana, M. Improving the ORS: Does glutamine have a role? *Am. J. Trop. Med. Hyg.* **1991**, *45*, 114–115.
50. Amankwah, E.N.; Adu, E.; Barimah, V.M.J.; Van Twisk, C. Amino acid profiles of some varieties of rice, soybean and groundnut grown in Ghana. *J. Food Process. Technol.* **2015**, *6*, 420–423.
51. Vesikari, T.; Isolauri, E. Glycine supplemented oral rehydration solutions for diarrhea. *Arch. Dis. Child.* **1986**, *61*, 372–376. [CrossRef]
52. Pizarro, D.; Levine, M.M.; Posada, G.; Sandi, L. Comparison of glucose/electrolyte and glucose/glycine/electrolyte oral rehydration solutions in hospitalized children with diarrhea in Costa Rica. *J. Pediatr. Gastroenterol. Nutr.* **1988**, *7*, 411–416. [CrossRef]
53. Ribiero, H.D.C., Jr.; Lifshitz, F. Alanine-based oral rehydration therapy for infants with acute diarrhea. *J. Pediatr.* **1991**, *118*, S86–S90.
54. Gutierrez, C.; Villa, S.; Mota, F.R.; Calva, J.J. Does an L-glutamine-containing, glucose-free, oral rehydration solution reduce stool output and time to rehydrate in children with acute diarrhea? A double-blind randomized clinical trial. *J. Health Popul. Nutr.* **2007**, *3*, 278–284.
55. Gore, S.M.; Fontaine, O.; Pierce, N. Impact of rice based oral rehydration solution on stool output and duration of diarrhea: meta-analysis of 13 clinical trials. *BMJ* **1992**, *304*, 28791. [CrossRef] [PubMed]
56. Mahalanabis, D.; Faruque, A.G.; Hoque, S.S.; Faruque, S.M. Hypotonic oral rehydration solution in acute diarrhea: A controlled clinical trial. *Acta Pediatr.* **1995**, *84*, 289–293. [CrossRef] [PubMed]
57. Davidson, G.P.; Barnes, G.L. Structural and functional abnormalities of the small intestine in infants and young children with rotavirus enteritis. *Acta Paediatr.* **1979**, *68*, 181–186. [CrossRef]

58. Navarro, H.; Arruebo, M.P.; Alcalde, A.I.; Sorribas, V. Effect of erythromycin on D-galactose absorption and sucrose activity in rabbit jejunum. *Can. J. Physiol. Pharmacol.* **1993**, *71*, 191–194. [CrossRef] [PubMed]
59. Rhoads, J.M.; MacLeod, R.J.; Hamilton, J.R. Diminished brush border membrane sodium-dependent L-alanine transport in acute viral enteritis in piglets. *J. Pediatr. Gastroenterol. Nutr.* **1989**, *9*, 225–231. [CrossRef]
60. Nalin, D.R.; Ally, K.; Hare, K.; Hare, R. Effects of cholera enterotoxin on jejunal osmoregulation of mannitol solutions in dogs. *J. Infect. Dis.* **1972**, *125*, 528–532.
61. Gray, G.M.; Ingelfinger, F.J. Intestinal absorption of sucrose in man: The site of hydrolysis and absorption. *JCI* **1965**, *44*, 399098. [CrossRef]
62. Mathews, C.J.; MacLeod, R.J.; Zheng, S.X.; Hanrahan, J.W.; Bennett, H.P.; Hamilton, J.R. Characterization of the inhibitory effect of boiled rice on intestinal chloride secretion in guinea pig crypt cells. *Gastroenterology* **1999**, *116*, 1342–1347. [CrossRef]
63. Macleod, R.; Bennett, H.; Hamilton, J. inhibition of intestinal secretion by rice. *Lancet* **1995**, *346*, 90–92. [CrossRef]
64. Alam, V.A.; Ahmed, T.; Khatum; Molla, A.M. Effect of food with two or four rehydration therapies: A randomized controlled clinical trial. *Gut* **1992**, *33*, 560–562.
65. Santosham, M.; Fyad, I.; Hashem, M.; Goepp, J.G.; Refaf, M.; Sack, B. A comparison of rice-based oral rehydration solute and early feeding for the treatment of acute diarrhea in infants. *J. Pediatr.* **1990**, *116*, 868–875. [CrossRef]
66. Clarke, A.M.; Miller, M.; Shields, R. Intestinal transport of sodium, potassium and water in the dog during sodium depletion. *Gastroenteritis* **1967**, *52*, 846–858. [CrossRef]
67. Houston, K.A.; Gibb, J.G.; Maitland, K. Oral rehydration of malnourished children with diarrhea: A systematic review (version 3). *Wellcome Open Res.* **2017**, *2*, 66. [CrossRef] [PubMed]
68. Arieff, A.I.; Ayus, J.C.; Fraser, C.I. Hyponatremia and death or permanent brain damage in healthy children. *BMV* **1992**, *304*, 1218–1222.
69. Rondon-Berrios, H.; Berl, T. Mild chronic hyponatremia in the ambulatory setting: Significance and management. *Clin. J. Am. Soc. Nephrol.* **2015**, *10*, 2268–2278. [CrossRef] [PubMed]
70. Shahrin, L.; Chistri, M.J.; Huq, S.; Nishath, T.; Christy, M.D.; Hannan, A.; Ahmed, T. Clinical manifestations of hyponatremia and hypernatremia in under-five diarrheal children in a diarrhea hospital. *J. Trop. Pediatr.* **2016**, *62*, 206–212. [CrossRef]
71. Khan, W.A.; Dhar, U.; Salam, M.A.; Griffiths, J.K.; Rand, W.; Bennish, M.L. Central nervous system manifestations of childhood shigellosis: Prevalence, risk factors and outcome. *Pediatrics* **1999**, *103*, E18. [CrossRef] [PubMed]
72. Mitra, A.K.; Khan, M.R.; Alam, A.N. Complications and outcome of disease in patients admitted to the intensive care unit of a diarrhoeal diseases hospital in Bangladesh. *Trans. Roy. Soc. Trop. Med. Hyg.* **1991**, *85*, 685–687. [CrossRef]
73. Chisti, M.J.; Pietroni, M.A.; Smith, J.H.; Bardhan, P.K.; Salam, M.A. Predictors of death in under-five chidren with diarrhea admitted to a critical care ward in an urban hospital in Bangladesh. *Acta Paediatr.* **2011**, *100*, e275–e279. [CrossRef] [PubMed]
74. Samadi, A.R.; Wahed, M.A.; Islam, M.R.; Ahmed, S.M. Consequences of hyponatraemia and hypernatraemia in children with acute diarrhea in Bangladesh. *BMJ Clin. Res. Ed.* **1983**, *286*, 671–673. [CrossRef]
75. Sazawal, S.; Black, R.E.; Bhan, M.K.; Bhandari, N.; Sinha, A.; Jalla, S. Zinc supplementation in young children with acute diarrhea in India. *NEJM* **1995**, *333*, 839–844. [CrossRef] [PubMed]
76. Phillips, R.A. Cholera in the perspective of 1966. *Ann. Int. Med.* **1966**, *65*, 922–930. [CrossRef] [PubMed]
77. Available online: www.alibaba.com/amino-acid-glycine-price (accessed on 18 December 2020).
78. Available online: www.alibaba.com/glucosepowder (accessed on 18 December 2020).
79. Khin-Maung-U; Bolin, T.D.; Duncombe, V.M.; Myo-Khin; Nyunt-Nyunt-Wai; Pereira, S.P.; Linklater, J.M. Epidemiology of small bowel bacterial overgrowth and rice carbohydrate malabsorption in Burmese (Myanmar) village children. *Am. J. Trop. Med. Hyg.* **1992**, *47*, 298–304. [CrossRef] [PubMed]
80. Khinmaungu; Nyuntnyuntwai; Myokhin; Mumukhin; Tinu; Thanetoe. Effect of boiled-rice feeding in childhood cholera on clinical outcome. *Hum. Nutr. Clin. Nutr.* **1986**, *40*, 249–254.
81. Fontaine, O.; Gore, S.M.; Pierce, N.F. Rice-based oral rehydration solution for treating diarrhea. *Cochrane Database Syst. Rev.* **1998**, CD001264. [CrossRef]
82. Eldridge, D.; Ledoux, M. Needs more salt: Old hydration habits are hard to break. *Lancet* **2014**, *385*, 1159–1160. [CrossRef]
83. Duke, T.; Molyneux, E.M. Intravenous fluids for seriously ill children: Time to reconsider. *Lancet* **2003**, *362*, 1320–1323. [CrossRef]
84. McNab, S.; Duke, T.; South, M.; Babl, F.E.; Lee, K.j.; Arnup, S.J.; Young, S.; Turner, H.; Davidson, A. 140 mmol/L of sodium versus 77 mmol/L. of sodium in maintenance intravenous fluid therapy for children in hospital (PIMS): A randomized controlled double-blind trial. *Lancet* **2015**, *385*, 1190–1197. [CrossRef]
85. Friedman, J.N.; Beck, C.E.; DeGroot, J.; Geary, D.F.; Sklansky, D.J.; Freedman, S.B. Comparison of isotonic and hypotonic intravenous maintenance fluids: A randomized clinical trial. *JAMA Pediatr.* **2015**, *169*, 445–451. [CrossRef] [PubMed]
86. Bhattachariya, S.K.; Dutta, P.; Dutta, D.; Chakraborti, M.K. Super ORS. *Indian J. Public Health* **1990**, *34*, 35–37.
87. Nalin, D.R. A spoonful of sugar. *Lancet* **1978**, *2*, 264. [CrossRef]
88. Nalin, D.R.; Cash, R.A. Oral or nasogastric maintenance for cholera patients in all age groups. *Bull. WHO* **1970**, *43*, 361–363.

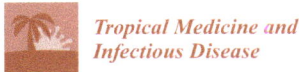 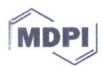

Correction

Correction: Nalin, D. Issues and Controversies in the Evolution of Oral Rehydration Therapy (ORT). *Trop. Med. Infect. Dis.* 2021, 6, 34

David Nalin

Albany Medical College, Albany, NY 12208-3478, USA; nalindavid@gmail.com

Error in Table

In the original publication [1], an error appears in Table 3 in the original article, in which the number 75 incorrectly appeared in the left hand column instead of the correct number 90. The corrected Table 3 appears below. The authors apologize for any inconvenience caused and state that the scientific conclusions are unaffected. The original publication has also been updated.

Table 3. How 4 ORS 90 packets could be dissolved in 3 L of water to make a solution more suitable for replacing cholera patients' electrolyte losses. Using ORS 75 packets with 2.6 g NaCl each, a similar solution could be prepared by dissolving four packets in 2.5 L of water.

ORS Suitable for Cholera Patients	
Dissolve 4 Packets of 90 ORS in 3 L Water	Resulting ORS Concentrations
	Na$^+$ 120 *
	K$^+$ 27 *
	Cl$^-$ 107 *
	Citrate 13@
	Glucose 147@

* mEq/L. @ mMol/L.

Reference

1. Nalin, D. Issues and Controversies in the Evolution of Oral Rehydration Therapy (ORT). *Trop. Med. Infect. Dis.* **2021**, *6*, 34. [CrossRef] [PubMed]

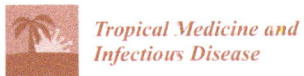

Article

Cholera and Pancreatic Cholera: Is VIP the Common Pathophysiologic Factor?

Farzana Afroze [1], Steven Bloom [2], Paul Bech [2], Tahmeed Ahmed [1], Shafiqul Alam Sarker [1], John D. Clemens [1], Farhana Islam [1] and David Nalin [3,*]

[1] International Centre for Diarrheal Disease Research (icddr,b), Dhaka 1212, Bangladesh; farzanaafroz@icddrb.org (F.A.); tahmeed@icddrb.org (T.A.); sasarker@icddrb.org (S.A.S.); jclemens@icddrb.org (J.D.C.); drfarhanaislam@icddrb.org (F.I.)
[2] North West London Pathology Consortium, Hammersmith Hospital, Imperial College London, Du Cane Road, London W12 0NN, UK; s.bloom@imperial.ac.uk (S.B.); p.bech@imperial.ac.uk (P.B.)
[3] Department of Immunology and Microbial Diseases, Albany Medical College, Albany, NY 12208, USA
* Correspondence: nalindavid@gmail.com; Tel.: +1-484-653-9945; Fax: +1-610-4301-6004

Received: 31 May 2020; Accepted: 30 June 2020; Published: 2 July 2020

Abstract: Background: Cholera remains a major global health problem, causing high output diarrhea leading to severe dehydration and shock in developing countries. We aimed to determine whether vasoactive intestinal polypeptide (VIP), the mediator of pancreatic cholera syndrome, has a role in the pathophysiology of human cholera. Methods: We conducted a prospective observational study of cholera cases hospitalized with severe dehydration. Plasma and stool water levels of VIP were measured just after admission, after complete rehydration (3–4 h), at 24 h post-rehydration and at discharge after diarrhea ceased. Results: In total, 23 cholera patients were examined between January and August 2018. The geometric mean of stool VIP (sVIP) and plasma VIP (pVIP) on admission were 207.67 and 8.34 pmol/L, respectively. pVIP values were all within the normal range (</= 30 pcmol/L); however, sVIP levels were very high at all timepoints, though less so just after rehydration. In multivariable GEE models, after adjustment for covariates, sVIP levels were significantly associated with duration of hospitalization ($p = 0.026$), total stool volume ($p = 0.023$) as well as stool output in the first 24 h ($p = 0.013$). Conclusions: The data suggest that VIP, which is released by intestinal nerves, may play an important role in human choleragenesis, and inhibitors of intestinal VIP merit testing for potential therapeutic benefits.

Keywords: VIP; cholera patients

Key Point's/Summary: Cholera patients during profuse watery diarrhea had very high levels of VIP in their stool water, while plasma VIP levels remained normal. This supports the role of VIP in human choleragenesis, as has previously been demonstrated in in vivo animal and in in vitro tissue models.

1. Introduction

In 1976, pursuing a possible shared mechanism between cholera and pancreatic cholera syndrome [1–3], an abstract described persistent elevated stool vasoactive intestinal polypeptide (sVIP) levels in Bangladeshi cholera patients and in U.S. volunteers contracting cholera or enterotoxigenic *Escherichia coli* diarrhea in vaccine development studies [4]. At admission, cholera patients in shock had elevated plasma VIP (pVIP) levels. These declined to normal levels after correction of shock and dehydration. No VIP was found in the small intestinal luminal fluids of the healthy volunteers. The full report was withheld from publication due to the analyst's death, with samples having been exhausted. Now, 44 years later, the study has been repeated in cholera patients to determine if the earlier results could be confirmed.

2. Background

Cholera patients have elevated intestinal mucosal cyclic amp (cAMP) levels [5], and cholera toxin raises cAMP in in vivo and in vitro animal models and in stripped tissue models [6]. In cats and rats, intraluminal cAMP in denervated intestinal loops also induces luminal secretion [7]. Much prior evidence suggests a role for VIP as a modulator of cAMP levels. VIP, like cholera toxin (CT), enhances tissue cAMP levels and active ion secretion [8]. In cat intestines, intraluminal CT and intra-arterial VIP led to elevated cAMP levels associated with reduced salt and water absorption in villi, but not in crypts, where most secretion into the lumen is believed to originate [9]. However this finding might be due to cAMP turnover being more important in crypt cells than cAMP concentration [10]. Splanchnic nerve stimulation lowers intestinal VIP, thereby reversing VIP-stimulated luminal fluid accumulation [11]. VIP can induce high cAMP levels but can also induce diarrhea without elevating cAMP [9]. The findings in cats linking cAMP, VIP and intestinal fluid accumulation are consistent with a predominant role of reduced unidirectional lumen to plasma sodium and water fluxes found in CT-treated intact in vivo canine jejunal loops (but not in Thiry-Vella loops, in which the plasma to lumen flux was dominant both before and after CT) (D. Nalin and R. Hare, unpublished data). The apparent affinity of VIP for cAMP activation is raised by CT [12] and, in studies of rabbit and human ileal mucosa in vitro, VIP promptly increased cAMP levels, in contrast to no increase after nine other hormones thought to be associated with gut secretion—pentagastrin, glucagon, calcitonin, secretin, carbachol, GIP, serotonin, bradykinin and vasopressin [8]. Substance P affects gut fluid transport by releasing VIP [13]. Luminal 5-hydroxytryptamine induced gut luminal fluid accumulation and its release from enterochromaffin cells was stimulated by CT, but not by the related *E. coli* LT toxin [9,14–16]. VIP also has other effects possibly associated with intestinal fluid accumulation, such as raising aquaporin three levels after a 3 h delay [17], similar to the delay between CT exposure and onset of fluid accumulation [18].

While many studies have established that cAMP-mediated changes in net intestinal water and electrolyte secretion is present in cholera, changes in paracellular permeability, such as those caused by the zonula occludens toxin (ZOT) and accessory cholera enterotoxin (ACE) [19], and other possible mechanisms, have been noted [20]. On the other hand, clinical and animal studies of intestinal permeability and vascular flow have not succeeded in identifying such mechanisms in cholera patients [21]. VIPergic pathways actually reduce epithelial paracellular permeability [22].

In vivo studies have the advantage over experimental models like inverted intestinal sacs or biopsied stripped tissues [6,7] of better matching the complete intact pathophysiologic environment by maintaining normal neural and vascular connections. In vivo studies of VIP were conducted in normal human volunteers, in whom intravenously administered VIP induced a decreased absorption of water and electrolytes whilst increasing chloride secretion [23], and induced secretory diarrhea [24,25]. Paradoxically, elevations of cAMP after CT [26] or forskolin [27] are also associated with increased absorption of substrates of the active transport of sodium, such as glucose and glycine, suggesting that all or part of the cAMP elevation (or alterations in cAMP isoform variants) might represent a compensatory mechanism, aimed at overcoming the absorptive defect exemplified by the failure of absorption of plain saline solutions seen in cholera patients [28]. The mechanisms by which cAMP and VIP produce their effects are highly complex and beyond the scope of this report, but have been detailed in recent publications [22,29].

The growing body of evidence relating CT to VIP and gut fluid accumulation leading to diarrhea led us to repeat the earlier unpublished study to confirm a possible VIP role in human cholera pathogenesis. Since diarrhea can be caused by raising VIP levels in either plasma, as in pancreatic cholera syndrome, or by release from nerve endings in the intestinal mucosa, we measured VIP levels in both plasma and cholera rice-water stool water.

3. Study Design and Settings

Per protocol, four plasma and concurrent rectal catheter stool sampling points were chosen: the first, following just after correction of shock with intravenous rehydration, but before complete rehydration; the second when rehydration was complete (targeted at 4 h after admission); the third at 28 h, signifying 24 h after completing rehydration, during ongoing maintenance therapy replacing continuing diarrhea; the fourth in convalescence when diarrhea had stopped, though some patients' stools were still soft, using the findings for comparison with the same patient's acute phase data. Based on data from the earlier unpublished study, it was anticipated that plasma levels in specimens obtained during or shortly after correcting shock with intravenous hydration would show elevations of pVIP attributable to dehydration and/or shock itself [30]. The rapid return to stable normal pVIP values seen after correcting shock with intravenous rehydration in the earlier study was anticipated as a likely event, for which, the second and third plasma specimens were considered potentially useful in evaluating whether pVIP in cholera patients remained elevated after rehydration during ongoing diarrhea. A return to normal pVIP levels along with continued elevation of sVIP after rehydration during ongoing diarrhea would suggest a local mucosal neuronal VIP source rather than a systemic plasma source, such as seen in pancreatic cholera syndrome. Stool volumes and diarrhea rates were monitored in anticipation of possible correlations with sVIP levels over the course of illness. Diarrhea volumes and rates in cholera are well documented to follow a pattern of steady decline over time, when patients maintain normal hydration [31], and even more strikingly when adjunct appropriate antibiotics are given [32].

4. Study Population and Site

The study was conducted at the Dhaka Hospital of the icddr,b (International Centre for Diarrhoeal Disease Research, Bangladesh) between January and August, 2018. The study was approved by the Research Review Committee and the Ethical Review Committee of the icddr,b (Project identification code: PR#17008). Written informed consent was obtained from the participant or caregiver of each participant before enrollment. Patients aged 18–64 years were included if hospitalized with severe dehydration (with absent or impalpable peripheral pulses and lethargic or obtunded mental status) due to acute rice-water diarrhea of <24 h duration, with diagnosis later confirmed by rectal swab culture positive for Vibrio *cholerae* 01 or 0139. Patients with preadmission antibiotic therapy or complicating comorbidity were excluded.

On admission, patients' respiratory and circulatory statuses were assessed, and intravenous rehydration was started within ninety seconds. Patients received an initial bolus of 30 mL/kg of isotonic fluid (normal saline or acetate solution) [33] over 30 min, followed by 70 mL/kg over the next 2.5–3.5 h, to replace fluid deficit equivalent to ≥10% body weight within 3–4 h. Patients were kept on cholera cots and ongoing stool volumes collected into calibrated buckets were monitored q2h and recorded q4h. Urine output was collected and measured separately. After initial rehydration, ongoing losses were matched with isotonic fluid (normal saline or acetate) for the first 24 h, after which, ongoing stool losses were replaced with oral rehydration solution [34,35]. Single dose oral azithromycin (1 g) was administered after intravenous rehydration with abatement of vomiting, based on a local antibiogram.

Parameters observed included diarrhea duration and volume, plasma parameters of hydration and electrolyte status and glucose to monitor diarrhea-associated hemoconcentration, bicarbonate loss and associated acidosis and potassium abnormalities, and hypoglycemia. As noted above, VIP levels in both plasma and diarrhea stool water were monitored to detect any elevations originating either systemically or produced by neurons in the intestinal mucosa.

5. Stool and Blood Samples for VIP Assay

We obtained stool and blood specimens at the following timepoints: just after enrolment into the study and initial stabilization of patients (time 0); 3–4 h (after full rehydration with replacement of fluid deficit equivalent to ≥10% body weight); 24 h after complete rehydration, during ongoing diarrhea in the presence of normal vital signs; at time of discharge.

The 30 mL rectal catheter specimens of rice-water stool were obtained and placed immediately into tubes containing 0.15 TIU of chilled aprotinin/mL of stool water (Trasylol, Sigma-Aldrich, Activity: 3–8 TIU/mg solid). Pre-discharge, freshly passed non-liquid stool specimens were treated with chilled distilled water (1:3 dilution) in a tube containing chilled aprotinin equivalent to 2% of the total volume of stool plus distilled water. Stool samples were cold centrifuged at 13,523 g, and the supernatant was retrieved in a disposable syringe to filter through a 0.2 micron Millipore filter (Whatman 25 mm GD/X syringe filter, Sigma-Aldrich). Small volumes of filtered supernatant from the enrolment samples were re-cultured to ensure removal of vibrios. Venous blood samples were collected and cold centrifuged in lithium heparin tubes containing 0.15 TIU of chilled aprotinin/mL blood. We processed all specimens within 15 min after collection and kept them frozen (−80 °C) until they were shipped in dry ice to the UK for RIA assay [36]. We also collected 5 mL blood to measure electrolytes, plasma specific gravity, glucose and blood urea nitrogen.

6. Statistics

To plot the distribution of stool and plasma VIP values after natural log transformation on admission, rehydration completion, 24 h post-rehydration and discharge, we used dot plots. The stool water and plasma VIP levels did not follow a normal distribution as depicted by box and whisker plots, Q–Q plots (quantile–quantile plots) and Shapiro–Wilk tests, but followed normal distribution after log transformation. Therefore, we reported mean as geometric mean (GM) with a 95% confidence interval. We applied generalized estimating equation (GEE) models with an exchangeable correlation and Gaussian family structure to compare longitudinal variations in stool water and plasma VIP concentrations at four different timepoints for each patient, while adjusting for possible intra-subject correlations. Application of ordinary regression analysis may confer biased results for repeated measures data, whereas GEE methodology indicates how the mean of an outcome variable of a participant changes with covariates while adjusting intra-subject correlations related to repeated measures outcome data [37]. GEE is the best model for repeated measures and gives more robust results than ANOVA. In the GEE model, stool water VIP was the outcome variable, while independent variables were both time-varying covariates as well as non-time-varying covariates. As we included log transformed variables in the GEE model, so as to interpret our results, we applied the exponential (inverse of a log) function in the GEE models. In multivariable models, potential covariates with $p < 0.2$ in the bivariate analysis were included. A p-value < 0.05 was considered statistically significant. We analyzed data using Stata version 13.1 (Statacorp LP, College Station USA).

7. Results

We included 23 cholera cases for analysis; stool specimens of twenty-two (96%) cases grew Vibrio *cholerae* O1 biotype El Tor serotype and one (4%) *V. cholerae* 0139 biotype. Patient characteristics are shown in Table 1.

sVIP and pVIP concentrations and sVIP distribution are shown in Table 2 and Figure 1. The geometric means (GM) of sVIP and pVIP on admission were 207.67 and 8.34 pmol/L, respectively (Table 2). pVIP values were all within the normal range (</= 30 pcmol/L), though pVIP levels after partial rehydration were significantly higher than post-rehydration levels ($p = 0.001$).

In both bivariable and multivariable models, sVIP concentration after complete rehydration at the 4 h timepoint (replacement of fluid deficit equivalent to ≥10% body weight) was considered as the reference category. As some patients reached complete rehydration by 3 h post-admission, the 4 h timepoint represents a range of 3–4 h post-admission. In addition, some patients' diarrhea ceased by 24 h post-rehydration, so those values were considered as discharge values in the analytic models. In fact, the geometric means were virtually identical whether using data from patients contributing four specimen sets or from those whose diarrhea terminated at 24 h post-rehydration. At all timepoints, sVIP levels were far higher than pVIP levels, though unadjusted models revealed that the 4 h sVIP level was lower than at the other timepoints (Figure 1).

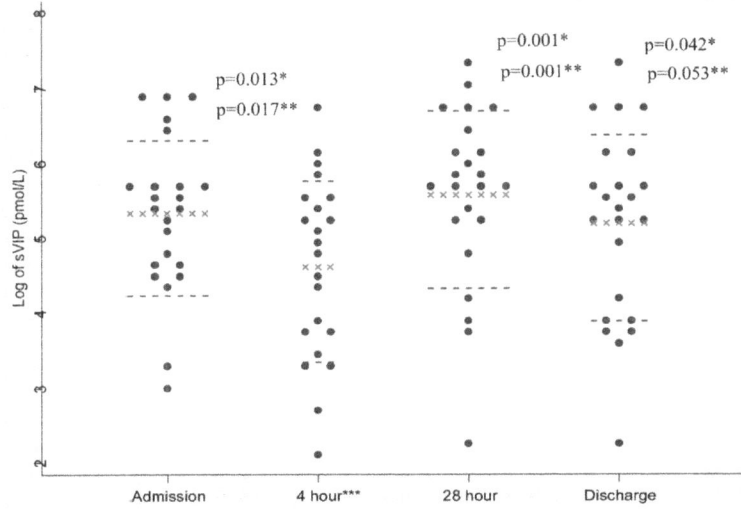

Figure 1. Distribution of average values of stool VIP after log transformation. Dot plot: Stool VIP concentrations are presented separately for admission, 4 h, 28 h and discharge samples. Bar representing mean ± SD. * p values derived from the bivariable GEE models. ** p values derived from the multivariable GEE models. *** 4 h time point is the reference category.

In multivariable (adjusted) GEE models, after adjusting other covariates, the comparison of discharge sVIP levels with 4 h levels did not reach significance. In multivariable models, after adjustment for covariates, sVIP levels were significantly associated with duration of hospitalization, total stool volume as well as stool output in the first 24 h (Table 3).

Net sVIP losses in cholera diarrhea were estimated based on ten patients with complete specimen sets and based on diarrhea output most closely matched in time with the time of specimen collection. For the admission timepoint, it was assumed that a mean of 1.0 L of diarrhea fluid remained unexpelled in the intestine on admission. The values at 0, 4, 28 and discharge timepoints were, respectively (pcg, mean ± s.d.): 308 ± 267, 422 ± 244, 749 ± 1126 and 188 ± 225.

Table 1. Clinical and laboratory characteristics of cholera patients with severe dehydration/hypovolemic shock in Dhaka, Bangladesh.

Characteristics	Total ($n = 23$)
Age (in years)	33 ± 10
Male (n, %)	20/23 (87)
Diarrhea duration (h)	41 ± 19
Emesis duration (h)	2 (1,3)
Abdominal pain (n, %)	4/23 (17)
Total stool volume (mL/kg)	141 (109, 191)
Urine output (mL/h)	136 ± 67
Stool output in 1st 24 h (mL/day)	8000 (5500, 10,500)
Total intravenous fluid (mL/kg/h)	11 (8.4, 12.75)
Duration of hospital stay (h)	63 ± 23
Admission blood glucose level (mmol/L)	8 (6,10) (4.2–7.8)
Admission plasma sp.gr.	1.0480 ± 0.006 (1.0232–1.0279)
Admission serum.Na^+ (mmol/L)	133.28 ± 2.30 (135–146)
Admission serum. K^+ (mmol/L)	5.16 ± 1.15 (3.5–5.3)
Admission serum. Cl^- (mmol/L)	102.26 ±3.06 (97–106)
Admission serum TCO_2 (mmol/L)	18.14 ± 4.63 (23–30)
Anion gap (mmol/L)	17.95 ±3.82 (7–21)
BUN (mmol/L)	14.80 ±4.80 (5–20)
Urine Sp. gr. at 4 h *	1.04 ± 0.005 (1.005–1.030)
Serum Na+ (mmol/L) at 4 h *	135 ± 2.76
TCO2 (mmol/L) at 4 h *	22.5 ± 3.57
Blood glucose level (mmol/L) at 4 h *	5.4 (4.88, 7.39)
Mean stool VIP (pmol/L)	307 (168,410)
Peak stool VIP (pmol/L)	591 (283,855)
Vibrio cholerae 01, El Tor	22/23 (96)
Vibrio cholerae 0139	1/23 (4)
Vibrio cholerae 01, El Tor Ogawa	17/22 (74)
Vibrio cholerae 01, El Tor Inaba	5/22 (22)

Data are presented as n (%), mean ± SD, or median (IQR). * Measured after complete rehydration. Abbreviations: VIP—vasoactive intestinal polypeptide; Total intravenous fluid (mL/kg/h)—replacement of fluid deficit equivalent to ≥10% body weight and ongoing loss. Normal reference values in brackets.

Table 2. Variations of stool and plasma VIP concentrations (pmol/L) over four timepoints before and after rehydration among cholera patients.

VIP Measurement Time Points	Stool VIP (pmol/L)		Plasma VIP (pmol/L)	
	Geometric Mean *	95% CI	Geometric Mean *	95% CI
Admission (0 h)	207.67	132.74, 324.90	8.34	5.53, 12.59
At 4 h (after complete rehydration)	101.55	59.40, 173.60	3.84	2.59, 5.67
At 28 h	265.97	159.17, 444.41	2.67	1.82, 3.92
At discharge	181.40	105.17, 310.63	3.31	2.26, 4.83

* Mean of stool and plasma VIP concentrations after log transformation.

Table 3. Associations of stool water VIP (pmol/L) in patients with cholera and severe dehydration/hypovolemic shock at four different timepoints before and after rehydration using generalized estimating equations models.

Characteristics		Unadjusted exp (Coefficient) * with 95% CI	p-Value	Adjusted exp (Coefficient) * with 95% CI	p-Value
Duration of hospital stay (h)		1.01 (0.992, 1.022)	0.161	1.01 (1.001, 1.023)	0.026
Total stool volume (mL/kg)		1.00 (0.993, 1.000)	0.087	1.01 (1.002, 1.025)	0.023
Stool output in first 24 h (mL)		1.00 (0.999, 1.000)	0.075	1.00 (0.999, 0.999)	0.013
Total IVF (mL/kg/h)		0.93 (0.864, 1.007)	0.077	0.94 (0.875, 1.021)	0.157
Stool VIP (pmol/L) measurement time points	4 h	ref		ref	
	Admission	2.01 (1.174, 3.762)	0.013	2.03 (1.136, 3.640)	0.017
	28 h	2.69 (1.504, 4.818)	0.001	2.60 (1.455, 4.662)	0.001
	Discharge	1.83 (1.026, 3.287)	0.042	1.77 (0.992, 3.179)	0.053

* Ratio of geometric mean: ratio of admission/28 h/discharge value to reference value.

8. Discussion

This is the first full prospective report of plasma and stool VIP levels in cholera patients. The findings confirm that in cholera patients, sVIP levels are elevated. The findings are consistent with earlier in vivo animal and in vitro tissue studies suggesting a neural mechanism of pathogenesis, though those studies did not measure sVIP. The current study shows a clear link bridging prior work to stool VIP in cholera patients. This underlines the possibility of new treatments aimed at interrupting the diarrheagenic process and shortening disease duration more than what is possible with antibiotics and fluid replacement alone.

The slightly higher pVIP levels, which fell after rehydration and correction of shock, probably represent a residual of dehydration and the recent correction of shock [30]. In any case, all pVIP values were within the normal range, ruling out any systemic pVIP elevation during cholera diarrhea. In contrast, the persistent high sVIP levels during the course of cholera diarrhea indicate that cholera diarrhea is associated with enhanced intestinal VIP production. The luminal VIP levels may have a direct mucosal effect or may represent the overflow from neural production in the mucosa. Intestinal VIP is neuronally controlled [7,11] and luminal VIP levels are not the product of direct transfer from plasma. In any case, pVIP levels before and after rehydration were within the normal range and were far below sVIP levels, even after rehydration. Slightly elevated blood peptide hormone levels have been reported in patients with presumed infectious or AIDS-related diarrhea [38,39], though stool volumes, diarrhea rates and stool water VIP levels were not reported. The relationship of these slightly high pVIP levels to sVIP levels in cholera patients is unclear, and may possibly have been due to dehydration levels, which were also not reported.

Sorting out the relative importance of VIP per se or in concert with other neuronally generated mediators of intestinal water and salt loss [7,12,13] awaits further study, but the bulk of evidence suggests that VIP may play a dominant role. Further study is also need to determine whether, in cholera patients, VIP's effects on cAMP activity influence the cAMP-enhanced absorption of actively transported sugars and amino acids [26], and superior absorption of oral rehydration solutions with glucose plus glycine [28] or with rice [40], rich in starch and amino acids [41,42]. This effect is not seen in diarrheal illnesses caused by other pathogens [43], in which VIP and cAMP may play a lesser role.

9. Limitations of this Study

While the results clearly confirm that cholera patients have elevated sVIP, the associations with total and 24 h stool volumes and diarrheal duration do not prove a causal relationship. To explore this possibility, the effects of VIP inhibitors or antagonists on cholera toxin-induced intestinal fluid losses in suitable animal models, such as the dog [44] or cat [45] cholera models, are warranted, elevated VIP levels in intestinal venous blood having already been demonstrated in the latter. The presence of sVIP levels exceeding plasma levels in convalescence may represent residual luminal VIP reaching the lower bowel after antibiotic therapy eradicates vibrios, stopping cholera toxin production. The correlations between sVIP and diarrhea duration and volume are notable, but this study was not designed to monitor diarrheal production rate and simultaneous luminal VIP levels in the small intestine. sVIP levels reflect production at the intestinal level at a prior timepoint, depending on intestinal transit time, influenced variably by intestinal motility. Studying these variables would require the intubation technique in cholera studies in human volunteers such as those previously reported in cholera vaccine pilot studies [46].

10. Conclusions

This study is the first fully documented report of high sVIP levels in cholera patients. High VIP levels in cholera patients' stool water may reflect an important role of VIP in the pathophysiology of cholera diarrhea. The findings suggest that human cholera diarrhea may be mediated by heightened intestinal neural production of VIP and luminal release of VIP, consistent with earlier in vitro and in vivo animal model studies suggesting participation of a neural/hormonal mechanism in pathogenesis.

11. Authors' Translational Perspective

While lidocaine and tetrodotoxin given after CT reduce its diarrheagenic effects [47], their neurologic and cardiovascular toxicities preclude use in cholera patients. Studies have demonstrated the effectiveness of somatostatin and methionine-enkephalin in antagonizing VIP's diarrheagenic activity when delivered intra-arterially [48], but the intestinal intra-arterial route is not clinically feasible, and intravenous administration of somatostatin had no effect on stool output in cholera patients [49]. Other VIP antagonists have also shown activity when administered I.V. immediately after cholera toxin [50,51], but the applicability of this to the clinical situation, when patients are seen long after diarrhea has been established, is not known. The identification of highly potent somatostatin-receptor agonists capable of inhibiting secretion after luminal mucosal surface application [52] suggests that these agents merit studies in appropriate animal cholera models such as the dog or cat to evaluate their possible suitability for human trials. It is striking that despite several decades of research pointing to a VIP role in choleragenesis, no translational study has appeared demonstrating a clinical benefit of antagonists or other compounds with antihormonal activity. Hopefully, the current confirmation of a VIP role in cholera patients may reawaken interest in such studies, including testing newer highly potent and mucosally active compounds to determine if they can safely interrupt the diarrheagenic process and shorten disease duration more than what is possible with antibiotics and fluid replacement alone.

Author Contributions: Conceptualization, D.N., S.B., F.A., T.A., S.A.S., P.B.; methodology, F.A., S.B., D.N. and P.B.; validation, T.A., S.A.S., J.D.C. and P.B., formal analysis, D.N. and F.A.; investigation, F.A. and F.I.; resources, D.N., J.D.C., S.B.; data curation, D.N. and F.A.; writing—original draft preparation, D.N.; writing—review and editing, D.N., F.A., S.A.S.; supervision, D.N., F.A., T.A. project administration, F.A., J.D.C, F.I. and T.A.; funding acquisition, D.N., J.D.C., S.B. All authors have read and agreed to the published version of the manuscript.

Funding: This study was made possible by a grant from the Child Health Foundation, Baltimore MD and the Capacity development fund of BMGF; and by clinical and laboratory support from the icddr,b and Imperial Hospital, London. No external funding was received.

Conflicts of Interest: The authors declare no conflict of interest.

References

1. Bloom, S.R.; Polak, J.M.; Pearse, A.G. Vasoactive intestinal peptide and watery-diarrhoea syndrome. *Lancet* **1973**, *2*, 14–16. [CrossRef]
2. Said, S.I. Vasoactive intestinal polypeptide (VIP) as a mediator of the watery diarrhea syndrome. *World J. Surg.* **1979**, *3*, 559–563. [CrossRef] [PubMed]

3. Editorial. VIP and diarrhea. *Lancet* **1984**, *28*, 202.
4. Bloom, S.R.; Nalin, D.R.; Mitchell, S.J.; Bryant, M.G. High Levels of Vip in Cholera Stool Water. *Gut* **1976**, *17*, 817.
5. Chen, L.C.; Rohde, J.E.; Sharp, G.W. Intestinal adenyl-cyclase activity in human cholera. *Lancet* **1971**, *1*, 939–941. [CrossRef]
6. Field, M. Intestinal Secretion—Effect of Cyclic Amp and Its Role in Cholera. *N. Engl. J. Med.* **1971**, *284*, 1137–1144.
7. Eklund, S.; Cassuto, J.; Jodal, M.; Lundgren, O. The involvement of the enteric nervous system in the intestinal secretion evoked by cyclic adenosine 3′5′-monophosphate. *Acta Physiol. Scand.* **1984**, *120*, 311–316. [CrossRef]
8. Schwartz, C.J.; Kimberg, D.V.; Sheerin, H.E.; Field, M.; Said, S.I. Vasoactive intestinal peptide stimulation of adenylate cyclase and active electrolyte secretion in intestinal mucosa. *J. Clin. Investig.* **1974**, *54*, 536–544. [CrossRef]
9. Eklund, S.; Brunsson, I.; Jodal, M.; Lundgren, O. Changes in cyclic 3′5′-adenosine monophosphate tissue concentration and net fluid transport in the cat's small intestine elicited by cholera toxin, arachidonic acid, vasoactive intestinal polypeptide and 5-hydroxytryptamine. *Acta Physiol. Scand.* **1987**, *129*, 115–125. [CrossRef] [PubMed]
10. Loeschke, K.; Farack, U.M.; Gerzer, R.; Keravis, T. Evidence That the Turnover Rather Than the Concentration of Camp Determines Cholera-Toxin Induced Fluid Secretion in Rat Intestine. *Z. Fur Gastroenterol.* **1987**, *25*, 388.
11. Sjoqvist, A.; Fahrenkrug, J.; Jodal, M.; Lundgren, O. The effect of splanchnic nerve stimulation and neuropeptide Y on cholera secretion and release of vasoactive intestinal polypeptide in the feline small intestine. *Acta Physiol. Scand.* **1988**, *133*, 289–295. [CrossRef] [PubMed]
12. Bennett, V.; Morg, L.; Cuatrecasas, P. Mechanism of activation of adenylate cyclase by Vibrio cholerae enterotoxin: Relations to the mode of activation by hormones. *J. Membr. Biol.* **1975**, *24*, 107–129. [CrossRef]
13. Brunsson, I.; Eklund, S.; Fahrenkrug, J.; Jodal, M.; Lundgren, O.; Sjoqvist, A. Effects of substance P on intestinal secretion, blood flow, motility and release of vasoactive intestinal polypeptide in vivo in the rat and cat. *J. Physiol.* **1995**, *483*, 727–734. [CrossRef] [PubMed]
14. Cassuto, J.; Jodal, M.; Tuttle, R.; Lundgren, O. 5-hydroxytryptamine and cholera secretion. Physiological and pharmacological studies in cats and rats. *Scand. J. Gastroenterol.* **1982**, *17*, 695–703. [CrossRef] [PubMed]
15. Nilsson, O.; Cassuto, J.; Larsson, P.A.; Jodal, M.; Lidberg, P.; Ahlman, H.; Dahlstrom, A.; Lundgren, O. 5-Hydroxytryptamine and cholera secretion: A histochemical and physiological study in cats. *Gut* **1983**, *24*, 542–548. [CrossRef]
16. Mourad, F.H.; O'Donnell, L.J.D.; Dias, J.A.; Ogutu, E.; Andre, E.A.; Turvill, J.L.; Farthing, M.J.G. Role of 5-hydroxytryptamine type 3 receptors in rat intestinal fluid and electrolyte secretion induced by cholera and Escherichia coli enterotoxins. *Gut* **1995**, *37*, 340–345. [CrossRef] [PubMed]
17. Itoh, A.; Tsujikawa, T.; Fujiyama, Y.; Bamba, T. Enhancement of aquaporin-3 by vasoactive intestinal polypeptide in a human colonic epithelial cell line. *J. Gastroenterol. Hepatol.* **2003**, *18*, 203–221. [CrossRef]
18. Carpenter, C.C.; Greenough, W.B. Response of the canine duodenum to intraluminal challenge with cholera exotoxin. *J. Clin. Investig.* **1968**, *47*, 2600–2607. [CrossRef]
19. Perez-Rector, D.; Jana, V.; Pavez, L.; Navrante, P.; Garcia, K. Acceessory toxins of vibrio pathogens and their role in epithelial disruption during infection. *Front. Microbiol.* **2018**, *9*, 2248. [CrossRef]
20. Camilleri, M.; Nullens, S.; Nelsen, T. Enteroendocrine and neuronal mechanisms in pathophysiology of acute infectious diarrhea. *Dig. Dis. Sci.* **2012**, *57*, 19–27. [CrossRef]
21. Barua, D.; Burrows, W. *Cholera*; Saunders: Philadelphia, PA, USA, 1974; pp. 18–23.
22. Iwasaki, M.; Akiba, Y.; Kaunitz, J.D. *Recent Advances in Vasoactive Intestinal Peptide Physiology and Pathophysiology: Focus on the Gastrointestinal System*; F1000Research: London, UK, 2019.
23. Davis, G.R.; Santa Ana, C.A.; Morawski, S.G.; Fordtran, J.S. Effect of vasoactive intestinal polypeptide on active and passive transport in the human jejunum. *J. Clin. Investig.* **1981**, *67*, 1687–1694. [CrossRef] [PubMed]
24. Kreis, G.J.; Fordtran, J.S.; Fahrenkrug, J.; Schaffalitzky, D.E.; Muckadell, O.B.; Fischer, J.E.; Humphrey, C.S.; Said, S.I.; Walsh, J.H.; Shulkes, A.A. O'dorisio TMA, Effect of VIP infusion in water and ion transport in the human jejunum. *Gastroenteritis* **1980**, *78*, 722–727.
25. Kane, M.G.; O'Dorisio, T.M.; Krejs, G.J. Production of secretory diarrhea by intravenous infusion of vasoactive intestinal polypeptide. *N. Engl. J. Med.* **1983**, *309*, 1482–1485. [CrossRef] [PubMed]

26. Wright, E.M.; Hirsch, J.R.; Loo, D.D.; Zampighi, G.A. Regulation of Na+/glucose cotransporters. *J. Exp. Biol.* **1997**, *200*, 287–293. [PubMed]
27. Reymann, A.; Braun, W.; Woermann, C. Proabsorptive properties of forskolin: Disposition of glycine, leucine and lysine in rat jejunum. *Naunyn Schm. Arch. Pharmacol.* **1986**, *334*, 110–115. [CrossRef] [PubMed]
28. Nalin, D.R.; Cash, R.A.; Rahman, M.; Yunus, M. Effect of glycine and glucose on sodium and water adsorption in patients with cholera. *Gut* **1970**, *11*, 768–772. [CrossRef] [PubMed]
29. Robichaux, W.G.; Xiaodong, C. Intracellular cAMP sensor EPAC: Physiology, pathophysiology and therapeutics development. *Physiol. Rev.* **2018**, *98*, 919–1053. [CrossRef] [PubMed]
30. Sakio, H.; Matsuzaki, Y.; Said, S.I. Release of Vasoactive Intestinal Polypeptide during Hemorrhagic-Shock. *Fed. Proc.* **1979**, *38*, 1114.
31. Hirschhorn, N.; Kinzie, J.L.; Sachar, D.B.; Northrup, R.S.; Taylor, J.O.; Ahmad, S.Z.; Phillips, R.A. Decrease in net stool output in cholera during intestinal perfusion with glucose-containing solutions. *N. Engl. J. Med.* **1968**, *279*, 176–181. [CrossRef]
32. Alam, N.H.; Ashraf, H. Treatment of infectious diarrhea in children. *Paediatr. Drugs* **2003**, *5*, 151–165. [CrossRef]
33. Cash, R.A.; Toha, K.M.; Nalin, D.R.; Huq, Z.; Phillips, R.A. Acetate in the correction of acidosis secondary to diarrhoea. *Lancet* **1969**, *2*, 302–303. [CrossRef]
34. World Health Organization. *Programme for the Control of Diarrhoeal Diseases: A Manual for the Treatment of Diarrhoea for Use by Physicians and Other Health Workers*; Geneva World Health Organization: Geneva, Switzerland, 1990.
35. World Health Organization. *The Treatment of Diarrhoea: A Manual for Physicians and Other Senior Health Workers*; World Health Organization: Geneva, Switzerland, 2005.
36. Mitchell, S.J.; Bloom, S.R. Measurement of fasting and postprandial plasma VIP in man. *Gut* **1978**, *19*, 1043–1048. [CrossRef] [PubMed]
37. Zeger, S.L.; Liang, K.Y.; Albert, P.S. Models for longitudinal data: A generalized estimating equation approach. *Biometrics* **1988**, *44*, 1049–1060. [CrossRef] [PubMed]
38. Besterman, H.S.; Christofides, N.D.; Welsby, P.D.; Adrian, T.E.; Sarson, D.L.; Bloom, S.R. Gut hormones in acute diarrhoea. *Gut* **1983**, *24*, 665–671. [CrossRef]
39. Manfredi, R.; Vezzadini, P.; Costigliola, P.; Ricchi, E.; Fanti, M.P.; Chiodo, F. Elevated plasma levels of vasoactive intestinal peptide in AIDS patients with refractory idiopathic diarrhoea. Effects of treatment with octreotide. *AIDS* **1993**, *7*, 223–226. [CrossRef] [PubMed]
40. Molla, A.M.; Sarker, S.A.; Hossain, M.; Molla, A.; Greenough, W.B. Rice-powder electrolyte solution as oral-therapy in diarrhoea due to Vibrio cholerae and Escherichia coli. *Lancet* **1982**, *1*, 1317–1319. [CrossRef]
41. Amankwah, E.N.; Adu, E.; Barimah, V.M.J.; Van Twisk, C. Amino acid profiles of some varieties of rice, soybean and groundnut grown in Ghana. *J. Food Process. Technol.* **2015**, *6*, 420–423. [CrossRef]
42. Kalman, D.S. Amino Acid Composition of an Organic Brown Rice Protein Concentrate and Isolate Compared to Soy and Whey Concentrates and Isolates. *Foods* **2014**, *3*, 394–402. [CrossRef]
43. Vesikari, T.; Isolauri, E. Glycine supplemented oral rehydration solutions for diarrhoea. *Arch. Dis. Child.* **1986**, *61*, 372–376. [CrossRef]
44. Nalin, D.R.; Ally, K.; Hare, R.; Hare, K. Effect of cholera toxin on jejunal osmoregulation of mannitol solutions in dogs. *J. Infect. Dis.* **1972**, *125*, 528–532. [PubMed]
45. Cassuto, J.; Fahrenkrug, J.; Jodal, M.; Tuttle, R.; Lundgren, O. Release of vasoactive intestinal polypeptide from the cat small intestine exposed to cholera toxin. *Gut* **1981**, *22*, 958–963. [CrossRef] [PubMed]
46. Levine, M.M.; Nalin, D.R.; Craig, J.P.; Hoover, D.; Bergquist, E.J.; Waterman, D.; Holley, H.P.; Hornick, R.B.; Pierce, N.P.; Libonati, J.P. Immunity of cholera in man: Relative role of antibacterial versus antitoxic immunity. *Trans. R. Soc. Trop. Med. Hyg.* **1979**, *73*, 3–9. [CrossRef]
47. Cassuto, J.; Jodal, M.; Tuttle, R.; Lundgren, O. On the role of intramural nerves in the pathogenesis of cholera toxin-induced intestinal secretion. *Scand. J. Gastroenterol.* **1981**, *16*, 377–384. [CrossRef] [PubMed]
48. Eklund, S.; Sjoqvist, A.; Fahrenkrug, J.; Jodal, M.; Lundgren, O. Somatostatin and methionine-enkephalin inhibit cholera toxin-induced jejunal net fluid secretion and release of vasoactive intestinal polypeptide in the cat in vivo. *Acta Physiol. Scand.* **1988**, *133*, 551–557. [CrossRef]
49. Molla, A.M.; Gyr, K.; Bardhan, P.K.; Molla, A. Effect of Intravenous Somatostatin on Stool Output in Diarrhea Due to Vibrio-Cholerae. *Gastroenterology* **1984**, *87*, 845–847. [CrossRef]

50. Banks, M.R.; Farthing, M.J.; Robberecht, P.; Burleigh, D.E. Antisecretory actions of a novel vasoactive intestinal polypeptide (VIP) antagonist in human and rat small intestine. *Br. J. Pharmacol.* **2005**, *144*, 994–1001. [CrossRef] [PubMed]
51. Mourad, F.H.; Nassar, C.F. Effect of vasoactive intestinal polypeptide (VIP) antagonism on rat jejunal fluid and electrolyte secretion induced by cholera and Escherichia coli enterotoxins. *Gut* **2000**, *47*, 382–386. [CrossRef]
52. Emery, P.T.; Higgs, N.B.; Warhurst, A.C.; Carlson, G.L.; Warhurst, G. Anti-secretory properties of non-peptide somatostatin receptor agonists in isolated rat colon: Luminal activity and possible interaction with P-glycoprotein. *Br. J. Pharmacol.* **2002**, *135*, 1443–1448. [CrossRef]

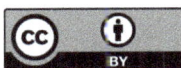

© 2020 by the authors. Licensee MDPI, Basel, Switzerland. This article is an open access article distributed under the terms and conditions of the Creative Commons Attribution (CC BY) license (http://creativecommons.org/licenses/by/4.0/).

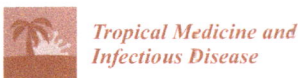

Editorial

Eliminating Cholera Incidence and Mortality: Unfulfilled Tasks

David Nalin

Center for Immunology and Microbial Diseases, Albany Medical College, Albany, NY 12203, USA; ralindavid@gmail.com

Citation: Nalin, D. Eliminating Cholera Incidence and Mortality: Unfulfilled Tasks. *TMID* 2022, 7, 69. https://doi.org/10.3390/tropicalmed7050069

Received: 23 March 2022
Accepted: 6 May 2022
Published: 9 May 2022

Publisher's Note: MDPI stays neutral with regard to jurisdictional claims in published maps and institutional affiliations.

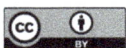

Copyright: © 2022 by the author. Licensee MDPI, Basel, Switzerland. This article is an open access article distributed under the terms and conditions of the Creative Commons Attribution (CC BY) license (https://creativecommons.org/licenses/by/4.0/).

Impressive advances have been made in new cholera vaccine development and vaccination control strategies. Possible future goals in this field could extend these advances by developing vaccines with higher efficacy and longer duration of protection, particularly in young children and individuals from non-endemic areas. The identification of more vibrio antigens may lead to confirmation of protective immune responses as surrogates of protection, a need arising from evidence that the traditionally monitored vibriocidal response, while paralleling evidence of protection, is not the protective mechanism. Such further developments could overcome current limitations, including the occurrence of cholera outbreaks in war-torn areas in which short-term vaccination programs often prove impracticable.

The advances in understanding of cholera immunology, bioecology, vaccine innovation and therapy presented in this series of articles have led to ambitious goals for controlling the incidence and the mortality of cholera, which persists in affected areas. The discussion would not be complete without noting areas not included or given priority in the current goals, but which may prove to be of value for achieving them.

First, there is too much talk and too little pressure brought to bear on the need for action to provide safe chlorinated drinking water and sanitary waste disposal to unserved areas. More effort is required to reframe national priorities so that adequate funds for these essential elements of modern public health are provided in both urban and rural environments, along with the educational and motivational components to ensure their effective usage. International standards and regulations governing urban development in the age of global urbanization [1] are essential if the Global Task Force on Cholera Control's goal of ending cholera by 2030 is to have any chance of succeeding.

Second, insufficient attention has been given to the etiologies and prevention, nutritional and otherwise, of tropical hypochlorhydria [2], which is widespread in the developing nations and renders their populations highly susceptible to cholera and other pathogens sensitive to gastric acid. Based on human volunteer studies [3], which established that even enormous numbers of *V. cholerae* fail to cause disease in normochlorhydric subjects, it is likely that elimination of tropical hypochlorhydria would greatly reduce cholera incidence in affected areas and potentially make vaccines significantly more protective.

Third, far too little research funding has been directed at discovering safe and effective anti-cholera medicines capable of quickly stopping cholera diarrhea. No mass screening of compounds likely to have such efficacy has been undertaken despite an abundance of potential candidates. Recent advances in cholera pathophysiology, such as confirmation of the role of VIP in human cholera [4], suggest a number of potential high-value targets which merit inclusion in such a screening program in animal models leading to clinical trials.

Finally, the continued high cholera case-fatality rates despite established highly effective and widely available treatment modalities demand renewed focus on the gaps preventing therapy from reaching patients.

References

1. Bollyky, T.J. Oral Rehydration Salts, Cholera, and the Unfinished Urban Health Agenda. *Trop. Med. Infect. Dis.* **2022**, *7*, 67. [CrossRef]
2. Nalin, D.R.; Levine, R.J.; Levine, M.M.; Hoover, D.; Bergquist, E.; McLaughlin, J.; Libonati, J.; Alam, J.; Hornick, R.B. Cholera, non-vibrio cholera and stomach acid. *Lancet* **1978**, *2*, 856–859. [CrossRef]
3. Cash, R.A.; Music, S.I.; Libonati, J.P.; Snyder, M.J.; Wenzel, R.P.; Hornick, R.B. Response of man to infection with *Vibrio cholerae*. I. Clinical, serologic, and bacteriologic responses to a known inoculum. *J. Infect. Dis.* **1974**, *129*, 45–52. [CrossRef] [PubMed]
4. Afroze, F.; Bloom, S.; Bech, P.; Ahmed, T.; Sarker, S.A.; Clemens, J.D.; Islam, F.; Nalin, D. Cholera and Pancreatic Cholera: Is VIP the Common Pathophysiologic Factor? *Trop. Med. Infect. Dis.* **2020**, *5*, 111. [CrossRef] [PubMed]

MDPI
St. Alban-Anlage 66
4052 Basel
Switzerland
Tel. +41 61 683 77 34
Fax +41 61 302 89 18
www.mdpi.com

Tropical Medicine and Infectious Disease Editorial Office
E-mail: tropicalmed@mdpi.com
www.mdpi.com/journal/tropicalmed

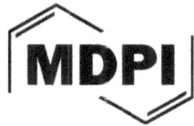